Developmental-Behavioral Disorders

Selected Topics

VOLUME 2

CRITICAL ISSUES IN DEVELOPMENTAL AND BEHAVIORAL PEDIATRICS

SERIES EDITOR: MARVIN I. GOTTLIEB, M.D., Ph.D.
Hackensack Medical Center
Hackensack, New Jersey
and University of Medicine and Dentistry of New Jersey–
New Jersey Medical School
Newark, New Jersey

DEVELOPMENTAL-BEHAVIORAL DISORDERS: Selected Topics
Volumes 1 and 2
Edited by Marvin I. Gottlieb, M.D., Ph.D., and John E. Williams, M.D.

Developmental-Behavioral Disorders

Selected Topics

VOLUME 2

EDITED BY

MARVIN I. GOTTLIEB, M.D., Ph.D.

Director, Institute for Child Development
Hackensack Medical Center
Hackensack, New Jersey
Professor, Department of Pediatrics
University of Medicine and Dentistry of New Jersey–
New Jersey Medical School
Newark, New Jersey

AND

JOHN E. WILLIAMS, M.D.

Chief, Section of Developmental Pediatrics
Associate Director, Institute for Child Development
Hackensack Medical Center
Hackensack, New Jersey
Clinical Assistant Professor, Department of Pediatrics
University of Medicine and Dentistry of New Jersey–
New Jersey Medical School
Newark, New Jersey

PLENUM MEDICAL BOOK COMPANY
NEW YORK AND LONDON

Library of Congress Cataloging in Publication Data

(Revised for volume 2)

Developmental–behavioral disorders.

(Critical issues in developmental and behavioral pediatrics)
1. Developmental disabilities. 2. Child psychiatry. 3. Pediatrics—Psychological aspects. I. Gottlieb, Marvin I. II. Williams, John E. (John Edward), 1951– III. Series.
RJ135.D475 1988 618.92′89 88-171674
ISBN 0-306-43124-6

Dedicated in memory of Nathan H. Gottlieb,

a kind and generous man whose love, wisdom,

and encouragement made dreams a reality.

233 Spring Street, New York, N.Y. 10013

Plenum Medical Book Company is an imprint of Plenum Publishing Corporation

Printed in the United States of America

Contributors

GLEN P. AYLWARD, PH.D. • Director, Division of Developmental and Behavioral Pediatrics, Departments of Pediatrics and Psychiatry, Southern Illinois University School of Medicine, Springfield, Illinois 62794-9230

RITA BENEZRA-OBEITER, M.D. • Staff Developmental Pediatrician, Institute for Child Development, Hackensack Medical Center, Hackensack, New Jersey 07601

STEPHEN H. BILLER, J.D. • Attorney at Law, Heiskell, Donelson, Bearman, Adams, Williams and Kirsch, Memphis, Tennessee 38138

WILLIAM B. CAREY, M.D. • Clinical Associate Professor of Pediatrics, Department of Pediatrics, University of Pennsylvania School of Medicine, Division of General Pediatrics, Children's Hospital of Philadelphia, Philadelphia, Pennsylvania 19104

EDWARD R. CHRISTOPHERSEN, PH.D. • Professor of Pediatrics, Chief, Department of Behavioral Pediatrics, The Children's Mercy Hospital, Kansas City, Missouri 64108

ISABEL DETRIZIO-CAROTENUTO, M.D. • Formerly Senior Fellow, Developmental Pediatrics, Institute for Child Development, Hackensack Medical Center, Hackensack, New Jersey 07601

RICHARD DONN, M.B.A. • Vice President, Systems Development, Hackensack Medical Center, Hackensack, New Jersey 07601

MARION P. DOWNS, M.A., D.H.S. • Department of Otolaryngology, University of Colorado Health Sciences Center, Denver, Colorado 80262

PAUL H. DWORKIN, M.D. • Associate Professor, Department of Pediatrics, Head, Division of General Pediatrics, University of Connecticut Health Center, Farmington, Connecticut 06032

MARVIN I. GOTTLIEB, M.D., PH.D. • Director, Institute for Child Development, Hackensack Medical Center, Hackensack, New Jersey 07601; and Professor of Pediatrics, Department of Pediatrics, University of Medicine and Dentistry of New Jersey–New Jersey Medical School, Newark, New Jersey 07103

MORRIS GREEN, M.D. • Perry W. Lesh Professor of Pediatrics, Chairman, Department of Pediatrics, Indiana University School of Medicine, and James Whitcomb Riley Hospital for Children, Indianapolis, Indiana 46223

SUSAN GUGENHEIM, M.S. • Department of Otolaryngology, University of Colorado Health Sciences Center, Denver, Colorado 80262

JONATHAN J. HALPERT, PH.D. • Director of Psychological Services, Camelot Community Residence Program, Port Jefferson Station, New York 11776

MARCEL KINSBOURNE, M.D. • Director, Department of Behavioral Neurology, Eunice Kennedy Shriver Center for Mental Retardation, Brandeis University, Waltham, Massachusetts 02154; and Harvard Medical School, Boston, Massachusetts 02115

JUDITH R. MATHEWS, M.A. • Department of Behavioral Pediatrics, University of Kansas Medical Center, Kansas City, Kansas 66103

JERRY L. NORTHERN, PH.D. • Head, Audiology Division, Professor of Otolaryngology, Department of Otolaryngology, University of Colorado Health Sciences Center, Denver, Colorado 80262

KAREN N. OLNESS, M.D. • Professor of Pediatrics, Chief, Division of General Academic Pediatrics, Case Western Reserve University School of Medicine, and Department of Pediatrics, Rainbow Babies and Childrens Hospital, Cleveland, Ohio 44106

HAROLD PERL, M.D. • Director, Neonatal Intensive Care Unit, Hackensack Medical Center, Hackensack, New Jersey 07601

ANNETTE L. ROSETTI-CARTAXO, M.D. • Consultant, Developmental Pediatrics, Institute for Child Development, Hackensack Medical Center, Hackensack, New Jersey 07601

N. PAUL ROSMAN, M.D. • Professor of Pediatrics and Neurology, Tufts University School of Medicine, and Chief, Division of Pediatric Neurology, Floating Hospital for Infants and Children, New England Medical Center Hospitals, Boston, Massachusetts 02111

FREDRICK T. SHERMAN, M.D. • Clinical Associate Professor of Medicine, Health Sciences Center, State University of New York at Stony Brook, Stony Brook, New York 11794; and Huntington Hospital, Huntington, New York 11743

DEWEY WALKER, M.D. • Department of Otolaryngology, University of Colorado Health Sciences Center, Denver, Colorado 80262

Preface

The Preface to the first volume of *Developmental–Behavioral Disorders: Selected Topics* outlined, in addition to the philosophy and objectives of such a text, the justification for an annual volume devoted to issues in developmental pediatrics:

> *Developmental–Behavioral Disorders: Selected Topics* was designed as a timely publication to meet the particular informational needs of concerned professionals. Unlike standard subspecialty textbooks, *Selected Topics* is not constrained by the necessity of presenting basic/fundamental text material and restating established theme-related doctrines. Indeed the editors of *Selected Topics* enjoy the liberty of presenting a menu of issues that encompasses: (1) the more recent developments and breakthroughs within the field; (2) the controversial issues of the day, viewed from various perspectives; (3) reviews of special interests; (4) state-of-the art management guidelines; and (5) a broad variety of topics in the field, from medical–legal issues to basic research studies. . . . It is an updating supplement, a companion, to standard reference texts.

The publication of a second volume of *Developmental–Behavioral Disorders: Selected Topics* suggests that this initial "editorial assumption" was indeed appropriate. The continued professional and public interest in developmental pediatrics, as a subspecialty area, has been manifested by a proliferation of themes-related, continuing medical education programs, journal articles, society growth and activities, and continued popularization of developmental–behavioral issues in the communications media.

Selected Topics, Volume 2, continues to reflect the increasing and varied responsibilities of pediatric developmental–behavioral health care professionals. Federal legislation, as designated by PL 94-142 (enacted in 1975) and more recently by PL 99-457, specifically focuses attention on developmental and behavioral issues. These landmark legislations have in effect served to dramatically enlarge and redefine the scope and depth of traditional "comprehensive health care" for infants, children, and adolescents.

The first volume of this series was based on some of the cogent problems presented at an annual conference, Developmental–Behavioral Disorders: Update, jointly sponsored by the Hackensack Medical Center's Institute for Child Development and the Division of Continuing Medical Education. This current volume was similarly constructed, representing a collection of selected timely topics which were presented by several nationally recognized experts participating in the 1987 annual conference.

The broad spectrum of issues presented in this volume (e.g., role of autorelaxation and mental imagery in developmental pediatrics; graduates of the neonatal intensive care unit; self-destructive behaviors in children and adolescents; office screening for communication disorders; outcome of the high-risk infant; the learning-disabled child; the child who fails to speak; child and adolescent depression; impact of television viewing on development; enhancing pediatric compliance in primary care) is once again representative of the myriad of developmental and behavioral issues confronting general pediatricians, family practitioners, pediatric subspecialists, and allied health care professionals.

Volume 3, currently in preparation, further underscores the diverse and challenging spectrum of disorders encountered under the generic classification of developmental–behavioral pediatrics. Some of the provocative topics to be discussed include:

- The fetal alcohol syndrome and its effects
- Hearing loss—early detection and intervention
- Early physical signs of developmental delay
- The sexually active adolescent
- Interview and intervention strategies for adolescents
- Movement disorders and paroxysmal behaviors
- Controversial therapies in developmental disabilities
- The child with cancer: Psychosocial issues confronting child and family
- Neuropsychological complications of therapy in acute lymphocytic leukemia
- Youth suicide
- Learning disabilities and juvenile delinquency
- Ethical issues in developmental pediatrics

The program for Developmental–Behavioral Disorders: Update 1989 has been again designed with major input from the previous conference participants. In essence, topics (as well as faculty) are selected from the expressed concerns of these professionals. The range of subjects suggested by participating conference attendees represents a myriad of concerns in developmental pediatrics: ethical/legal issues; current trends in management of attention-deficit disorders; the impact of PL 99-457 on services to be offered by primary health care providers; early intervention programs—pros and cons; teenage pregnancy; sleep and eating disorders; counseling adolescents; predictive value of screening inventories. This is a sample of some of the issues which confront primary health care providers *and* pediatric subspecialists.

From the above, past, current, and projected "menus" of developmental–behavioral issues, it appears that several generalizations can justifiably be formulated:

1. Primary and tertiary health care providers have literally been bombarded with disorders, dysfunctions, and delays in child/adolescent neurodevelopment.
2. There is a continuing need to provide professionals with materials to enhance their basic knowledge in developmental medicine.
3. Health care providers are eager to become involved in developmental problems, but appear to need practical screening and diagnostic inventories to assess children *and* adolescents in developmental–behavioral jeopardy.
4. There is a critical need to define and refine office intervention strategies for managing developmental issues, both for primary health care providers and pediatric subspecialists (recognizing professional capabilities and limitations).
5. It is critical to enhance familiarity with the interdisciplinary ("team") approach to management of developmental problems, as well as those skills necessary in coordinating professional interventions.
6. Quality research in this pediatric subspecialty is essential in providing a substantive basic fund of knowledge of etiology, identification, management, and prognosis for the child and adolescent at risk.
7. The issues addressed in these volumes can effectively serve, in part, as a guideline for the construction of a core curriculum in developmental pediatrics for medical students, residents, and fellows.

The subspecialty of developmental pediatrics has unquestionably experienced meteoric growth, in both its scope and degree of sophistication. There is, however, much more to be learned about child and adolescent development and behavior. Perhaps this series will help contribute to that learning process.

Once again, we express our appreciation to Mr. John P. Ferguson (President/Chief Executive Officer of Hackensack Medical Center), Dr. William C. Black (Vice President of Medical Affairs/Director of Medical Education at Hackensack Medical Center), and the Board of Governors of the Hackensack Medical Center. Their continued support and encouragement in various academic activities in developmental pediatrics will ultimately be measured in the improved quality of life for many children.

Marvin I. Gottlieb, M.D., Ph.D.
John E. Williams, M.D.

Hackensack, New Jersey

Contents

Chapter 1

Child/Adolescent Depression: Guidelines for Office Management

GLEN P. AYLWARD

1. Introduction ... 1
2. Diagnosis ... 1
3. Epidemiology ... 7
4. Risk Factors ... 7
5. Biological Indicators ... 8
6. Biochemical Treatment ... 9
7. Developmental Concerns ... 10
8. Office Management ... 11

References ... 12

Chapter 2

Outcome of the High-Risk Infant: Fact versus Fiction

GLEN P. AYLWARD

1. Introduction ... 15
2. Low Apgar Scores (Asphyxia) and Outcome ... 16
3. Seizures ... 19
4. Subependymal Germinal Matrix Hemorrhage (SEH)/ Intraventricular Hemorrhage (IVH) ... 21
5. Hypoxic–Ischemic Encephalopathy (HIE) ... 22
6. Very Low Birthweight (VLBW) ... 23
7. Summary ... 25

References ... 27

CHAPTER 3

Syndrome Synopsis: AIDS Embryopathy, Cerebral Gigantism (Sotos's Syndrome), Fragile X Syndrome, and Tourette's Syndrome

RITA BENEZRA-OBEITER, ISABEL DETRIZIO-CAROTENUTO, AND ANNETTE L. ROSETTI-CARTAXO

1. AIDS Embryopathy 29
2. Cerebral Gigantism (Sotos's Syndrome) 31
3. Fragile X Syndrome 33
4. Tourette's Syndrome 36
References 37

CHAPTER 4

Juvenile Delinquency: The Interface between Pediatrics and the Law

STEPHEN H. BILLER

1. Introduction 41
2. The Concept of Fixed Sentencing 41
3. Founding Principles of the Juvenile Court 43
4. Court-Appointed Expert Witnesses 44
5. Due Process Rights of Juvenile Offenders 45
   5.1. Right to Notice and an Opportunity to Be Heard 45
   5.2. The Right to Counsel 46
   5.3. Confrontation of Adverse Witnesses 46
   5.4. The Right to Proof of Guilt beyond a Reasonable Doubt 46
   5.5. The Dispositional Process 47
   5.6. The Needs and Desires of the Juvenile 47
   5.7. Privacy of Juvenile Records 47
   5.8. Miscellaneous Considerations 47
6. Conclusion 48
References 48

CHAPTER 5

Temperament and Its Role in Developmental–Behavioral Diagnosis

WILLIAM B. CAREY

1. Introduction 49
2. Basic Issues 49

2.1. Definition 49
2.2. Measurement 52
2.3. Origins and Stability 53
2.4. Clinical Importance 53
3. Temperament in the Diagnostic Process: An Algorithm 54
3.1. Concern 56
3.2. Agreement 57
3.3. Developmental or Physical Problem? 58
3.4. Severe Behavioral Adjustment Problems 59
3.5. Minor Behavioral Adjustment Problems 59
3.6. Moderate Behavioral Adjustment Problems Related to Temperament–Environment Interactions 60
3.7. Moderate Behavioral Adjustment Problems Related to Other Factors 61
3.8. Other Management Problems 62
4. Summary 63
References 64

CHAPTER 6

Managed-Care Plans: An Update

RICHARD DONN

1. Introduction 67
2. Preferred Provider Organization 67
2.1. Provider-Sponsored PPOs 68
2.2. Insurer-Sponsored PPOs 69
2.3. Investor–Entrepreneurial-Sponsored PPOs 69
3. HMOs 69
4. Selection of Managed-Care Plans by Physician Providers 70
5. Evaluation of the HMO Quality 71
5.1. Access to Care 71
5.2. The Management Structure 71
5.3. Miscellaneous Factors 72
6. Evaluating Competitive Dimensions of Private Practice 72
7. Conclusions 73
References 74

CHAPTER 7

The Learning-Disabled Child: Pediatric Roles in Assessment and Management

PAUL H. DWORKIN

1. Introduction 75
1.1. The Concept of Specific Learning Disabilities 75

1.2. Factors Molding Pediatric Roles 77
2. Pediatric Assessment: Beyond Basic Competency 78
2.1. An Overview of Pediatric Assessment 78
2.2. Clinical Correlates of Learning Disabilities 79
2.3. Guidelines for Pediatric Assessment 82
2.4. One Pediatric Model 83
3. Management of Learning Disabilities: Effective or Elusive? 85
3.1. An Overview of Pediatric Roles in Management 85
3.2. Specific Intervention Strategies 87
4. Summary 89
References 90

CHAPTER 8

Television Viewing: Impact on Child and Adolescent Development

MARVIN I. GOTTLIEB

1. Introduction 93
2. General Epidemiological Considerations 94
2.1. Quantitative Considerations 96
2.2. Qualitative Considerations 97
3. Developmental–Behavioral Implications: Negative Effects 97
3.1. Television and Aggressive/Violent Behaviors 98
3.2. Television and Youth Suicide 99
3.3. Television and Pediatric Health Practices 100
3.4. Television and Reading/Learning Skills 103
4. Guidelines for Management of Television Practices 104
5. Summary 105
References 107

CHAPTER 9

Self-Destructive Behaviors in Children and Adolescents: Intermediary Levels of Intervention by Parents, Peers, and Pediatricians

MARVIN I. GOTTLIEB

1. Introduction 111
2. The Adolescent Crisis 112

3. Youth Suicide ... 114
3.1. Epidemiological Considerations ... 114
3.2. Depression and Suicide ... 116
3.3. Cluster Suicides (The Werther Effect) ... 120
3.4. Myths and Misconceptions ... 122
3.5. Childhood Suicide ... 124
3.6. Adolescent Suicide ... 125
3.7. Contributing Factors and Warning Signs ... 132
4. Self-Destructive Behaviors: "The Slow Lane" ... 135
4.1. Drug and Alcohol Abuse ... 136
4.2. Inappropriate Adolescent Behaviors ... 138
5. Intermediary Levels of Intervention ... 141
5.1. Role of Parents ... 141
5.2. Role of Peers ... 143
5.3. Role of Primary-Care Physicians ... 144
6. The Survivors ... 146
7. Summary ... 147
References ... 147

CHAPTER 10

Developmental–Behavioral Pediatrics: Past, Present, and Future

MORRIS GREEN

1. A Time of Change ... 153
2. Fashioning a New Identity ... 158
3. Pediatrics and Adaptation ... 159
4. The Adaptation of the Pediatrician ... 160
5. The Need for New Pediatric Ambulatory Care Models ... 162
6. Looking to the Future ... 165
Suggested Reading ... 167

CHAPTER 11

Long-Range Management Strategies for Adolescents and Adults with Developmental Disabilities

JONATHAN J. HALPERT

1. Introduction ... 169
2. Intermediate Care Facility ... 169

2.1. General Goals of an ICF 170
2.2. Impact of an ICF on Health Care Delivery 171
2.3. Resolving Problems: Possible Strategies 174
3. Summary 175
References 175
Suggested Reading 176

CHAPTER 12

Right Brain, Left Brain: Practical Implications from Infancy to Adulthood

MARCEL KINSBOURNE

1. Introduction 177
2. Two Intelligences 180
3. The Structure of the Intellect 181
4. Specializations of the Hemispheres 182
5. Is a Hemisphere Used as a Whole? 184
6. Hemisphere Styles 185
7. Hemispheric Profiles of Mental Abilities 187
8. Summary 189
References 189

CHAPTER 13

Enhancing Pediatric Compliance in Primary Care

JUDITH R. MATHEWS AND EDWARD R. CHRISTOPHERSEN

1. Introduction 193
2. Child and Adolescent Compliance 194
2.1. Compliance with Medical Procedures 194
2.2. Noncompliance with Medical Regimens 195
3. Strategies for Enhancing Child and Adolescent Compliance 196
3.1. Improving Compliance with Medical Procedures 196
3.2. Improving Compliance with Medical Regimens 205
4. Suggestions for the Medical Community 206
4.1. Medical Personnel 206
4.2. Organizational Changes 207
5. Conclusion 207
References 209

CHAPTER 14

Office Screening for Communicative Disorders in Young Children

JERRY L. NORTHERN, DEWEY WALKER, MARION P. DOWNS, AND SUSAN GUGENHEIM

1. Introduction 213
2. Otitis Media in Children 216
   2.1. General Epidemiological Considerations 217
   2.2. Middle Ear Effusions in Neonates 217
   2.3. Persistent Middle Ear Effusion 218
3. Normal Speech Development 218
4. Screening Speech, Language, and Hearing 220
5. Guidelines for Hearing and Language Screening of Young Children in Physicians' Offices 221
   5.1. Hearing Screening 224
   5.2. Language Screening 227
6. Additional Guidelines for Following Children with Middle Ear Effusion 228
7. Home Language Stimulation 228
8. Hearing Aid Placement 230
   References 230

CHAPTER 15

Relaxation Imagery Training: Applications to Developmental–Behavioral Pediatrics

KAREN N. OLNESS

1. Introduction 233
2. The New Pediatrics and Self-Regulation Strategies 234
   2.1. Applications to Child Health Professionals 235
   2.2. Applications in Hospital Settings 236
   2.3. Applications in School Settings 237
   2.4. Applications in Athletics, Arts, and Music 238
   2.5. Applications in Third-World Child Health 239
3. Methods 239
4. Decision Making Regarding Appropriate Therapy 240
5. Research Findings 242
6. The Future 243
7. Appendix 245
   References 245

Chapter 16

Graduates of the Neonatal Intensive Care Unit

HAROLD PERL

1. Introduction 247
2. Incidence 247
3. Sequelae 248
   3.1. Intraventricular Hemorrhage 248
   3.2. Bronchopulmonary Dysplasia 249
   3.3. Retinopathy of Prematurity 250
   3.4. Hearing Problems 251
4. Summary 251
   References 252
   Suggested Reading 252

Chapter 17

Pediatrics, Neurology, and Psychiatry—A Common Ground: The Child Who Fails to Speak

N. PAUL ROSMAN

1. Introduction 253
2. Levels of Language 254
3. Speech 254
   3.1. Normal Speech Development 254
   3.2. Speech Delay and Deficits 255
   3.3. Speech Disorders Sometimes Associated with Speech Delay 255
   3.4. Major Causes of Speech Delay in Children 256
4. Summary 263
   References 264
   Suggested Reading 265

Chapter 18

Developmental–Behavioral Disorders: Need the Geriatrician Be Concerned?

FREDRICK T. SHERMAN

1. Aging of America 267
   1.1. Demographic Changes of All Populations 267

1.2. Demography of Developmentally Disabled Populations 268
2. Normal Senescence 268
3. Common Geriatric Problems 269
3.1. Ageism 269
3.2. Underreporting and Nonreporting 270
3.3. Nonspecific Indicators of Serious Illness 270
4. Clinical Problems in Aging MR/DD Populations 271
4.1. Medical Problems 271
4.2. Psychiatric Problems 272
5. Prevention 275
6. Conclusion 276
References 277

Index 279

CHAPTER 1

Child/Adolescent Depression

Guidelines for Office Management

GLEN P. AYLWARD

1. Introduction

One of the most common reasons for referral of children and adolescents to mental health professionals is suspected depression. The concept of childhood depression has gained increased recognition over the last 20 years. Although there continues to be debate as to whether childhood and adolescent depression (particularly childhood) are a reflection of normal variation in mood; a symptom (dysphoric mood) that may occur with other conditions; a syndrome with a cluster of cognitive, psychomotor, and biological manifestations that occur together regularly; or an illness having a characteristic cause, clinical course, history, and response to treatment. It is reasonable for the primary-care physician to view childhood depression as a constellation of factors that resemble a syndrome. This constellation consists of a persistent mood disorder (dysphoria) and dysfunctional behavior that interfere with the child's day-to-day activities. The manifestations vary according to the age of the child and other factors such as family dynamics.

2. Diagnosis

A major problem facing professionals who deal with depression in childhood and adolescence is assessment and diagnostic techniques. No

GLEN P. AYLWARD • Division of Developmental and Behavioral Pediatrics, Departments of Pediatrics and Psychiatry, Southern Illinois University School of Medicine, Springfield, Illinois 62794-9230.

single measure is used predominantly, although the DSM-III criteria are quite popular. Assessment techniques include self-report measures, interviews, and rating scales. Generally, self-report scales and structured interviews are used most frequently (Table 1). These techniques have three possible functions: (1) identification of children with clinically significant depression, (2) provision of a psychiatric diagnosis, or (3) measurement of the degree of response to a therapeutic intervention. It appears that identification of depressed children would be a major diagnostic challenge for the primary care physician.

Self-report scales such as the Childhood Depression Inventory (Kovacs and Beck, 1977) or the Children's Depression Scale (Tischer and Lang, 1983) are attractive for use in office practice, since the child or adolescent is given a form to complete, thereby maximizing time efficiency. Unfortunately, this approach reflects the bias that childhood depression is similar to the adult form and therefore may be adequate for adolescents but may not be for younger children. Younger children utilize denial and answer questions inaccurately, especially if the face validity of the question is high. Further, language and cognitive skills may not be well developed in the child, thereby influencing the interpretations of the questions. Cognitive functioning could be hampered by depressive symptoms, decreasing the child's ability to interpret questions or respond accurately. For example, the Children's Depression Scale contains items such as, "often I feel I am not getting anywhere," and "often I feel dead inside." As a result, self-report measures are sometimes presented in interview format. Though interviews circumvent some of these problems, the child's interpretation of the questions may still confuse the results. Further, interviews and self-report measures are generally useful only in children older than six years of age. The practitioner must also consider that interviews will usually take at least 30 minutes. Nonetheless, to screen for depression in children, pediatricians are advised to use information from multiple sources, including short, structured interviews with the child [e.g., Poznanski *et al.*'s (1984) Children's Depression Rating Scale-R] and parents [e.g., Petti's (1978) Belleview Index of Depression], as well as school reports and psychological testing. Psychological testing should include projective techniques in prepubertal children; projective techniques and the Minnesota Multiphasic Personality Inventory could be used in older adolescents.

Several caveats need to be emphasized. Mildly to moderately depressed adolescents perceive themselves as more depressed than do experienced raters. They also tend to report biological symptoms less often than psychosocial symptoms. Adolescents from lower socioeconomic backgrounds tend to score higher on self-report measures. With younger children, there is often little correspondence between parent and

Table 1. Popular Assessment Instruments/Diagnostic Criteria in Childhood and Adolescent Depression

	Author	Applicable age range
Self-Rating		
Children's Depression Inventory (CDI)[a,b]	Kovacs and Beck, 1977	6–13
Reynolds Adolescent Depression Scale (RADS)	Reynolds, 1984	12–18
Children's Depression Scale (CDS)[a,b]	Tischer and Lang, 1983	9–16
Short Children's Depression Inventory (S-CDI)[b]	Carlson and Cantwell, 1979	7–17
Modified Zung Depression Scale (M-ZUNG)[b]	Lefkowitz and Tesiny, 1980	>12
Beck Depression Inventory-Adolescents (BDI-A)[b]	Chiles *et al.*, 1980	>12
Interview Schedules		
Interview Schedule for Childern (ISC)[b]	Kovacs, 1981	8–17
Schedule for Affective Disorder and Schizophrenia for School-Age Children (K-SADS-E[a,b]; K-SADS-P)[b]	Orvaschel and Puig-Antich, 1986	6–17
Diagnostic Interview for Children and Adolescents (DICA)[b]	Herjanic and Reich, 1982	6–17
Children's Depression Rating Scale (Revised) (CDRS; CDRS-R)[a,b]	Poznanski, 1979, 1984	6–12
Bellevue Index of Depression (BID)[a,b]	Petti, 1978	6–16
Interview Schedules		
School Age Depression Listed Inventory (SALDI)[b]	Petti and Law, 1982	6–13
Symptom Checklist for Major Depressive Disorders (DSM-III-CL)[b]	Kashani *et al.*, 1982	6–17
Child Assessment Schedule (CAS)[b]	Hodges *et al.*, 1981	7–16
Other (diagnostic criteria, group assessment)		
Peer Nomination Inventory for Depression (PNID)[b]	Lefkowitz and Tesiny, 1980	≥8
Weinberg Diagnostic Criteria	Weinberg *et al.*, 1973	—
Research Diagnostic Criteria (RDC)[b]	Spitzer *et al.*, 1978	—
Diagnostic and Statistical Manual of Mental Disorders (DSM-III)[a]	American Psychiatric Association, 1980	—

[a]Used more frequently than other instruments.
[b]Discussed in: National Institute of Health, 1985, Rating scales and assessment instruments for use in pediatric psychopharmacology research, *Psychopharm. Bull.* **21**:951–998.

child ratings, with children underestimating depression. The higher the child's IQ, the greater the discrepancy. Fathers have also been reported to give lower ratings of depression than mothers.

The DSM-III criteria for major depression (Table 2) are used frequently. The primary manifestation concerns dysphoric mood or anhe-

Table 2. DSM-III Criteria for Major Depression[a]

Dysphoric mood (or loss of interest in most activities)
At least four of the following present almost daily ≥2 weeks:
Poor appetite/weight loss, weight gain[b]
Insomnia/hypersomnia[b]
Psychomotor agitation or retardation (hypoactivity)[b]
Apathy[b]
Loss of energy/fatigue
Feelings of worthlessness, self-reproach, guilt
Diminished ability to think or concentrate
Recurrent thoughts of death, suicidal ideation, suicide attempt

[a]The more recent DSM-III–R criteria are quite similar although the degree of the child's current state is graded mild, moderate, and severe.
[b]In children under 6 years of age, three of the first four criteria.

donia (loss of interest in most usual activities and pastimes), which has to be present daily for a period of at least 2 weeks. Children under six years of age should have at least three of the first four criteria, and hyperactivity and signs of apathy are also expected. There has been some recent evidence that symptoms of the disorder can last longer than the period of time during which the episode meets the full diagnostic criteria. Further, in a recent study of preschoolers (Kashani *et al.*, 1986) it was noted that a significant proportion manifested a high number of depressive symptoms that were of concern to teachers and parents. They did not, however, meet the DSM-III criteria necessary for the clinical diagnosis of depression. Anger (versus sadness) is often the predominant feeling of depressed preschoolers.

The diagnosis of a "dysthymic disorder" (previously called depressive neurosis) is sometimes used with children and adolescents when the symptoms persist in an intermittent but chronic fashion for a year or more. Depressive manifestations could be separated by periods of normal mood, lasting from several days to more than a few months at a time (Table 3). There is considerable overlap between major depression and dysthymia.

Some National Institute of Mental Health criteria (developed in 1977) are basically similar to those of DSM-III, although the minimum duration of the disorder is considered to be four weeks. Further, in these criteria, it is emphasized that developmental levels should be considered in making the diagnosis of depression (i.e., ≤8 years; >8 years).

The concept of "masked depression," with its attendant "depressive equivalents," which originated in the mid-to-late 1960s, deserves mention. Although not a formal diagnosis per se, this controversial concept became increasingly accepted following the publication of Cytryn and

Table 3. DSM-III Criteria for Dysthymic Disorder

For the past 2 years, depressive symptoms of insufficient intensity and duration to meet criteria for major depression
Depressive symptoms may be intermittent[a]
Prominent depressed mood or loss of interest in usual activities during depressed periods[a]
During depressed periods at least three of the following present:
- Insomnia/hypersomnia[a]
- Low energy level, chronic tiredness[a]
- Feelings of inadequacy, loss of self-esteem, self-depreciation[a]
- Decreased effectiveness or productivity at school or home
- Decreased attention, concentration, or ability to think clearly[a]
- Social withdrawal
- Loss of interest in or enjoyment of pleasurable activities (anhedonia)
- Irritability or excessive anger (in children, expressed toward parents or caretakers)
- Inability to respond with apparent pleasure to praise or rewards
- Less active or talkative than usual/slowed down, restless
- Pessimistic attitude toward the future; brooding about past events[a]
- Tearfulness or crying
- Recurrent thoughts of death or suicide

[a]In DSM-III-R, these criteria are indicated, in addition to poor appetite or overeating. Duration for children and adolescents is only one year and social interactions are particulary impaired.

McKnew's (1972) three-part operational classification. The proposed classification included: *acute depression,* seen in previously well-adjusted children with minimal family psychopathology; *chronic depression,* which usually occurs in conjunction with a depressed parent and a poor premorbid adjustment in the child; and *masked depression,* which is associated with severe family psychopathology. In masked depression, the depressive symptoms are not obvious and take the form of hyperactivity, aggressiveness, school refusal, or somatic complaints. In all likelihood the patient with masked depression is an "externalizer" whose behavior pattern obscures the depression and who may strongly deny feeling depressed. Support for this particular concept has generally waned. There is evidence, however, that one quarter to one third of adolescents and prepubertal children with conduct disorders, or those who are involved with correctional systems, have major depressive disorders. The onset of depression tends to precede the conduct disorder in the vast majority of patients. Treatment with antidepressant medication generally has facilitated disappearance of the conduct problems.

Differential Diagnosis

A responsibility of the primary-care physician is to identify children with clinically significant depression. The DSM-III criteria are generally helpful. A large number of children (2.5% to 17.4%), however, will exhibit depressive symptoms, but not of a sufficient magnitude to warrant this diagnosis. Some investigators have characterized these criteria as being too restrictive. Table 4 contains a listing of those symptoms that appear consistently across various diagnostic criteria. In determining whether a child is depressed, duration, precipitating causes, premorbid adjustment, family history, and the child's developmental stage should be considered. In addition, there should be a significant change from the previous emotional status of the child and this change should be sustained from two to four weeks.

Several other disorders are similar to a major depressive disorder in childhood and adolescence. An adjustment disorder with depressed mood is a maladaptive reaction to an identifiable psychosocial stressor. The symptoms usually occur within three months of the onset of stress and generally remit once the stressor is removed. Uncomplicated bereavement, where the focus is on the death of a loved one, is also sometimes confused with major depression. A separation anxiety disorder (anxiety involving separation from persons to whom the child is at-

Table 4. Primary and Associated Symptoms of Depression in Children

Primary symptoms
Depressed affect/sadness (dysphoric mood)
Anhedonia (loss of pleasure)
Self-deprecatory ideation
Tearfulness/frequent crying
Psychomotor retardation/fatigue
Low sense of self-worth/self-esteem
Social withdrawal
Impairment of schoolwork
Difficulty with biological functions (sleeping, eating)
Morbid ideation/suicide attempts
Associated symptoms
Irritability
Moodiness (emotional lability)
Social interactive difficulties
Pathological guilt
Somatic complaints
Anxiety, decreased concentration
Obsessive rumination and thoughts
Attention deficit
Feelings of helplessness/hopelessness
Aggressive and explosive behaviors
Enuresis/encopresis

tached), learning disabilities, or sadness associated with a physical illness also may be misconstrued as major depression of childhood. It should be noted that anxiety disorders, attention deficit disorders, and conduct disorders have been found to coexist with major depression. Also, a significant number of severely depressed preadolescents may exhibit hallucinations, particularly of an auditory type.

3. Epidemiology

The samples of children studied, their ages, and the diagnostic criteria used preclude agreement as to the prevalence of depression in childhood and adolescence. Rates of depression have varied from 0.8% to almost 60%; children in these studies have included inpatients, outpatients, and children from the general population. The prevalence of major depressive disorder (using DSM-III criteria) appears to be slightly less than 2% of the general population. Rates of depression in samples of child psychiatry inpatients or children referred to an educational diagnostic center approach 60%. Therefore, higher rates of depression exist in clinical versus epidemiologic surveys. Since the sample of children typically brought to the pediatrician's office is heterogeneous and the reasons for referral vary, it is reasonable to estimate a prevalence rate somewhat higher than that found in the general population studies. Perhaps 5–8% warrant the formal diagnosis of depression, with many more children having a number of associated symptoms, but not sufficient for the diagnosis.

4. Risk Factors

Risk factors for major depression in childhood or adolescence may be genetic, psychosocial, or both. There is evidence for clustering of depression in families, but genetic and environmental influences are difficult to separate in such a relationship.

There are generally two types of genetic studies: offspring studies and twin studies. In the former, a strong correlation exists between unipolar (major depression) or bipolar (manic–depressive illness) in parents and the same disorder in children. A higher rate of depressive symptoms (11 to 19%) has been reported in children of depressed parents. If one parent has a depressive disorder, a morbidity risk of 27% may be present in the children; with two affected parents, the risk increases to 74% (Gershon *et al.*, 1982). An increase in the incidence of *cyclothymic* disorders (an attenuated form of a bipolar disorder) and *dysthymic* disorders has been reported to occur in children of bipolar parents. It also appears that cyclothymic and dysthymic disorders may later evolve into other affective disorders. Therefore, genetic risk factors include a family history of alcoholism, suicide, or affective disorder. Further, the stronger the family history of depression, the increased probability that childhood depression would occur at an earlier age.

In twin studies, the concordance rate for affective disorders is reported to be 65 to 76% among monozygotic twins and 14 to 19% in dyzygotic twins. A 67% concordance rate has been reported in a small sample of monozygotic twins raised apart. Thus there appears to be a genetic risk for depression, although the mode of transmission is speculative with some evidence supporting a polygenetic basis.

Psychosocial risk factors for child/adolescent depression include a loss of any type. Such a loss could be the death of a parent or close relative, parental rejection, a geographic move, divorce, abuse or neglect, foster placement, or long-term hospitalization. Loss of self-esteem or self-image is also a risk factor that may be affected by learning disabilities, chronic illness, or physical deformity. Losses may be real, perceived, or could potentially occur. Affective illness in the parents may also be a psychosocial risk factor, as this depression could disrupt the parent/child interaction and lead to development of symptoms in the child. Depressed mothers have been reported to be less positive in regard to their responses to children, exhibiting more critical and rejecting behaviors. Rigid, disengaged, or uncompromising parents may precipitate the onset of depression in the child.

5. Biological Indicators

There is much interest in the investigation of biological correlates of depression in adults, an interest that has recently been extended to children.

Cortisol hypersecretion, a neuroendocrine measure, is an area of investigation in children made popular by the focus on the dexamethasone suppression test (DST) in the diagnosis of adult depression. The procedure involves the hypothalamic–pituitary–adrenal axis, with exogenous dexamethasone administration suppressing normal increases in diurnal plasma cortisol and 17-hydroxycorticosteroid levels for 24 hr. Typically, a 0.5- to 1.5-mg dosage is given orally at 11:00 PM, and blood is drawn at 4:00 PM the next day. In preadolescents, sensitivity rates in the 50 to 60% range and specificity rates of 85 to 90% have been reported (Petty *et al.*, 1985). Lower sensitivity rates (e.g., 14.4%) or limited specificity, however, have been reported in other studies (Geller *et al.,* 1983). Similar figures have been reported in adolescents, indicating that approximately one half of the significantly depressed adolescents failed to show positive DST findings. Generally, the numbers of subjects in most studies have been small; samples typically consisted of inpatients and the methodologies differed (e.g., dosage of dexamethasone). Further, children and adolescents with anxiety disorders and dysthymia have also shown positive DST findings (perhaps reflecting the similarity in the diagnostic criteria). Therefore, the DST should be considered experimental in children and of limited use for the practitioner at this time.

Depressed children have demonstrated hyposecretion of growth hormone after injection of exogenous insulin (Puig-Antich *et al.,* 1984). They also secrete more growth hormone during sleep compared with controls. These phenomena may reflect a functional hypothalamic–serotonin deficit.

Other areas of biological investigation of depression in children and adolescents include decreased urinary metabolites of norepinephrine in depressed children (thereby suggesting decreased levels of norepinephrine in the depressed patients) and sleep studies. In the latter, depressed children did not display any of the polysomnographic characteristics generally found in adult depression, such as a decrease in slow-wave sleep, decrease in sleep efficiency, or alteration of rapid eye movement sleep.

6. Biochemical Treatment

Drug studies, evaluating the efficacy of medication in the treatment of child and adolescent depression, contain numerous methodological problems. Many are uncontrolled, sample sizes are small, different diagnostic criteria are used, the length of treatment and dosage vary, and improvement is measured in a variety of ways. Imipramine (Tofranil) and amitriptyline (Elavil), both tricyclic antidepressants, are the two drugs used most frequently in the treatment of childhood depression. A greater variety of drugs (besides imipramine and amitriptyline) are used in adolescents, including amoxapine (Ascendin), nortriptyline (Aventyl), desipramine (Norpramin), and the so-called "second-generation" tetracyclics (Ludiomil). Pediatricians and family practitioners are probably more familiar with the use of Tofranil, as this drug is also used in the treatment of enuresis. The Food and Drug Administration regards the use of imipramine and other antidepressants as investigational in the treatment of emotional disorders in children younger than 12 years of age.

Data from the better-controlled studies of tricyclic antidepressants (particularly imipramine) suggest that 60 to 80% of prepubertal children respond, whereas approximately one third of the adolescents improve. The key to efficacy appears to lie in plasma levels: plasma levels in the range of 125 to 155 ng/ml are associated with a positive response, with 200 to 225 mg/ml being optimal (Weller *et al.,* 1982). It appears that although a response can occur at less than 125 mg/ml, it takes longer. Plasma monitoring is also indicated by the fact that a sixfold rate of between-patient variability in steady-state plasma drug concentrations has been found with a fixed 75-mg dose of imipramine. A recommended regimen consists of a maximum of 5 mg/kg per day administered in three roughly equivalent doses (Puig-Antich, 1984). This regimen, however, is typically used on an inpatient basis, where compliance can be monitored closely. Other clinicians prefer administration of one evening dose to decrease the daytime sedative effect that some patients experience during the first few weeks of treatment. A trial of at least 4 to 6 weeks is necessary in order to determine efficacy. There are various precautionary measures that need to be taken when imipramine is prescribed (Rauber and Maroncelli, 1984). The incidence of less serious side effects was found not to be related to plasma drug concentrations; this suggests that complaints about side effects may not be useful in titrating medications to avoid toxicity. The use of monoamine oxidase inhibitors and lithium in the treatment of depression in children and adolescents is reported; however, the data are inconclusive and the risks of complications do not currently support the use of these medications.

7. Developmental Concerns

The issue of whether depression is the same in children and adolescents is controversial and has obvious implications in the area of diagnosis. During childhood and adolescence, symbolism, language, and cognitive development undergo change; it therefore appears logical that manifestations and perhaps causes of depression would change as well (Phillips, 1979). At younger ages there is a more direct cause–effect relationship between stressors and depression, with manifestations being more physiological or organic. With development, the relationship between stressful environmental events and depression becomes less clear and reactions become more cognitively complex and less physiological.

Depression in infancy takes the form of biologic, deprivation syndromes, with symptoms including feeding problems, growth retardation, sleep difficulties, social withdrawal, or apathy. Excessive irritability and lethargy are also noted. When depression occurs in infancy, the problem is assumed to be related to disruptions in the mother–infant interaction and failure to thrive or rumination are common.

In early childhood, depression is displayed as abnormal motor activity. Symptoms include high levels of activity (often prompting referral for evaluation of hyperactivity), physical aggressiveness, and other manifestations of anger. Enuresis, encopresis, social withdrawal, separation problems, and sleep or eating problems are also frequently found. Emotional lability is more commonly observed.

Depression during middle childhood (ages 5 through 8 years) becomes more obvious and episodes of sadness appear to be more sustained. Children are generally unable to verbalize their reasons for the dysphoric mood. Symptoms include somatization disorders, psychogenic pain, social withdrawal, accident proneness, oppositional behavior, and acting out behavior such as lying, stealing, and physical aggression. Academic underachievement is frequently found. Self-esteem issues become prominent and a poor self-concept, self-blame, and guilt become major problems as well.

During late childhood (ages 9 to 12 years), depression more frequently involves low self-esteem and a child's disappointment with self. Prominent symptoms include obvious sadness, apathy, a sense of helplessness, somatization disorders, psychogenic pain, irritability, anhedonia, anxiety, school problems, and an inability to concentrate. Suicidal ideation or attempts are also found.

Depression in adolescents is reported to resemble that found in adults. This disorder is more frequent at this age, the incidence in 14-year-old patients being three to four times higher than that found with 10-year-old children. Hopelessness or a fear of the future become paramount and the adolescent often views options in an inflexible, all-or-none manner. The sense of futility or hopelessness is reflected in the increased prevalence of suicides in this age group. Other symptoms include somatization disorders, psychogenic pain, anorexia nervosa, excessive drug/alcohol abuse, antisocial behavior, and social withdrawal.

It therefore appears that depression exists at all ages of childhood; however, the manifestations of dysphoria and the resultant dysfunctional behavior in children are probably age-specific (Aylward, 1985).

8. Office Management

Pediatricians and family practitioners are usually the first professionals to be contacted by parents when they become concerned about the behavior of their child. There are several steps that the practitioner may follow. First, a history should be obtained from caretakers, using one of the instruments listed in Table 1 or the diagnostic criteria found in Tables 2–4. Second, the use of a structured interview with the child, such as Poznanski's CDRS-R, is advisable. If possible, additional information from the teachers and other sources should be obtained. This procedure, coupled with information concerning risk factors, often enables the practitioner to determine whether the child may be depressed. The physician may assume the primary role of case manager or coordinator. A working relationship with pediatric psychologists, child psychiatrists, or other mental health professionals is recommended to assist in further diagnosis and treatment. The primary-care physician typically has a good relationship with the family and can support the parents, helping them overcome fears or misgivings concerning mental health interventions. Although the informed practitioner can manage a medication regimen, additional therapeutic interventions are typically required, and these interventions are usually time consuming. Thus pediatricians and family practitioners, while still remaining case managers, may opt for more interdisciplinary follow-up and in so doing continue to provide a valuable service to their young patients and their families.

References

Aylward, G. P., 1985, Understanding and treatment of childhood depression, *J. Pediatrics* **107:**1.

Cytryn, L., and McKnew, D. H., 1972, Proposed classification of childhood depression, *Am. J. Psychiatry* **129:**149.

Diagnostic and Statistical Manual of Mental Disorders (DSM-III), 1980, American Psychiatric Association, Washington, D.C.

Diagnostic and Statistical Manual of Mental Disorders–Revised (DSM-III-R), 1987, American Psychiatric Association, Washington, D.C.

Geller, B., Pirel, J. M., Knitter, E. F., *et al.*, 1983, Nortriptyline in major depressive disorder in children: Response, steady state plasma levels, predictive kinetics and pharmacokinetics, *Psychopharmacol. Bull.* **19:**62.

Gershon, E. S., Hamovit, J., and Guroft, J. J., 1982, A family study of schizoaffective, bipolar I, bipolar II, unipolar, and normal control probands, *Arch. Gen. Psychiatry* **39:**1157.

Kashani, J. H., Holcomb, W. R., and Orvaschel, H., 1986, Depression and depressive symptoms in preschool children from the general population, *Am. J. Psychiatry* **143:**1138.

Kovacs, M., and Beck, A. T., 1977, An empirical clinical approach towards a definition of childhood depression, in: *Depression in Children* (J. G. Schulterbrandt and A. Raskin, eds.), pp. 1–25, Raven Press, New York.

National Institute of Health, 1985, Rating scales and assessment instruments for use in pediatric psychopharmacology research, *Psychopharm. Bull.* **21:**951–998.

Petti, T. A., 1978, Depression in hospitalized child psychiatry patients: Approaches to measuring depression, *J. Am. Acad. Child Psychiatry* **17**:49.

Petty, L. K., Asarnow, J. R., Carlson, G. A., *et al.*, 1985, The dexamethasone suppression test in depressed, dysthymic, and non-depressed children, *Am. J. Psychiatry* **142**:631.

Phillips, I., 1979, Childhood depression: Interpersonal interactions and depressive phenomena, *Am. J. Psychiatry* **136**:511.

Poznanski, E. O., Freeman, L. N., and Mokros, H. B., 1984, Children's Depression Rating Scale-Revised, *Psychopharm. Bull.* **21**:979.

Puig-Antich, J., 1984, Clinical and treatment aspects of depression in childhood and adolescence, *Pediatr. Annu.* **13**:37.

Puig-Antich, J., Novacenko, H., Davies, M., *et al.*, 1984, Growth hormone secretion in prepubertal children with major depressive episode, *Arch. Gen. Psychiatry* **41**:455.

Rauber, A., and Maroncelli, R., 1984, Prescribing practices and knowledge of tricyclic antidepressants among physicians caring for children, *Pediatrics* **73**:107.

Tischer, M., and Lang, M., 1983, The Children's Depression Scale: Review and further developments, in: *Affective Disorders in Childhood and Adolescence* (D. P. Cantwell and G. A. Carlson, eds.), pp. 181–203, SP Medical and Scientific Books, New York.

Weinberg, W. A., Rutman, J., Sullivan, L., *et al.*, 1973, Depression in children referred to an educational diagnostic center, *J. Pediatr.* **83**:1065–1072.

Weller, E. B., Weller, R. A., Preskorn, S. H., *et al.*, 1982, Steady-state plasma imipramine levels in prepubertal depressed children, *Am. J. Psychiatry* **139**:506.

CHAPTER 2

Outcome of the High-Risk Infant

Fact versus Fiction

GLEN P. AYLWARD

1. Introduction

Investigation of the contribution of perinatal factors to subsequent cognitive, motor, and neurologic outcome is an important but difficult task. Follow-up of at-risk infants is necessary to evaluate the efficacy of innovative medical procedures, to provide an immediate diagnosis and a baseline to compare change in status, and to identify babies who will require intervention. This issue becomes more important with increased survival rates and the potential for an increased number of children who will have what are termed high-prevalence, low-severity disabilities. As a result, this issue extends more and more into the realm of the practitioner who, in addition to providing continuing medical care to these infants, must determine the possibility of sequelae and provide feedback and prognostic information to parents. Unfortunately, outcome data from perinatal investigations often are not clear, being hampered by sampling issues, multiple factors converging to influence outcome, and problems in definition.

Developmental neuropsychological processes are complex and involve plasticity and modifiability. The nervous system of the infant adjusts to environmental influences by the subtractive, retrogressive mech-

GLEN P. AYLWARD • Division of Developmental and Behavioral Pediatrics, Departments of Pediatrics and Psychiatry, Southern Illinois University School of Medicine, Springfield, Illinois 62794-9230.

anisms of cell death and process elimination (Prechtl, 1984). Damage, which is often termed neurodevelopmental deficit, is typically due to loss of neural tissue (necrosis) or malformations due to developmental arrest, abnormalities of cell migration, or unsuccessful attempts at repair. Further, interactions between perinatal factors, race, socioeconomic status, and education are extremely difficult to separate and may affect cognitive, motor, and neurologic function differently (Aylward *et al.*, 1987). Therefore, outcome after the occurrence of any single potentially hazardous perinatal event is extremely difficult to predict. Furthermore, short-term evaluation allows for greater follow-up compliance and better inference regarding the relationships between the perinatal complication and outcome; however, early assessment instruments have many limitations. Later follow-up enables more detailed assessment of higher-order cognitive functioning and school achievement, but environmental influences may obscure any effects attributable to the original perinatal problem. Several perinatal complications have been selected for review in this chapter, with the acknowledgment that they are highly interrelated: asphyxia as determined by Apgar scores, seizures, intraventricular hemorrhage (IVH), hypoxic ischemic encephalopathy (HIE), and very low birthweight (VLBW).

2. Low Apgar Scores (Asphyxia) and Outcome

Asphyxia, a biochemical increase in blood carbon dioxide, is the result of a decrease in oxygen. Asphyxia is not a single causative factor; in addition to lowered oxygen and increased carbon dioxide there is also a decrease in blood pH, depressed respiration, cyanosis, and involvement of other organ systems besides the brain. The substrate on which asyphyxia is applied will also influence outcome. Low Apgar scores have a different relevance to preterm and full-term infants. Apgar scores have been shown to be related to gestational age, and respiratory effort, muscle tone, and reflex irritability are the major determinants of a decreased score (Catlin *et al.*, 1986). Thus the significance of a low Apgar score is dependent on the severity and duration of asphyxia, as well as the infant's gestational age. Although asphyxia has been indicated to be the single most influential event causing adverse developmental sequelae, data from longitudinal studies are inconclusive.

Much of our current understanding of the relationship between asphyxia and outcome is derived from the National Collaborative Perinatal Project (NCPP) data, where enrollment occurred from 1959 to 1966. Cognitive and motor development were assessed at 8 months, neurologic function at 1 and 7 years, and cognitive function was evaluated at 4 and 7 years.

At 8 months, ten signs of anoxia accounted for 2–3% of the variance on the developmental indexes of the Bayley Scales of Infant Development, with the Apgar at 1 min having no significant association. Birthweight and gestational age were the largest contributors (Broman, 1979). Apgar scores at 5 min were associated with neurobehavioral outcome (neurologic abnormality, motor retardation, aberrant muscle tone) at 12 months.

The relationship was weak between asphyxia and intellectual development at 4 years as measured by the Stanford-Binet Intelligence Test (Broman *et al.*, 1975). Neonatal variables (which included Apgar scores) accounted for only 1–2% of the variance.

By the age of 7 years, approximately 25% of the cases of poor neurologic outcome could be attributed to asphyxia. However, duration of asphyxia versus simple presence appears to be the critical factor. The incidence of neurologic problems in surviving children with Apgar scores of 0 to 3 at 5 min was 1%; however, it was 9% in those with 0 to 3 scores at 15 min and 57% in those babies with Apgar scores of 0 to 3 at 20 min. Of the original 45,559 children enrolled in the NCPP study, 189 had cerebral palsy (CP) at age 7 years. Of these, 40 children had neurologic dysfunction and one or more clinical signs of asphyxia. Fifty-eight percent of these children had additional predictors of neurologic dysfunction which were present before the onset of labor, most typically a major congenital malformation (Nelson and Ellenberg, 1986). Also at age 7 years, perinatal asphyxia explained less than 1% of the variance on the Wechsler Intelligence Scale for Children (WISC) IQ. Asphyxia was not predictive of visual–motor integration as measured by the Bender Gestalt Test. The question of whether so-called minimal brain dysfunction (MBD) was caused or influenced by asphyxia has also been addressed (Nichols and Chen, 1981). Analyzing data from 30,000 children from the NCPP at 7 years of age, these investigators found three factors: learning difficulties, hyperkinetic–impulsive behavior, and neurologic "soft signs." In general, indicators of asphyxia were poor predictors of any of these three factors.

A high mortality rate occurred in the NCPP infants who had severe birth asphyxia. Paneth (1986) reported that of approximately 45,000 children who were evaluated at age 7, 122 had Apgar scores ≤3 at 10 min. Approximately 270 of 390 babies with Apgar scores of <3 at 10 min or later died before their first birthday. The possibility was raised that this high mortality rate prevented many children, who had significant early asphyxia, from contributing to the number of children later found to have sequelae. It was inferred that if more asphyxiated infants survived, these survivors might have an increased incidence of sequelae compared with the general population.

In an attempt to evaluate this hypothesis, we analyzed data from the five-center National Institute of Health–National Heart, Lung, and Blood Institute Collaborative Antenatal Steroid study (where enrollment occurred between 1977 and 1981). The study consisted of 739 babies and evaluations were performed at 40 weeks and 9, 18, and 36 months. Follow-up assessments included: (1) the Prechtl Neurologic Examination at 40 weeks; (2) the Bayley Scales of Infant Development and a neurological examination at 9 and 18 months; and (3) the McCarthy Scales of Children's Abilities (MSCA) and a neurologic examination at 36 months. A total of 11 asphyxia variables were correlated with outcome at 9, 18, and 36 months. The correlations were found to range from $r = .08$ to .30 ($\leq .05$) (see Table 1). The best predictors were Apgar scores at 1 and 5 min and the presence of seizures. However, the Apgar scores at 1 and 5 min accounted for 1% of the variance at 9 months and 2% of the variance at 18 months. Neither variable was predictive by 36 months. Seizures accounted for 4–7% of the variance at 9 months and 5% of the variance at 18 months. This variable was not associated with MSCA outcome at 36 months. More variables correlated with the Prechtl neurobehavioral examination at 40 weeks than with later measures, suggesting that there is a fading of influence of perinatal variables over time, particularly asphyxia. Of particular significance is the fact that these data support the findings that have been reported previously.

Current data do *not* support earlier opinions that asphyxia is the major cause of cerebral palsy and mental retardation. The relationships between low Apgar scores and outcome have been weak and usually

Table 1. Asphyxia Variables

Severe variable decelerations	Initial heart rate
Meconium stained	Initial pH
Apgar at 1 min[a]	Initial PACO
Apgar at 5 min[a]	Initial PAO
Infant resuscitated	Seizure[a]
Unassisted respiration	

[a]Best predictors.

apply only to prediction of function during infancy. The so-called "continuum of reproductive casualty," where a small degree of a hazardous perinatal factor was considered to yield minimal impairment and more significant perinatal complications were construed to cause more severe sequelae, is probably not accurate. More likely, a threshold phenomenon exists where a certain level or duration of a perinatal complication such as hypoxia must be reached before damage becomes evident (Task Force on Assessment of Prenatal and Perinatal Factors Associated with Brain Disorders, 1985). Clinically significant asphyxia depends on duration and degree of asphyxia, the infant's immediate response to the asphyxia (Apgar score), and the baby's ability to repair and recover from the hypoxic injury as evidenced by behavioral characteristics during the neonatal period. Recent evidence suggests that an Apgar score of ≤ 5 at 10 min is the most sensitive Apgar measure predicting adverse outcome. There is evidence that prolonged partial asphyxia may be worse than acute periods of more complete asphyxia, the former causing damage to the cortex and basal ganglia, whereas the latter has more implications for brain stem damage. Further, since postpartum asphyxia is treated almost immediately with resuscitation, in all likelihood it is the prolonged prenatal or perinatal asphyxia (not measured by Apgar scores) that contribute to compromised outcome. It should be emphasized that there is no doubt that children with low Apgar scores are at greater risk for sequelae than babies with higher scores; however, the influence on outcome attributed to this factor may be excessive.

3. Seizures

Neonatal seizures may also negatively influence the outcome of babies at risk. Seizures are neurologic signs that indicate acute brain disturbance. Seizures have been associated with asphyxia, intracranial hemorrhage, infection, congenital malformations, metabolic disorders, or drug withdrawal. Some investigators suggest that neonatal seizures may be better indicators of asphyxia than Apgar scores. The actual seizure activity, which occurs in the neonate during neuronal differentiation and neurodevelopmental processes, can cause destruction of neurons, reorganization of the remaining neuronal circuits, and brain metabolic effects. Because temporal lobe and subcortical structures are more maturationally advanced, these areas display more epileptic activity. Therefore, clinical manifestations are more subtle and differ between neonates and older children. Of note is the fact that seizures due to asphyxia usually have their onset 6 to 18 hr after birth, increasing in frequency over the first 24 to 48 hr. Onset generally occurs after 48 hr, if the etiology is intracranial infection; seizures attributable to congenital malformations occur 7 to 10 days after birth. Thus the timing of seizure onset, the frequency, and etiology of seizures (not simply the presence of seizures per se) have prognostic significance.

The NCPP data have provided us with much of the current knowledge about the outcome of babies who manifested seizures during the perinatal and postnatal period. In a report of the 7-year outcome of 181 survivors with neonatal seizures, 13% had cerebral palsy, 19% had a WISC IQ less than 70 (another 15% had borderline scores), and 13% had combined cerebral palsy, mental retardation (MR), or epilepsy (Holden *et al.,* 1982). Infants with seizures were 55 to 70 times more likely to have handicapping CP than babies without seizures, 5.3 times more likely to have MR, and 18 times more likely to have epilepsy than infants who did not have seizures. Prediction was increased with inclusion of low Apgar scores at 5 min (<7), longer seizure duration (>30 min), and an increased number of days over which seizures occurred. Nevertheless, 70% of those infants with neonatal seizures were normal at 7 years. Brann (1986) summarized additional NCPP data and reported that 30% of the significantly handicapped infants had seizures during the neonatal period, whereas 1% of the neurologically intact survivors had neonatal seizures. In other later-born cohorts, morbidity and mortality have been reported to be as high as 50%. Moderate neurologic impairment was found in more than 50% of the survivors, whereas 85% of those infants who had seizures spanning over a 4-day interval were severely impaired.

Few reports of specific long-term neuropsychological sequelae due to early seizures are available. This may be due to problems in the detection of seizures or the fact that seizures may simply be an indication of other more potent factors such as asphyxia or intracranial hemorrhage. It is therefore difficult to separate the effects of these precursors from the sequelae that are due specifically to seizures.

Infants who have seizures during the neonatal period are definitely at increased risk for developmental sequelae such as cognitive deficits and neuromotor impairment. However, at least 50% of those babies with seizures do not exhibit sequelae. Babies are at increased risk with seizures that occur in conjunction with low Apgar scores or those with prolonged seizure events (seizures occurring over more than a 4-day time span), significant intraventricular hemorrhage, or tonic seizures. There is a definite need for additional studies to identify specific types of deficit that may be attributable to seizures, covarying onset, duration, frequency, and presence of other hazardous perinatal factors.

4. Subependymal Germinal Matrix Hemorrhage (SEH)/Intraventricular Hemorrhage (IVH)

Germinal matrix and choroid plexus bleeding (SEH/IVH) typically occur in the preterm infant. Periventricular leukomalacia (PVL), a lesion in the white matter in the periventricular region, is found in both preterm and full-term infants. Necrotic cortical lesions (HIE) typically occur in full-term babies. SEH/IVH is related to gestational age and the birth process, although asphyxia has also been implicated as a causative factor. Asphyxia bears a strong relationship to the latter two brain disorders and is often used interchangeably with HIE. Awareness of the incidence of IVH has increased within the last decade. At present, SEH/IVH occurs in 40–50% of infants weighing less than 1500 g; hydrocephalus is a frequent sequelae. SEH/IVH generally occurs 30–36 hr after birth and affects central areas of the brain, sparing the cortical mantle. Accurate diagnosis with CT and ultrasound is a fairly recent phenomenon, and as a result, SEH/IVH was not addressed in the NCPP. The lack of accuracy in detection of IVH by clinical indicators is underscored in several studies (Ahmann *et al.*, 1980) that report that only 50% of the infants with IVH detected by CT scan were diagnosed clinically as having IVH. Therefore, long-term data on neuropsychological deficits are inconclusive.

Papile *et al.* (1978), using brain imaging, developed a classification scheme for IVH that appears to have some prognostic utility. Grades I and II are classified as mild IVH (no change in ventricular size), whereas grades III and IV are considered moderate and severe (with ventricular dilatation and parenchymal hemorrhage). The grade of IVH is therefore a major determinant of the degree of sequelae. Approximately 11% of babies with IVH of grades I or II display severe neurodevelopmental sequelae, this number being comparable to control infants who do not have IVH. However, 36–53% of infants with grade III and 76–86% of babies with grade IV IVH have major handicaps including neuromotor dysfunction, mental retardation, and hydrocephaly. There is also some evidence that Bayley motor scores are particularly affected.

Presently, most of the follow-up studies are short-term; one exception is a 3.5-year follow-up of 29 IVH babies (Williamson *et al.,* 1983). These infants, born between 1977 and 1978, were administered the McCarthy Scales of Children's Abilities (MSCA) and neurologic evaluations. Only 34% of these children had a normal neurologic outcome and 48% had a normal MSCA General Cognitive Index. Of these IVH children, 41% were involved in some type of special education program. Grade of hemorrhage and birthweight were identified as predictive variables. The CT scan may also be useful as a follow-up assessment. It appears that the more aberrant the CT scan is at term conceptional age, the worse the outcome will be on the Bayley over the first 18 months. The severity of parenchymal involvement on ultrasound has been related to significant mortality and neurologic deficits.

To summarize, severe IVH is associated with significant motor and intellectual deficits. Ventricular dilatation, found in moderate and severe IVH, produces axonal stretching and loss, gliosis, loss of protein and lipids, and alteration of cerebral vessels. It is likely that the degree of parenchymal involvement is a more critical factor than the amount of intraventricular blood; the degree of initial insult to the parenchyma also appears to be more influential than the effects of subsequent hydrocephalus. The outcome of infants with mild-to-moderate IVH (grades II and III) is not as clear, although these infants also appear to be at risk for sequelae. Again, the outcome studies are confusing due to varying definitions of poor outcome. It is quite likely that minor neurodevelopmental problems would be more prevalent. Motor problems, particularly diplegia, have been linked to IVH and most likely are due to damage in the white matter below the central sulcus, which contains the corticospinal system. With IVH, however, cells bordering the lesion, which otherwise might degenerate, are spared. Therefore, diffuse, neonatal connections would remain between structures and once stabilized, these diffuse connections could project to inappropriate structures or fail to segregate normally within a structure. The caudate involvement in IVH has possible long-range implications due to major connections with the prefrontal cortex, perhaps impairing subsequent delayed response or attentional behavior.

5. Hypoxic–Ischemic Encephalopathy (HIE)

HIE, found primarily in full-term infants, is due to asphyxia in approximately 90% of the cases, but is also associated with respiratory failure and cardiovascular disease. HIE refers to structural changes in the brain, manifest in neurologic signs, with the diagnosis typically being established on the basis of clinical findings. It also refers to damage in the peripheral and dorsal areas of the cerebral cortex, with necrotic lesions of the gyri at the depths of the sulci, the neuronal nuclei of the basal ganglia, and the brain stem (Brann, 1986). Thus there are neuroanatomic and neurologic signs. The neurologic signs that occur after birth were described by Sarnat and Sarnat (1976): in stage I, the infant displays hyperalertness and hyperreflexia; in stage II there is lethargy, obtundation, and hypotonia; whereas in stage III stupor occurs.

Data from NCPP were based on the clinical appearance of HIE. In infants with neurologic signs indicative of HIE, 53% died and 16% of the survivors had neuromotor dysfunction. In infants having HIE and seizures there was a 30–75% likelihood of sequelae. In another sample, 35% of the HIE babies either died or were handicapped, whereas in a later follow-up 16% were moderately and 26% were mildly impaired based on diagnoses from combined neurologic and developmental data (obtained at approximately 2 years of age). It appears that the degree of damage was directly related to the severity of neurologic signs after birth. Data from 167 infants evaluated with a battery of tests at 3½ years of age have been reported. Of those infants with moderate HIE (stage II), 21% had one or two handicaps and 15–18% had more than a 6-month delay in gross motor and/or fine motor skills. Visual–motor integrative and language problems were also noted. In those infants with severe HIE (stage III), 75% died and all survivors displayed one to four major handicaps; deficits were global and included compromised IQ scores, deficiencies in visual–motor integration, and receptive and expressive language.

When HIE has been documented with CT scans, surviving infants who had diffuse and global areas of decreased density (changes in density reflecting hypoxic–ischemic injury) had an 89% and 100% incidence of major handicap during the first 2 years, respectively. Infants with so-called "patchy" areas of decreased density (thus signifying less damage) had a 25% incidence of minor handicap.

In summary, HIE, whether determined clinically or by CT, places an infant at significant risk for subsequent dysfunction. Presently, most studies have described short-term outcome with one exception, which reports 3.5-year data. Infants reaching Sarnat's and Sarnat's (1976) stages II and III are at significant risk for various neurodevelopmental deficits, as are those infants with diffuse or global areas of decreased brain density identified by CT scan. The magnitude of the problem is great, as HIE typically involves full-term infants, with damage occurring in the cortical areas (in contrast to central brain areas in IVH). The areas of damage would therefore be more likely to yield subsequent higher-order processing deficits at later ages.

6. Very Low Birthweight (VLBW)

The earliest reviews of the outcome of VLBW infants contained reports of a high incidence of mental retardation and neurologic disorders. Subsequently, neonatal intensive care units came into existence, but iatrogenic problems contributed to a high incidence of serious sequelae. There is a wide degree of variability in regard to the definition of VLBW, but the general trend has been toward a decrease in weight criteria (i.e., ≤2500 g, ≤1500 g, ≤1250 g, ≤1000 g, and more recently ≤750 g). At present, the consensus is that ≤1500 g is considered VLBW, whereas ≤1000 g is considered very-very-low birthweight or extremely low birthweight.

VLBW comprises a heterogeneous group and consists of at least three categories of infants: (1) extremely premature babies with appropriate gestational age (AGA) birthweight; (2) less premature babies with SGA (small for gestational age) birthweight; and (3) older preterm and term infants with an extreme SGA birthweight (Touwen, 1986). Extremely premature infants with very low birthweight (SGA) have a poorer prognosis.

Further, many other variables influence outcome: (1) perinatal and neonatal course (presence of IVH, asphyxia, seizures, respiratory distress syndrome), (2) postnatal growth, (3) the causes of premature birth or low birthweight, (4) different treatment regimens, (5) varying definitions of morbidity, (6) the age at evaluation, and (7) differences in the manner in which outcome is measured. Other potential variables include whether the study is prospective or retrospective, if babies are inborn or outborn, the end point for assessment, and the method in which environmental/psychosocial factors are treated. Therefore, results of studies may often be of importance to individual centers in their evaluation of new methods of treatment, but applicability to other centers is limited.

A survey of the world literature concerning mortality and neurologic morbidity in VLBW infants between 1960 and 1977 has documented a decrease in mortality, whereas neurologic morbidity did not change. Other surveys report similar findings. In contrast, some studies suggest that the incidence of severe neurologic sequelae has decreased or that severe neurologic sequelae has decreased but the incidence of minor neuromotor dysfunction has not changed. Generally, there appears to be a decrease in major handicaps. However, the incidence of "soft" neurologic signs, minor neurodevelopmental abnormalities, learning disorders, or problems in school performance have been evaluated less adequately.

There is evidence that gestational age and postnatal complications (Calame *et al.*, 1986) are the two most important variables influencing outcome in studies of VLBW infants. Duration of hospitalization has been identified as another significant variable. At this time the incidence of major neurologic/intellectual handicap in VLBW samples is in the

5–15% range, a marked decline from the 50% rates reported in the early to mid-1960s. In terms of less severe sequelae, several areas of deficit are reported fairly frequently, including poor visual–motor integration, deficits in spatial relations, reading problems, and language disorders. Estimates vary from 25 to 50% of VLBW infants having some type of learning disability. There are also reports of an increased incidence of borderline IQ. VLBW infants also have a reported increased incidence of classroom behavior problems, such as hyperactivity, irritability, and a short attention span. A higher proportion of VLBW infants require special educational help than their heavier birthweight peers, with estimates ranging from 25 to 60%.

The question has been raised as to whether differences in scores have actual clinical relevance or if they can explain differences in functional adaptation to the environment. In actuality, numerous reports on the outcome of VLBW infants contain either equivocal findings or questionable interpretations of results, with statistically lower mean test scores being interpreted as a significant deficit. Frequently, VLBW babies' scores are somewhat lower than those of control groups, but still are well within normal limits. Therefore, such differences may be statistically significant but clinically meaningless.

To summarize, VLBW babies are at risk for both major and minor sequelae; still, most VLBW babies will have a relatively positive outcome. A host of problems make interpretation of the data difficult and often contradictory. In addition to CNS damage described as occurring with IVH and asphyxia, neuropathological studies of VLBW babies have also revealed microscopic areas of necrosis in the gray and white matter, including superficial cortical and deep basal brain structures. These necrotic areas may be postulated to be precursors of later neurodevelopmental abnormalities, learning disabilities, and behavioral disorders. Future studies with MRI scans, cerebral blood flow, and brain metabolic measurements may hopefully help to clarify this issue.

7. Summary

Previous sections of this chapter have accented many issues involved in the developmental follow-up of high-risk infants. It is apparent that a multitude of variables converge to affect outcome. The designs of many studies do not take this into account. Further, most investigations refer to group versus individual prediction. Therefore, outcome data must be interpreted cautiously.

The outcome of infants having asphyxia, as documented by low

Apgar scores, is not clear. Low Apgar scores per se appear to have minimal long-term predictive utility, particularly those obtained at less than 10 min. Augmenting low Apgar scores with other variables (seizures, clinical manifestations of HIE) improves predictability somewhat. It is likely that prenatal asphyxia, which is *not* documented by Apgar scores, is more influential in regard to outcome. In fact, the low Apgar score may not be the cause of subsequent sequelae, but rather, it may be the result of some earlier insult.

In regard to seizures, the etiology, duration, and frequency must be considered. Infants who had neonatal seizures are at risk for cerebral palsy and epilepsy. The effects of seizures cannot be isolated readily from the influence of other variables such as IVH or asphyxia.

Infants who meet Papile *et al.*'s (1978) grades I and II classification of IVH are at moderate risk for significant sequelae, whereas infants with grades III and IV are at increased risk. It is not clear, however, whether it is IVH or other perinatal factors occurring in conjunction with IVH that place the infant in jeopardy. Since documentation of IVH (particularly less severe cases) is relatively recent, the long-term outcome of these babies is not clear.

HIE of a moderate to severe stage (Sarnat and Sarnat's stages 2 and 3) typically places an infant at significant risk for sequelae. The degree of dysfunction corresponds to increased stage of HIE; more global deficits occur at higher stages, whereas more subtle problems are related to lower stages of HIE. Documentation with CT scans may improve predictive accuracy.

Studies of VLBW infants contain many methodological flaws. Although major neurologic sequelae have decreased in frequency, it is not clear what the incidence of long-term, less severe disabilities will be. This becomes a critical issue, given increased survival rates. It must be emphasized that VLBW does not occur in isolation; thus there are VLBW groups with and without various perinatal complications. Nevertheless, these infants have an increased incidence of problems in visual–motor integration, spatial relations, reading, language development, and behavior.

Most likely, a specific threshold (in terms of intensity, duration, or both) of a perinatal complication must be reached before damage becomes evident. The ultimate impact that such a complication will have on outcome depends on the infant's age, prenatal and perinatal care, biological endowment, and environmental/psychosocial variables. Social factors can exacerbate or ameliorate the influence of neonatal problems. It must be emphasized, however, that many poor outcomes have no definable cause.

A recommended follow-up protocol should contain the three categories of VLBW infants: (1) extremely premature babies with appropriate birthweight; (2) less premature infants with SGA birthweight; and (3) older preterm and term infants with extreme SGA birthweight. Environmental/psychosocial and medical/biological variables (pre-, peri-, and postnatal) must be controlled either statistically or by subject stratification. In so doing, the effects of a specific perinatal variable could be better evaluated. In addition, better consensus will need to be reached regarding age at testing, types of assessments used, diagnostic categories, definitions of nonoptimal perinatal factors, and correction for prematurity. Finally, cognitive, motor, and neurologic function should be evaluated separately. There is a differential influence of medical and environmental background variables at different times, depending on the functional area that is assessed (Aylward *et al.*, 1987). Unfortunately, the influence of the environment may subsequently overshadow the effects of any treatment or potentially hazardous perinatal factor.

References

Ahmann, P., Lazarra, A., Dykes, F. D., *et al.*, 1980, Intraventricular hemorrhage in the high-risk preterm infant: Incidents and outcome, *Ann. Neurol.* **7:**118–124.

Aylward, G. P., Gustafson, N., Verhulst, S. J., *et al.*, 1987, Consistency in the diagnosis of cognitive, motor, and neurologic function over the first three years. *J. Pediatr. Psychol.* **12:**77–98.

Brann, A. W., 1986, Hypoxic ischemic encephalopathy, *Pediatr. Clin. N. Am.* **33:**451–463.

Broman, S. H., 1979, Prenatal anoxia and cognitive development in early childhood, in: *Infants Born at Risk* (T. M. Field, S. Goldberg, and H. H. Shuman, eds.), pp. 29–52, Spectrum Publications, New York.

Broman, S. H., Nichols, P. L., and Kennedy, W. A., 1975, *Preschool I.Q. Prenatal and Early Developmental Correlates,* Lawrence Erlbaum, Hillsdale, NJ.

Calame, A., Fawer, C. L., Claeys, V., *et al.*, 1986, Neurodevelopmental outcome and school performance of very-low-birth-weight infants at 8 years of age, *Eur. J. Pediatr.* **145:**461–466.

Catlin, E. A., Carpenter, M. W., Brann, B. S., *et al.*, 1986, The Apgar score revisited: Influence of gestational age, *J. Pediatr.* **109:**865–868.

Holden, K. R., Mellets, E. D., and Freeman, J. M., 1982, Neonatal seizures. I. Correlation of prenatal and perinatal events with outcome, *Pediatrics* **70:**165–176.

Nelson, K. B., and Ellenberg, J. H., 1986, Antecedents of cerebral palsy: Multivariate analysis of risk, *N. Engl. J. Med.* **315:**81–86.

Nichols, P. L., and Chen, T., 1981, *Minimal Brain Dysfunction: A Prospective Study,* Lawrence Erlbaum, Hillsdale, NJ.

Paneth, N., 1986, Brain and the origins of cerebral palsy, *N. Engl. J. Med.* **315:**124–126.

Papile, L. A., Burstein, J., Burstein, R., *et al.*, 1978, Incidence and evolution of subependymal and intraventricular hemorrhage: A study of infants with birthweight less than 1500 g, *J. Pediatr.* **92:**529–534.

Prechtl, H. F. R., 1984, Continuity and change in early neural development, in: *Continuity of Neural Functions from Prenatal to Postnatal Life* (H. F. R. Prechtl, ed.), pp. 1–15, Spastic International Medical Publications, London.

Sarnat, H. B., and Sarnat, M. S., 1976, Neonatal encephalopathy following fetal distress. A clinical and electroencephalographic study, *Arch. Neurol.* **33:**696–705.

Task Force on Joint Assessment of Prenatal and Perinatal Factors Associated with Brain Disorders, 1985, National Institutes of Health report on causes of mental retardation and cerebral palsy *Pediatrics* **76:**457–458.

Touwen, B. C. L., 1986, Very low birth weight infants, *Eur. J. Pediatr.* **145:**460.

Williamson, W. D., Desmond, M. M., Wilson, G. S., *et al.,* 1983, Survival of low birthweight infants with neonatal intraventricular hemorrhage, *Am. J. Dis. Child.* **137:**1181–1184.

CHAPTER 3

Syndrome Synopsis

AIDS Embryopathy, Cerebral Gigantism (Sotos's Syndrome), Fragile X Syndrome, and Tourette's Syndrome

RITA BENEZRA-OBEITER, ISABEL DETRIZIO-CAROTENUTO, AND ANNETTE L. ROSETTI-CARTAXO

1. AIDS Embryopathy

A new dysmorphic syndrome associated with intrauterine human immunodeficiency virus (HIV) infection has recently been described by the Departments of Immunology and Genetics at the Albert Einstein College of Medicine, Bronx, New York. In the initial study (Marion *et al.*, 1986), 25 infants and children of intravenous drug-abusing women with positive serology for HIV who met the case definition (as established by the Centers for Disease Control, Atlanta) for AIDS or AIDS-related complex (ARC) were evaluated by the same observers. The children were noted to have similar features. Seventy-five percent had growth failure (height and weight less than the third percentile for chronological age), which in five of the children was intrauterine in onset. Seventy percent had microcephaly [head circumference (HC) less than the third percentile for age]. Fifty percent had craniofacial abnormalities consisting of ocular hypertelorism (inner canthal and outer canthal distances equal to or greater than the 95th percentile for HC age). Seventy-five percent had prominent boxlike appearance of the forehead, and 70%

RITA BENEZRA-OBEITER, ISABEL DETRIZIO-CAROTENUTO, AND ANNETTE L. ROSETTI-CARTAXO • Institute for Child Development, Hackensack Medical Center, Hackensack, New Jersey 07601.

had a flat nasal bridge, which because of the prominent forehead appeared "scooped-out" in profile. Seventy-five percent had a mild upward or downward obliquity of the eyes and 60% had long palpebral fissures with blue sclerae. Sixty-five percent had a short nose with flattening of the columella and well-formed, triangular philtrum. Sixty percent had markedly patulous lips. The facial appearance was so distinct that casual observation in a crowded waiting area allowed the examiners to discriminate between affected and unaffected patients.

Not all children affected were equally stigmatized. However, those children who were more severely stigmatized tended to manifest clinical symptoms at a younger age. Transplacental transmission of the virus was implicated in all cases. In 87% of the patients, blood transfusions could not be incriminated. The concept of transplacental transmission was reinforced when the virus was cultivated from the brain, liver, and other organ systems of a 14-week-old fetus aborted by a woman with ARC (Editorial, Lancet, 1986).

Since the test group was composed of children born to women also known to abuse alcohol and numerous street drugs (as well as being at risk for infections with cytomegalovirus, *Toxoplasma gondi,* and Epstein–Barr virus), the stigmata of these environmentally induced embryopathies were examined and found to be quite distinct (Marion *et al.,* 1986).

The exact mechanism of transplacental transfer has not been defined. Discovery of monozygotic twins discordant for the HIV antibodies is even more perplexing (Menez-Bautistz *et al.,* 1986). The degree of expression of the features described may be related to the timing of viremia during fetal life, as has been reported in other congenital infections.

The diagnosis of HIV infection is sometimes difficult to establish in the first 6 months of life. The presence of antibodies to HIV may be reflective of maternally acquired, placentally transmitted IgG. Furthermore, immunologic aberrations may not be present in clinically ill children until after the first 6 months of life. Therefore, possible identification of affected individuals using external stigma would be beneficial.

To objectively evaluate the fetal-acquired immunodeficiency syndrome, a scoring system was developed based on the presence of the characteristic features previously reported (Marion *et al.,* 1987). In the scoring system the maximum score obtainable was 15. Two points were assigned for the presence of the features noted in 14 or more of the original 20 patients, including growth failure, microcephaly, forehead prominence, and flattening of the nasal bridge. One point each was given for the presence of hypertelorism as defined by Smith (1982), prominence of the eyes, flattening of the columella, and prominence of the philtrum and upper vermillion border. A score of 12 to 15 points was classified as severe; 9 to 11 points as moderate; and 0 to 9 as mild or not stigmatized.

A record of the second study group members were reviewed for age at onset of symptoms consistent with immunodeficiency and history of the presence of opportunistic infection. The results revealed that there was a statistically significant correlation between the severity of the dysmorphic features and the age at onset of symptoms of immunodeficiency, with the more severely stigmatized manifesting symptoms at a younger age ($p < .005$). There was, however, no correlation between the dysmorphism and either the presence of opportunistic infections or pulmonary lymphoid hyperplasia (PLH) at the time of the initial examination.

In summary, the scoring system method may be useful in early identification of infants infected with HIV.

2. Cerebral Gigantism (Sotos's Syndrome)

In 1964, Sotos *et al.* described a syndrome associated with cerebral gigantism. Sotos's original five patients were characterized by excessive growth during the first 4 years of life and advanced height, weight, and bone age. They had distinctive facies: high foreheads, frontal bossing, prominent jaw, hypertelorism, and downslanting palpebral fissures. In addition, there was a distinctive large dolichocephalic head, high-arched palate, increased arm span, and large hands and feet. Four of the five children were mentally retarded and clumsy. None of the patients, however, exhibited gross neurological abnormalities. Pneumoencephalography revealed enlarged ventricles in three of the patients. After ruling out all of the known causes of excessive growth, Sotos and his colleagues concluded that this pattern of clinical findings failed to conform to any of the recognized causes of tall stature. He suggested that the remarkable similarity among the cases justified their grouping as a syndrome.

After almost 25 years since the original description of Sotos's syndrome, several issues remain unsettled: Is cerebral gigantism a true syndrome? What are the features necessary for diagnosis? How and when does it originate? What are the prognostic and therapeutic implications?

There is perhaps more controversy today regarding delineation of cerebral gigantism as a true syndrome than when it was first described. To some, it represents a malformation sequence rather than a syndrome per se. It is postulated that the pattern of anomalies including macrocephaly, craniofacial abnormalities, mental retardation, language deficits, and large size may be derived from a single anomaly such as an enlarged cerebrum. There is also variability in the characteristic features in each case. Jaeken (1972) reviewed 80 patients diagnosed with Sotos's syndrome. The most common clinical findings included gigantism (100%), prominent forehead (96%), high-arched palate (96%), hypertelorism (91%), dolichocephaly (84%), developmental retardation (83%), large hands and feet (83%), pointed chin (83%), advanced bone age (74%), lack of fine motor control (67%), premature eruption of teeth (57%), and neonatal adaptation and/or feeding difficulties (44%) (Sotos and Dodge, 1977). Additional findings have been occasionally reported, such as musculoskeletal abnormalities, abnormal dermatoglyphic patterns, ocular abnormalities, and malignancies (Evans, 1971). Clumsiness in the absence of other abnormal findings is a relatively frequent finding. Other reported neurological signs include nystagmus, strabismus, increased deep tendon reflexes, hypotonia, and muscle weakness.

Wilson *et al.* (1980) reported several cases of thyrotoxicosis in which the diagnosis of cerebral gigantism clearly predated the onset of the thyroid disorder. In three cases, hypothyroidism had also been associated with cerebral gigantism. Pancreatic, adrenal, pituitary, gonadal, and thyroid function usually are normal, as are measurements of growth hormone and somatomedin (Wit *et al.*, 1985). Abnormal glucose tolerance tests have been noted with some frequency (14%). There is no satisfactory explanation for the overgrowth observed prior to and after birth, or for the advanced bone age. The growth velocity is particularly excessive in the first 2 to 3 years of life, and subsequently growth proceeds at a normal rate.

Abnormalities have been reported on computerized axial tomography (CAT) studies of the brain including enlarged ventricles (but rarely is progressive hydrocephalus noted), absence of the body of the corpus callosum; delayed opercularization, prominent cortical sulci, cavum septum pellucidum, and cavum velum interpositi (Barth *et al.*, 1980).

Most cases of cerebral gigantism have been sporadic, but familial occurrence has been documented. Zonana *et al.* (1977) reported three families with multiple affected members. Linear transmission of cerebral gigantism also was reported by Hansen and Friis (1976) and Halal (1982). It has been suggested that other cases reported as sporadic are in fact inherited. A parent may not have been diagnosed as a child and as an adult the distinguishing features may be less apparent. If cerebral gigantism is inherited as an autosomal dominant trait, as these case reports suggest, other sporadic cases may represent new mutations. A preponderance of sporadic cases is not unexpected in a rare autosomal dominant trait, especially one not easily recognized in adults. Autosomal recessive inheritance appearing in other pedigrees may represent (1) nonpenetrance, (2) gonadal mosaicism, or (3) genetic heterogenicity. Cerebral gigantism shares the diagnostic problem common to all syndromes that are defined by physical characteristics but lack a biochemical marker. Recent studies of metacarpophalangeal pattern profile analysis suggest that a particular pattern exists for Sotos's syndrome and may provide a more conclusive aid in diagnosis (Butler *et al.*, 1985).

In a review of over 100 cases, Sotos and Cutler (1977) estimated that five of six affected persons (approximately 83%) had some degree of mental retardation. Data reported by Bloom *et al.* (1983) suggest that this previously reported incidence of mental retardation associated with cerebral gigantism may be inflated. They reported several cases of children diagnosed with cerebral gigantism who exhibited auditory perceptual processing problems manifested by word-finding difficulties and very long latency response to verbally presented stimuli. The general impression was that these patients would have scored significantly lower on IQ tests if they were not allowed sufficient time to respond to verbal tasks.

The management of mental retardation in Sotos's syndrome is no different than for any other child with mental deficiency. Livingood and Borengasser (1981), however, suggest that children whose physical growth and stature far exceeds their chronological age are vulnerable to various psychological and social problems.

Excessive growth in patients with cerebral gigantism remains unexplained (Dodge *et al.*, 1983). We are hampered in our understanding of this phenomenon by our lack of knowledge of the intimate physiological mechanisms of growth. Regardless of the intermediary mechanisms, growth is genetically determined. Therefore, a genetic basis for the pattern of growth and bone development seen in cerebral gigantism is obviously plausible.

3. Fragile X Syndrome

A male predominance in the population of the mentally retarded has been reported in community surveys and data obtained from institutions (Leroy, 1983). In 1943, Martin and Bell described 11 mentally retarded males from one family, suggesting a pattern of X-linked inheritance. Approximately 20 years ago, Lehrke (1972) hypothesized that approximately 20% of all mental retardation is X-linked. A fragile site on the X chromosome (a constriction on the end of the long arm of the X chromosome at X q27) was described by Lubs in 1969 in four mentally retarded males and the heterozygous females (who were not retarded) from one family. Sutherland (1977) realized that the demonstration of the fragile site was dependent on culturing the chromosomes in folic acid and thymidine-restricted media. Turner *et al.* (1978) reported on the association of the fragile X marker chromosome and macroorchidism in mentally retarded males. In 1981, Richards *et al.* reviewed the Martin–Bell kindred and found the fragile X site in seven of the mentally retarded males available for study. They also noted macroorchidism, large ears, and prognathism in many of these patients.

Fragile X syndrome is felt to be second only to Down's syndrome in incidence of chromosomally based mental retardation. Fragile X is calculated to occur in 0.92/1000 males (Opitz, 1986).

The clinical features generally associated with fragile X syndrome are macroorchidism (generally found only after puberty), large or prominent ears, a relatively large head circumference, a high or prominent forehead, and mild prognathism (Turner *et al.*, 1980). It should be noted that fragile X can be identified in individuals with none of the "typical" facial features (Nielsen, 1983). Although prepubertal boys generally have normal testicular size, there have been case reports of prepubertal boys with macroorchidism (Carmi *et al.*, 1984). In addition to these physical features, certain behavioral characteristics have been described. Autistic behavior appears to be associated with fragile X syndrome; however, the incidence varies in different studies from 12 to over 50% in affected males (Hagerman *et al.*, 1986a–c; Brown *et al.*, 1986a,b). Mental retardation varies from mild to severe, and there are males with fragile X syndrome who are of normal intelligence. It is estimated that 30% of female heterozygotes and 80% of males with fragile X are mentally retarded.

Froster-Iskenius *et al.* (1986b) recently evaluated the pedigree data from six kindreds known to have members with fragile X syndrome. Fifteen unaffected males presumably passed the gene to their generally normal daughters and to a total of 51 mentally retarded grandsons and great-grandsons. Of the four transmitting males personally examined by the authors, none showed evidence of fragile X syndrome. However, there are also reports of males with apparently normal intelligence who test positive for fragile X syndrome. Only two of the 50 daughters of these 15 transmitting males were of subnormal intelligence, which is in agreement with previously published data. It had been previously found that the risk of mental retardation in siblings of transmitting males was very low. Unexpectedly, four of the 15 transmitting males had brothers who were mentally retarded. In view of this new data, women with *paternal* uncles with mental retardation due to fragile X may be at risk for transmitting the fragile X gene. The etiology of the differences in expression of the gene is unclear and several hypotheses are currently being evaluated.

The spectrum of clinical manifestations in fragile X women is broad and is only beginning to be investigated. It is interesting to note that only in females is the percentage of fragile X seen inversely correlated with IQ (Van Dyke and Weiss, 1986). As noted, only 30% of fragile X women are mentally retarded. Partington (1986) examined 83 women from 21 families with known fragile X. All 18 women who were mentally retarded and five other women were normal IQ's, identified by family members as being "less bright," were positive for fragile X on cytogenetic studies. Kemper *et al.* (1986) found significantly lower block design subtest scores in eight fragile X women who were compared with eight non-fragile X learning-disabled females with the same full-scale IQ scores. In another study (Fryns, 1986), 144 women who were "obligate carriers" of fragile X were examined. Twenty-eight percent exhibited facial stigmata, including a long face, prominent forehead, relative macrocephaly, and large everted ears. Phenotypic expression was more commonly seen in those who were retarded, as only 14% of those with normal intelligence had typical facies, whereas 41% of the retarded "carriers" did. Fifty percent of the carriers were negative for fragile X despite repeated testing. However, all those with partial clinical expression were positive for fragile X. Curiously, a fourfold increase in twinning was observed in all of these women. Psychiatric disorders (most frequently psychotic behavior) were seen in 10% of the cognitively normal and 20% of the mentally retarded heterozygous women. Autism has also been described in these women (Hagerman *et al.*, 1986).

Prenatal diagnosis has been attempted during the past few years and is still felt by many geneticists to be somewhat experimental. A report of 147 cases studies worldwide revealed that 31 fetuses (24 males, 7 females) were positive and were confirmed. At least one false negative and one false positive case have occurred. Amniocytes from one fragile X syndrome fetus were studied in three different laboratories and showed strikingly different frequencies of fragile X. Because of this, it was recommended that at least two different induction systems be used in order to prevent false negative diagnosis. In addition, fetal lymphocyte cultures for chromosomes yield a higher fragile X frequency than do amniocyte cultures. Although it would be impractical to recommend fetal lymphocyte cultures universally, some feel that it would be useful to confirm low-frequency positive results when an abortion is being considered (Jenkins *et al.*, 1986).

Folic acid treatment for fragile X has been tried with varying results.

Many studies have found no significant changes in behavior and/or IQ *overall.* When the results were further analyzed, however, it appeared that many prepubertal patients did benefit from treatment, both behaviorally and cognitively (Brown *et al.,* 1986a); Froster-Iskemius *et al.,* 1986a; Hagerman *et al.,* 1986a; Wells and Madison, 1986). Additional studies regarding the role of folic acid treatment is required in order to clarify the effects.

4. Tourette's Syndrome

Tourette's syndrome is a chronic, familial neuropsychiatric syndrome of unknown etiology. Diagnostic criteria include (1) onset between 2 and 15 years of age, (2) the presence of motor as well as multiple vocal tics, (3) the ability to suppress these tics for minutes to hours, (4) a variation in the intensity of symptoms over weeks or months, and (5) a duration of symptoms for more than 1 year to throughout life. There is usually a progression from simple to complex tics, which often have a compulsive or ritualistic quality. Tourette's syndrome was once thought to be quite rare. Estimates of the prevalence, however, have been reported to be as high as 1 per 2000, with males outnumbering females by approximately 3 to 1 (Price *et al.,* 1986).

Tourette's syndrome is now considered to be a hereditary disorder. There is frequently a family history of a tic syndrome (chronic motor tics or Tourette's syndrome) in the parents, grandparents, aunts, uncles, and siblings of affected children (Kurlan *et al.,* 1986). Studies of monozygotic twins suggest a genetic influence in both Tourette's syndrome and chronic motor tics, but the specific pattern of transmission within families has not been determined (Price *et al.,* 1985). Both single-major-locus and multifactorial patterns have been proposed. There appears to be a clearly sex-related threshold to the expression of tics and Tourette's syndrome. Girls with the syndrome tend to come from families with higher frequencies of tics of Tourette's syndrome than those of boys. It has been suggested that this indicates that females Tourette's syndrome patients may carry a heavier genetic "loading" before symptoms are expressed (Kidd *et al.,* 1980). At present, this observation is still controversial.

"A neurologic substrate for Tourette's syndrome is evidenced by a high incidence of electroencephalographic nonspecific abnormalities and soft signs on neurological examination." (Hoder and Cohen, 1983). Harcherik *et al.* (1985), however, failed to demonstrate any significant differences on CT scan in patients with Tourette's syndrome from the normal controls. Vocal tics, such as grunts, barks, yelps, throat clearing, or coughs, and various other noises subsequently become associated with motor tics. Ultimately echolalia (a repetition of one's own last words or phrases) and echokinesis (a repetition of another person's movements) may appear. Coprolalia, an irresistable urge to utter profanities, occurs in 40 to 53% of the cases.

A patient in whom Tourette's syndrome is suspected should first undergo neurological, psychological, and psychiatric investigation to rule out other movement disorders. Although the pressure to start treatment quickly is difficult to resist, pharmacologic treatment is usually begun when a child is emotionally distraught or unable to function normally because of his symptoms. Of all the treatment methods available, drug therapy seems to be the most effective. Haloperidol, a dopamine blocker, has been the most widely used neuroleptic drug and is considered the drug of choice at the present time (Shapiro *et al.*, 1983). Average improvement in tics for patients taking this medication is close to 75% (Freeman *et al.*, 1984; Goets *et al.*, 1984). Unfortunately, haloperidol may cause short-term side effects, such as weight gain, parkinsonian symptoms, intellectual blunting, anergy, sedation, dysphoria, school phobia, and depression (Linet, 1985). The long-term consequences, such as tardive dyskinesia, causes particular concern because of its disabling effects and its medicolegal implications. Only one third of patients continue to take haloperidol; the others choose to endure the symptoms rather than suffer the side effects. Treatment with pemozide, another antipsychotic drug, has been shown to be equally effective and may have fewer side effects. Clonidine hydrochloride, an antihypertensive drug, has also been reported to be effective in a minority of patients (Leckman *et al.*, 1985). Psychotherapy and counseling for the patient and the family, as well as contact with the school, are considered necessary adjuncts to medical treatment.

References

AIDS Embryopathy

Editorial, 1986, Transplacental transmission of human immunodeficiency virus, *Lancet* **20:**215–216.

Marion, R. W., Wiznia, A. A., Hutcheon, R. G., *et al.*, 1987, Fetal AIDS syndrome score, *Am. J. Dis. Child.* **141:**429–531.

Marion, R. W., Wiznia, A. A., Hutcheon, R. G., *et al.*, 1986, AIDS embryopathy: A new dysmorphic syndrome, *Am. J. Dis. Child.* **140:**638–640.

Menez-Bautista, R., Fikrig, S. M., Pahwa, S., *et al.*, 1986, Monozygotic twin discordant for the acquired immunodeficiency syndrome, *Am. J. Dis. Child.* **140:**678–679.
Smith, D. W., 1982, *Recognizable Patterns of Human Malformations,* W. B. Saunders Co., Philadelphia, PA.
Update: Acquired immunodeficiency syndrome (AIDS)—United States, 1984, *Morbid. Mortal. Weekly Rep.* **32:**688–691.

Cerebral Gigantism

Barth, P. G., Valsveld, L., and Valk, J., 1980, Unilateral delayed opercularization in a case of Sotos' syndrome (cerebral gigantism), *Neuroradiology* **20:**49–52.
Bloom, A. S., Reese, A., Hersh, J. H., *et al.*, 1983, Cognition in cerebral gigantism: Are the estimates of mental retardation too high? *J. Dev. Behav. Pediatr.* **4:**250–252.
Butler, M. G., Meaney, F. J., Kihur, S., *et al.*, 1985, Metacarpophalangeal pattern profile analysis in Sotos' syndrome, *Am. J. Med. Genet.* **20:**625–629.
Dodge, P. R., Holmes, S. J., and Sotos, J. F., 1983, Cerebral gigantism, *Dev. Med. Child Neurol.* **25:**248–252.
Evans, P. R., 1971, Sotos' syndrome (cerebral gigantism) with peripheral dysostosis, *Arch. Dis. Child.* **46:**199–202.
Halal, F., 1982, Male to male transmission of cerebral gigantism, *Am. J. Med. Genet.* **12:**411–419.
Hansen, F. J., and Friis, B., 1976, Case report familial occurrence of cerebral gigantism, Sotos' syndrome, *Acta Pediatr. Scand.* **65:**387–389.
Jaeken, J., vander Schueren-Lodeqeycks, M., and Eeckels, R., 1973, Cerebral gigantism syndrome: A report of four cases and review of the literature, *Z. Kinderheilkunde* **112:**332–346.
Livingood, A. B., and Borengasser, M., 1981, Cerebral gigantism in infancy: Implications for psychological and social development. *Child Psychiatry Hum. Dev.* **12:**46–53.
Sotos, J. E., and Cutler, E. A., 1977, Cerebral gigantism, *Am. J. Dis. Child.* **131:**625–627.
Sotos, J. F., Dodge, P. R., Muirhead, D., *et al.*, 1964, Cerebral gigantism in childhood, *N. Engl. J. Med.* **271:**109–116.
Sotos, J. F., and Dodge, P. R., 1977, Cerebral gigantism, *Am. J. Dis. Child.* **131:**625–627.
Wilson, T. A., Neufeld, M. R., Robinson, M., *et al.*, 1980, Cerebral gigantism and thyrotoxicosis, *J. Pediatr.* **96:**685–687.
Wit, J. M., Beemer, F. A., Barth, P. G., *et al.*, 1985, Cerebral gigantism (Sotos' syndrome): Compiled data of 22 cases, analysis of clinical features, growth and plasma somatomedin, *Eur. J. Pediatr.* **144:**131–140.
Zonana, J., Sotos, J. F., Romshe, C. A., *et al.*, 1977, Dominant inheritance of cerebral gigantism, *J. Pediatr.* **91:**251–256.

Fragile X Syndrome

Brown, W. T., Jenkins, E. C., Cohen, I. L., *et al.*, 1986a, High-dose folic acid treatment of fragile X males, *Am. J. Med. Genet.* **23:**263–271.
Brown, W. T., Jenkins, E. C., Cohen, I. L., *et al.*, 1986b, Fragile X and autism: A multicenter survey, *Am. J. Med. Genet.* **23:**341–352.

Carmi, R., Meryash, D. L., Wood, J., *et al.*, 1984, Fragile X Syndrome ascertained by the presence of macro-orchidism in a 5-month old infant, *Pediatrics* **74**:883–886.

Froster-Iskenius, U., Bodeker, K., Oepen, T., *et al.*, 1986a, Folic acid treatment in males and females with Fragile X syndrome, *Am. J. Med. Genet.* **23**:273–284.

Froster-Iskenius, U., McGillivrary, B. C., Dill, F. J., *et al.*, 1986b, Normal male carriers in the Fra (X) form of X-linked mental retardation (Martin–Bell syndrome), *Am. J. Med. Genet.* **23**:619–631.

Fryns, J. P., 1986, The female and the Fragile (X), *Am. J. Med. Genet.* **23**:157–169.

Hagerman, R. J., Jackson, A. W., Levitas, A., *et al.*, 1986a, Oral folic acid versus placebo in the treatment of males with Fra (X) syndrome, *Am. J. Med. Genet.* **23**:241–262.

Hagerman, R. J., Jackson, W., Leviyas, A., *et al.*, 1986b, An analysis of autism in 50 males with Fragile X syndrome, *Am. J. Med. Genet.* **23**:359–374.

Hagerman, R. J., Chudley, A. E., Knoll, J. H., *et al.*, 1986c, Autism in Fra (X) Females, *Am. J. Med. Genet.* **23**:375–380.

Jenkins, E. C., Brown, W. T., Wilson, M. G., *et al.*, 1986, The prenatal detection of Fragile (X) chromosome: Review of recent experience, *Am. J. Med. Genet.* **23**:297–311.

Kemper, M., Hagerman, R., Ahmad, R., *et al.*, 1986, Cognitive profiles and the spectrum of clinical manifestations in heterozygous Fra (X) women, *Am. J. Med. Genetics* **23**:139–156.

Lehrke, R. G., 1972, A theory of X-linkage of major intellectual traits, *Am. J. Ment. Defic.* **76**:611–619.

Leroy, J. G., 1983, Heredity, development and behavior, in: *Developmental-Behavioral Pediatrics* (M. D. Levine, A. C. Crocker, R. T. Gross, eds.), W. B. Saunders Company, Philadelphia, p. 318.

Lubs, H. A., 1969, A marker X chromosome, *Am. J. Hum. Genet.* **21**:231–244.

Martin, J. P., and Bell, J., 1943, A pedigree of mental defect showing sex linkage, *J. Neurol. Neurosurg. Psychol.* **6**:154–157.

Nielsen, K. B., 1983, Diagnosis of the Fragile X Syndrome (Martin–Bell Syndrome). Clinical findings in 27 males with the fragile site at Xq28, *J. Ment. Defic. Res.* **27**:211–226.

Opitz, V., 1986, Fra (X) retardation—A gene mutation? *Am. J. Med. Genet.* **21**:1–10.

Partington, M. W. L., 1986, Females in Fra X syndrome families, *Am. J. Med. Genet.* **23**:111–126.

Richards, B. W., Sylvester, P. E., and Brooker, C., 1981, Fragile X-linked mental retardation: The Martin–Bell syndrome, *J. Ment. Defic. Res.* **25**:253–256.

Sutherland, G. R., 1977, Fragile sites of human chromosomes: Demonstration of their dependence on the type of tissue culture medium, *Science* **197**:265–266.

Turner, G., Daniel, A., and Frost, M., 1980, X-linked mental retardation, macroorchidism and the Xq27 fragile site (1980), *J. Pediatr.* **96**:837–841.

Turner, G., File, R., and Daniel, A., 1978, Marker X chromosomes: Mental retardation and macroorchidism, *N. Engl. J. Med.* **299**:1427.

Van Dyke, D. L., and Weiss, L., 1986, Maternal effect in Fragile X, *Am. J. Med. Genet.* **23**:723–737.

Tourette's Syndrome

Freeman, R. D., Connolly, J. E., and Baird, P. A., 1984, Tourette's Syndrome: Update, *Can. Med. Assoc.* **130**:1554–1557.

Goets, C. G., Tanner, C. M., and Klawans, H. L., 1984, Fluphenazine and multifocal tic disorders, *Arch. Neurol.* **41:**271–272.

Harcherik, D. F., Cohen, D. J., Ort, S., *et al.*, 1985, Computed tomographic brain scanning in four neuropsychiatric disorders of childhood, *Am. J. Psychiatry* **142:**731–734.

Hoder, E., and Cohen, D. J., 1983, Repetitive behavior patterns in childhood, in: *Developmental–Behavioral Pediatrics* (M. D. Levine, W. B. Carey, A. C. Crocker, R. T. Gross, eds.), pp. 617–621, W. B. Saunders Company, Philadelphia.

Kidd, K. K., Prusoff, B. A., and Cohen, D. J., 1980, Familial pattern of Gilles de la Tourette syndrome, *Arch. Gen. Psychiatry* **37:**1336–1339.

Kurlan, R., Behr, J., Medved, L., *et al.*, 1986, Familial Tourette's syndrome: Report of a large pedigree of potential for linkage analysis, *Neurology* **36:**772–776.

Leckman, J. F., Detlor, J., Harcherik, D. F., *et al.*, 1985, Short and long term treatment of Tourette's syndrome with clonidine: A clinical perspective, *Neurology* **35:**343–351.

Linet, L. S., 1985, Tourette syndrome, priozide and school phobia: The neuroleptic separation anxiety syndrome, *Am. J. Psychiatry* **142:**613–615.

Price, R. A., Leckman, J. F., Pauls, D. L., *et al.*, 1986, Gilles de la Tourette's syndrome: Tics and central nervous system stimulants in twins and non-twins, *Neurology,* **36:**232–237.

Price, R. A., Kidd, K. K., Cohen, D. J., *et al.*, 1985, A twin study of Tourette syndrome, *Arch. Gen. Psychiatry* **42:**815–820.

Shapiro, A. K., Shapiro, E., and Eisenkraft, G. J., 1983, Treatment of Gilles de la Tourette syndrome with primizide, *Am. J. Psychiatry* **140:**1183–1186.

CHAPTER 4

Juvenile Delinquency

The Interface between Pediatrics and the Law

STEPHEN H. BILLER

1. Introduction

Today's more splintered life-styles, with fewer people living in families and more mothers working, have placed new pressures and demands on both parent and child. These changes in family dynamics have required that sociologists, educators, and the court system develop new methods to deal with the shift in children's values away from the family. The resulting increase in psychosocial pressures and weakening of values have further contributed to a rise in youth crime. To stem this rise in juvenile delinquency and crime, profiles have been developed to aid in the early detection, rehabilitation, and, if necessary, incarceration of the youthful offender. It would appear that the profile of a great number of delinquents is characterized by depressed socioeconomic environments, illegitimate births, single-parent (mother only) homes, experimentation with and abuse of drugs, a high percentage of teenage pregnancy, and a high rate of unemployment. To date, the sequential treatment ritual of children in trouble generally has been (1) probation, (2) home confinement, (3) residential facility, (4) training facility, and (5) state facility.

2. The Concept of Fixed Sentencing

A recent innovation in the methodology of sentencing in federal criminal adult jurisprudence is the "fixed-sentencing concept," which

STEPHEN H. BILLER • Heiskell, Donelson, Bearman, Adams, Williams and Kirsch, Memphis, Tennessee 38138.

was created by the U.S. Sentencing Commission as part of the Comprehensive Crime Control Act of 1984. The fixed-sentencing guidelines work on a complex assigned point value system, ranging in severity from 1 to 43. The judge is to add or subtract points based on the other acts committed with the crime. Specifically, the judge must add sentencing points for any crimes when the victim suffers psychological injury. The guidelines do not ordinarily permit the judges to take into account the defendant's age, community ties, family responsibilities, or previous employment record; these factors have mitigated in the past. The principal complaint of the guidelines is that the rules are too mechanical, leaving little or no discretion to the judge.

The guidelines took effect November 1, 1987, and apply only to crimes committed after November 1, 1987. Lawsuits, however, have been filed in San Diego, California and Nashville, Tennessee asserting that the Commission was improperly constituted and that the authority of the Commission violates the Constitution's separation of power.

The Rose Institute Study, conducted by the Advisory Board on Missing Children, reflects a growing belief that juveniles convicted of delinquent acts should also receive fixed sentences based on the severity of the delinquency and/or that police should be allowed to detain runaway or neglected children.

The Rose Institute Study also suggests a point system to determine punishment for juveniles. Simply stated, the sentence would depend on the delinquent act, and would be increased or decreased depending on the juvenile's age and offense history. In the terms of the report, "we wanted to move away from the notion of sanctioning based on prediction of further delinquent behavior, and [put more emphasis] on what the juvenile has actually done. . . . " Under the proposal, youths committing the least serious offenses could be required to make restitution or offer community service.

Both reports and studies criticize the present juvenile system as unjust, commenting that "Two juveniles can do the same thing and be charged with the same delinquent act. One juvenile, because he is viewed as amenable to treatment, might be put on probation. The other because he is viewed as obstreperous or because of his family background, might well be confined."

The National Counsel of Juvenile and Family Court Judges and the National Coalition of State Juvenile Justice Advisory Groups are critical of the fixed sentencing proposal. However, Ralph A. Rossum, author of the Rose Institute Study, states that fixed sentencing has been effective in the State of Washington since 1977 without overcrowding juvenile institutions, because less serious offenders are no longer held.

The basic criticism for the fixed sentencing concept is that it does away with the primary function of the juvenile justice system, which is to rehabilitate children and provide treatment. Furthermore, the fixed sentencing concept will result in more children going to prison and more children being held for longer periods of time. New York Judge M. Holt Meyer, President of the New York City Family Court Judges Association, states: "Very often, they're (children) products of neglect, abuse, and other kinds of deprivation. A whole host of services is necessary."

The American Bar Association's Juvenile Justice Project urges that legislatures should establish only maximum penalties and that the judges should use the least restrictive sentence that is appropriate.

3. Founding Principles of the Juvenile Court

The concept of a juvenile court system is predicated on the theory that the young criminal is by definition immature and subject to manipulation. The offending behavior of the juvenile delinquent, therefore, could be corrected or readjusted by concerned members of a justice system designed for the juvenile himself. Juveniles were viewed as not having committed crimes but as having engaged in unacceptable behavior because of the act itself or because of their status as a child. A "child" offense includes behaviors such as truancy, running away from home, not obeying parents or guardians, and curfew violations. If a child committed one of these "child offenses" and was "adjudicated" (not convicted), he/she was found to be a "person in need of supervision" or a "juvenile" or a "child in need of supervision." The sentencing process was not a court proceeding, but was regarded as a dispositional hearing. The juvenile was not confined in a "prison," but rather was sent to a "training school" or a "youth camp." This process avoided the placing of a criminal label on the child that would adversely affect the child's future relations with the public and the child's self-image.

The United States Supreme Court, in its decision in *McKeiver v. Pennsylvania,* 403 U.S. 528 (1971), held:

> Reprehensible acts by juveniles are not deemed the consequence of mature and malevolent choice, but environmental pressures (or lack of them) or other forces beyond their control. Hence, the state legislative judgment not to stigmatize the juvenile delinquent by branding him criminal; his conduct is not deemed so blameworthy that punishment is required to deter him or others.

The boundary between childhood and adulthood, for the purpose of the juvenile court system, is established by each state juvenile code.

Although age 17 years is the more biologically based demarcation, it is not unusual for a particular state to use numerous age cutoffs, within its own juvenile code, depending on the type of delinquent conduct involved. Usually, the difference in the benchmark within the same juvenile code is between a child who engages in acts that would be a criminal activity if engaged in by an adult and the more serious offenses such as rape and murder.

The juvenile court system itself is most commonly found in an administrative form, with judges, juvenile officers, and attorneys who represent the interest of the juvenile court and the various support personnel to run a court of law.

In 1974, the Congress of the United States passed The Juvenile Justice and Delinquency and Prevention Act of 1974, 42 U.S.C. 5601, *et seq.*, legislation that is predicated on the congressional findings that "understaffed, overcrowded juvenile courts, probation services, and correctional facilities" are not able to provide individual justice or effective help" to troubled youths, 42 U.S.C. 5601(a) (2). This act provides federal grants to state and local programs for education, prevention, diversion, and treatment and assists such entities in planning and implementing effective rehabilitative programs in order to prevent juvenile delinquency and to improve the juvenile justice system. To participate in these grants, the state must cease the practice of confining status offenders in secured detention centers and institutions as well as the practice of placing children in adult jails.

4. Court-Appointed Expert Witnesses

In recent years, judicial decisions involving children, which were once largely respected as given truths, are now subject to criticism, thereby increasing the role of the expert witness.

The major utilization of expert witnesses in cases involving children has occurred mostly in child custody cases. In some jurisdictions, such expert witnesses are publicly funded, reporting to the court at or before the trial. In most states, the courts struggle with the traditional, costly adversarial clash of opposing expert witnesses, each testifying for the party paying his or her witness fee.

Perhaps one of the paramount problems in utilizing a psychologist or psychiatrist, or seeking a psychological evaluation, is the delay it causes in a speedy adjudication of the problem. Further, in all psychological evaluations, whether court-ordered or voluntary, there is no purity. In a court-ordered evaluation, there is pressure placed on the person being evaluated because it is the court system itself which has compelled the evaluation. Within the traditional system of adversary witnesses, the psychologist is employed by the one being evaluated. Therefore, it is a friendly evaluation that substantially reduces tension. In the court ordered evaluation process, at the core of the responses by the person being evaluated is the involuntariness of that person. Thus, a diagnostic block is created that must be overcome; and of course fear of testing is heightened in an involuntary evaluation.

A practical problem for the psychologist is posed with every court-ordered referral. The referral is directed for evaluation and not counseling and/or therapy. Its purpose is to advance the knowledge of the court, rather than to advance the parenting skills of perhaps the principal litigants (parents). The psychologist or psychiatrist is usually expected to render a report on a family's status at a moment in time, so that a legal decision can be made martialing the future. Since a report is to be made, there is no privilege of confidentiality between the subject and the evaluator. The psychologist must, by necessity, emphasize the absence of confidentiality before the evaluation begins and do his or her best to factor that absence into the final report. The psychologist is realistically only a reporter and not an advocate. The report per se may create new problems. For example, it may provide one parent with a tool to exploit the other, or it may cause a progressing individual to retreat.

5. Due Process Rights of Juvenile Offenders

At times one may forget or overlook the fact that children and adolescents are entitled to the same protections of the law as that provided for adults. In the following sections the due process rights of youthful offenders are briefly reviewed.

5.1. Right to Notice and an Opportunity to Be Heard

Although seemingly an obvious legal protection, the right to be served notice and the right to have an opportunity to be heard are mandated by law.

In re Gault, 387 U.S. 33:

> Notice, to comply with due process requirements, must be given sufficiently in advance of scheduled court proceedings so that reasonable opportunity to prepare will be afforded, and it must set forth the alleged misconduct with particularity.

5.2. The Right to Counsel

Similarly, this protection is guaranteed by law [*in re Gault,* 387 U.S.1,41 (1967)]. The right to counsel for children and adolescents is not an exception. However, at what stage of the process is the right to counsel assured? The response to this question is sometimes not clearly defined for juvenile delinquents.

5.3. Confrontation of Adverse Witnesses

It required multiple court decisions to provide protection for juveniles in this right. *In re Gault,* 387 U.S. 56, the Court held:

> . . . confrontation and sworn testimony by witnesses available for cross-examination were essential for a finding of "delinquency" and an order committing the juvenile to a state institution for a maximum of six years.

This holding by the Supreme Court applies to the adjudicatory stage of the proceedings. The question is whether there is a right to confront and cross-examine at detention hearings, probable cause hearings, dispositional hearings, or waiver hearings. In the state of Tennessee (37-1-127), basic rights at a hearing include: (1) a party is entitled to the opportunity to introduce evidence and otherwise be heard in his own behalf and to cross-examine adverse witnesses; (2) a child charged with a delinquent act need not be a witness against or otherwise incriminate himself; (3) an extrajudicial statement, if obtained in the course of violation of this part or which would be constitutionally inadmissible in a criminal proceeding, shall not be used against him; (4) evidence illegally seized or obtained shall not be received over objection to establish the allegations made against him; and (5) a confession validly made by a child out of court is insufficient to support an adjudication of delinquency unless it is corroborated in whole or in part by other evidence.

5.4. The Right to Proof of Guilt beyond a Reasonable Doubt

The United States Supreme Court *in re Winship,* 397 U.S. 358 (1970), held that proof beyond a reasonable doubt at the *adjudication* stage of a delinquency proceeding was constitutionally required by the due process clause of the Fourteenth Amendment. The issue remains open as to whether this standard of proof is required at dispositional or waiver hearings. The issue at a *dispositional hearing* is whether or not the juvenile is in need of some type of treatment that the state can provide. The issue at a *waiver hearing* is whether a juvenile will be amenable to any type care and treatment that the juvenile court system may have to offer.

5.5. The Dispositional Process

The objective of the action is to determine if there is a need for rehabilitative treatment, and if so, what is the best course for securing these services. Unfortunately there is a lack of judicial guidelines relating to what is the best-interest-of-the-child standard and the best-interest-of-the-state standard. Options available to the Court: (1) probation; (2) restitution; (3) community service work; (4) out-of-home placement; (5) nonsecure facilities; and (6) secure facilities.

5.6. The Needs and Desires of the Juvenile

Once again, state statutes protect the rights of children and adolescents who are generically grouped as youthful offenders. The role of the juvenile court worker is required in obtaining a social investigation and social report (determining facts about the child's family, a psychological profile, the school situation, and history/nature of prior offenses). The reports and evaluations are made accessible to the juvenile, the parents, and the attorney. The attorney for the juvenile offender has the right to examine authors of the reports and evaluations. In addition, the child/adolescent's attorney is entitled to present witnesses and evidence on the child's behalf.

5.7. Privacy of Juvenile Records

Various issues have been raised as they apply to the privacy of a juvenile's records including police arrest records, fingerprints, photographs, social history, pleadings, and psychological studies. Similarly, considerations address the expungement of records and the sealing of records.

5.8. Miscellaneous Considerations

In addition to the topics cited, a variety of special legal issues, as they pertain to juveniles, are recognized: the right to be free of double jeopardy; intake detention and pretrial practice; trial procedures (role of parents; capacity of juveniles to plead; trial by jury; rules of evidence; social reports, and appeal).*

6. Conclusion

The basic criticism of the imposition or introduction of uniformity into the treatment of children, in the broadest sense of the word, is that it is the antithesis of the basic philosophy (individual) of medical treatment and education of children. Physicians must participate in the educational process because of the need to make lay educators aware of the multimedical conditions (medical, physical, neurological, and environmental) that impact on a child's ability to learn. Physicians must participate in the juvenile court process because fixed sentencing and the categorizing of children denigrates the primary function of the juvenile justice system which is to rehabilitate the offending child and to provide treatment for that offending child. Fixed sentencing will result in more children going to prison and more children being incarcerated for a longer period of time.

References

Biller, Stephen.: Legal and ethical considerations: Medical treatment of minors. Presented by the Hackensack Medical Center Institute for Child Development, April 11, 1984.

Gottlieb, Marvin I.: Teenage pregnancy, adolescence substance abuse, juvenile delinquincy, youth suicide: Challenges and strategies for primary health care providers. Presented by the Hackensack Medical Center Institute for Child Development, November 13, 1986.

*The reader may contact the author to secure specific legal codes addressing these issues.

CHAPTER 5

Temperament and Its Role in Developmental–Behavioral Diagnosis

WILLIAM B. CAREY

1. Introduction

Despite the increased interest in recent years about temperament differences in children, relatively little has been presented about how and when to use the concept in the practical clinical management of problems in children's development and behavior (Carey, 1985a; Chess and Thomas, 1986). The purpose of this chapter is first to present a brief review of our current understanding of temperament, and then to demonstrate by means of an algorithm just where and how this knowledge can fit into the diagnostic process.

2. Basic Issues

2.1. Definition

The term "temperament" has been used since ancient times, with varying descriptions and interpretations. The prevailing view defines temperament as "behavioral style." As Thomas and Chess (1977) have suggested, it is the "how" of behavior, rather than the "what" (abilities)

WILLIAM B. CAREY • Department of Pediatrics, University of Pennsylvania School of Medicine, Division of General Pediatrics, Children's Hospital of Philadelphia, Philadelphia, Pennsylvania 19104.

or "why" (motivations). They have subdivided temperament into nine characteristics: activity, biological rhythmicity, initial approach/ withdrawal, adaptability, intensity, mood, persistence/attention span, distractibility, and sensory threshold (Table 1). Most clinicians and many academicians have preferred this conceptualization because of its derivation from clinical descriptions and its established practical value.

The concept of difficult temperament was introduced by Thomas *et al.* (1968) in their New York Longitudinal Study. This study investigated the manner in which certain normal behavioral style traits interacted with features of the environment in the production of behavioral problems. These disorders were particularly likely to develop between the ages of 2 and 10 years among members of their middle-class population of New York City children, who were determined by parental interview during the first 5 years of life to be: (1) difficult (arrhythmic, low in approach and adaptability, intense and negative); (2) slow-to-warm-up (low in approach and adaptability, negative in mood, but low in activity and intensity), or (3) characterized by excessive persistence, distractibility, or activity.

This useful clinical concept was readily accepted by many child care professional persons but was rapidly generalized by various investigators far beyond its original scope to other ages, settings, and outcomes. Consequently, numerous problems have arisen both in practical and theoretical areas. Doubts as to the clinical appropriateness of this extension of the terminology were generated as additional data revealed that

Table 1. Temperament Characteristics

Activity: the amount of physical motion during sleep, eating, play, dressing, bathing, etc.
Rhythmicity: The regularity of physiologic functions such as hunger, sleep, and elimination
Approach/withdrawal: The nature of initial responses to new stimuli—people, situations, places, foods, toys, procedures
Adaptability: The ease or difficulty with which reactions to stimuli can be modified in a desired way
Intensity: The energy level of responses regardless of quality or direction
Mood: Amount of pleasant and friendly or unpleasant and unfriendly behavior in various situations
Persistence/attention span: The length of time particular activities are pursued by the child with or without obstacles
Distractibility: The effectiveness of extraneous environmental stimuli in interfering with ongoing behaviors
Sensory threshold: The amount of stimulation, such as sounds or light, necessary to evoke discernable responses in the child

(1) the stress-producing characteristics vary somewhat in differing age groups; (2) the same characteristics may be involved in rather different interactions in other cultures or subcultures; and (3) other characteristics may be more important for other outcomes, as persistence/ attention span is for school performance problems. An additional hazard emerged as some clinicians were tempted to use these terms for labeling children in discussions with their parents and researchers overutilized them for inappropriate data reduction (Carey, 1986).

A solution to these problems is the restriction of the concept of difficult temperament to its original meaning and the introduction of a more general term to cover any temperamental characteristics likely to be troublesome in certain settings. "Temperamental risk factors" is not a completely satisfactory description but would be an improvement (Carey, 1986).

Temperamental risk factors for "poor fit" (or incompatible relationship) are defined as any temperamental characteristics predisposing a child to excessive interactional stress and conflict with the caretakers, and to secondary clinical problems in the child's physical health, development, or behavior. It is important to be specific as to which characteristics place the child at risk for what outcome and under what circumstances. These characteristics are likely to be perceived and experienced as hard to manage by most caretakers in the specific set of circumstances.

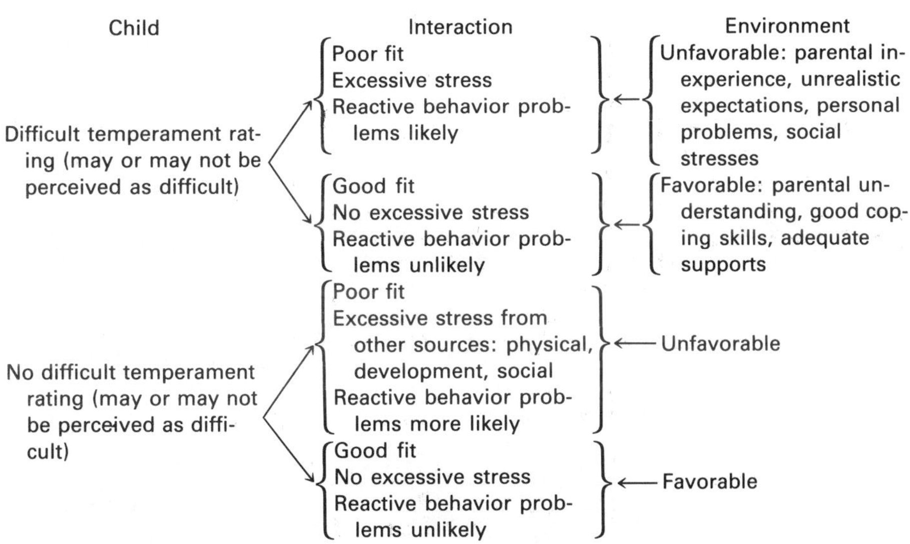

Figure 1. Interactions of difficult temperament. (From Carey, 1986.)

A problematic outcome is not inevitable but depends on the strength and durability of the characteristics and on the environmental stresses and supports (Carey, 1986).

Thus, difficult temperament, as defined by Thomas and Chess (1977), may be regarded as a temperament risk factor for poor fit in 2- to 10-year-old urban middle-class American children, possibly leading to social behavior problems during that time. The same is true for the slow-to-warm-up child. To these two groups, low task orientation, low flexibility, or high reactivity in elementary school children should be added, since they place children at risk for unacceptable scholastic performance (Keogh, 1982). In addition, low sensory threshold has been shown to increase the risk of "colic" and sleep disturbance in infants (Carey, 1985b). In fact, any characteristic regarded as abrasive or undesirable by the child's caretakers is a risk factor for poor fit. For example, a vigorous athletic parent may expect the same characteristics of his child and push him so relentlessly to be more active that the child becomes rebellious (see Fig. 1).

Outcomes of these interactions depend largely on the quality of the caretaking. Situations predisposing parents to problems in the handling of difficult traits include inexperience, unrealistic expectations or values, personal problems, and/or social stresses such as marital disharmony or financial straits. However, since some children are experienced as difficult by practically any parent, it should not be assumed that parents reporting difficulty are necessarily encumbered by personal problems. Furthermore, difficult traits may be stronger and more durable in some children than in others.

2.2. Measurement

Much has been written elsewhere on techniques currently available for the measurement of temperament and obviates the need for extensive description in this chapter (Carey, 1983).

There is no single definitive method for measuring temperament. Parental reports in interviews or questionnaires make use of their extensive knowledge of the child, but may be distorted by their various attitudes or feelings about the child. Professional observations in the office, home, or laboratory are thought to be more objective, but can be impaired by brevity, unrepresentative sampling, and/or various effects from the presence of the outsider.

Clinicians continue to rely primarily on the parents' reports of their children's behavior. However, the clinician must combine data from both history and physical examination, as well as prior experience with the child, in order to form an overall assessment of behavior. This is analogous to the principles involved in physical and developmental diagnosis. Temperament questionnaires remain a primary data source for the evaluation of temperament.

2.3. Origins and Stability

Temperamental characteristics appear to be partly genetically determined, partly determined through interaction with environmental forces, and also influenced by other factors as yet poorly understood, such as the physical state of the child and the nonhuman environment. In addition to the impact of the psychosocial environment, the child may alter the environment in three ways: (1) selecting certain aspects of it to deal with or avoid; (2) modifying the way it is experienced; and (3) actually causing caretakers to change. Thus, the child's temperament has an impact both on the child and his environment (Chess and Thomas, 1986).

There is evidence of stability of temperament and some of change. It is never either completely fixed or changeable. Apparently stability increases as children get older (McDevitt, 1986).

2.4. Clinical Importance

Temperament differences are important both in ordinary daily interactions and in certain clinical problems. Parents and teachers often misunderstand the nature and meaning of temperament variations. For example, fussiness in infants may be misinterpreted as milk allergy or the result of parental inadequacy. Teachers sometimes believe that difficult children are "immature" or that slow-to-warm-up children are "insecure." The primary health care professional, committed to the general welfare of his or her patients, will find much to do in helping parents understand and deal appropriately with these normal variations of behavior.

The other clinical importance of temperamental risk factors is that the stress and conflict they can generate in interpersonal interactions may lead to an increased incidence of a variety of clinical problems. It has been documented that relationships exist between certain temperament characteristics and various aspects of children's physical health, development, and behavior. In addition to problems in social behavior and academic performance, there are variations in growth and development, accidents, "colic," functional abdominal pain, sleep disturbances, and enuresis. A role of temperament in child abuse and failure to thrive has also been suspected, but is difficult to prove because of methodological problems. Difficult infants, for example, are more likely to be "colicky" or have accidents, whereas difficult children experience more academic and behavior problems in school. Apart from its role in predisposing to the incidence of various conditions temperament may also affect the child's reaction to an illness (Carey, 1985b).

3. Temperament in the Diagnostic Process: An Algorithm

Three principal areas of the clinical use of temperament data have been previously described (Carey, 1985a). First, general educational discussions with parents may help them increase their awareness and understanding of the phenomenon. Second, it is sometimes useful to identify a specific child's temperament profile in order that the clinician and parents can get a clearer picture of the child's contribution to the parent–child interaction Third, it may be possible to influence the temperament/environment interaction when its dissonance has produced excessive stress and reactive symptoms in the child.

Some clinicians have expressed uncertainty that these general principles do not demonstrate how to incorporate the concept of temperament in the management of specific concerns about children's behavior. In response to these inquiries, the author has developed an algorithm, or decision tree, to clarify the process (see Fig. 2).

There are three components to a clinical algorithm: clinical states, diagnostic decisions, and recommended therapy (Margolis, 1983). In broad outline, the process of this algorithm involves two preliminary diagnostic decisions, then three major substantive ones. First, one must determine whether the parents wish to become involved in the diagnostic process and whether there are significant developmental or physical elements to the problem. The remaining decisions are based on determinations of (1) whether a behavioral adjustment problem is present; (2) how severe it is, if present; (3) the role of the child's temperament in creating the concern; whether or not there is a behavior adjust-

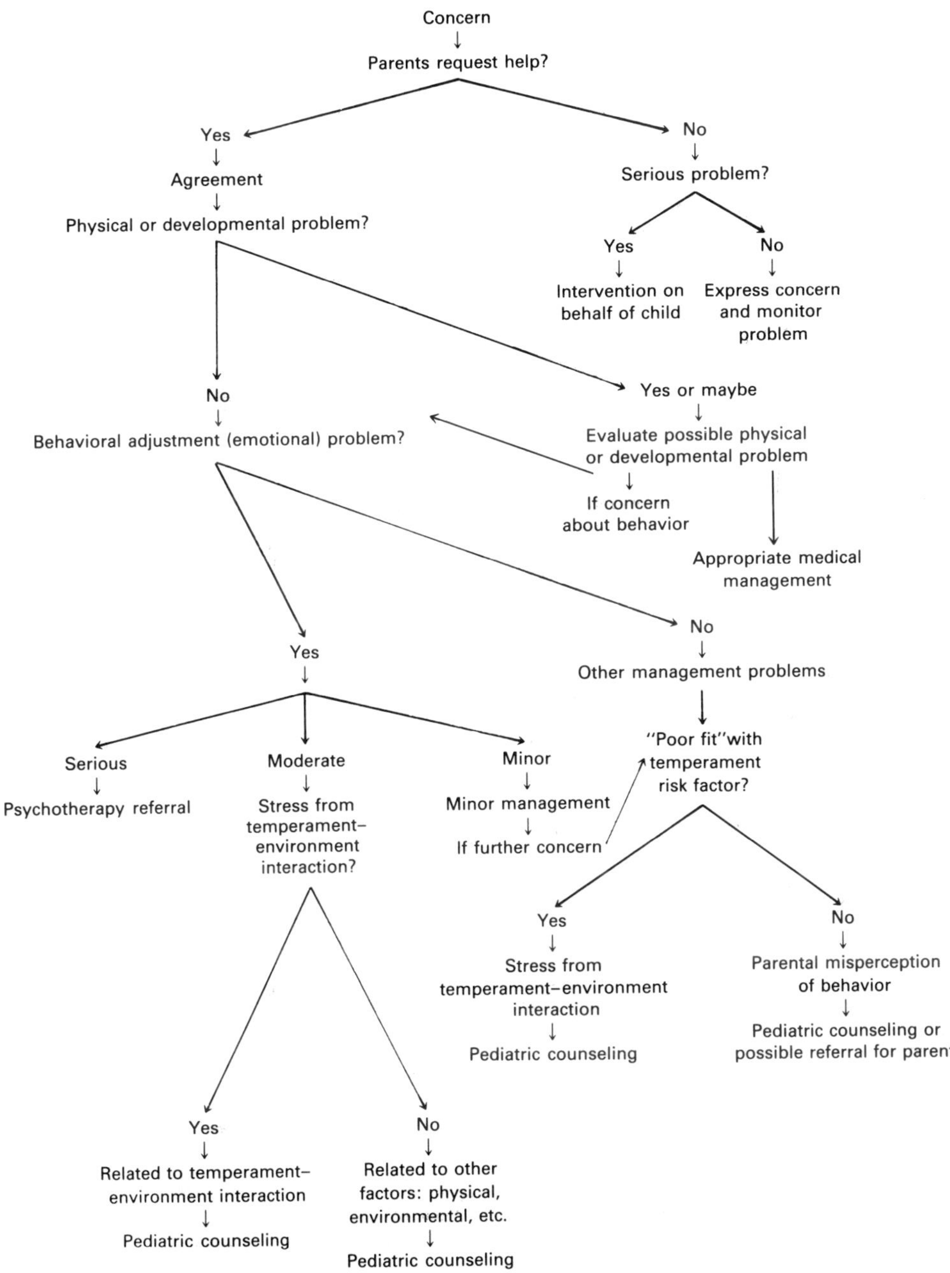

Figure 2. Pediatric algorithm for behavior management problems.

ment problem. Only by presenting the entire algorithm can the timing and method of the use of temperament data be fully explained.

3.1. Concern

The diagnostic process begins with someone's concern about the child; i.e., the parent, patient, outside referral (e.g., the school), or from the pediatrician's own observations. It may involve the child's behavior, development, or physical function. The intensity of the concern may range from casual mention to insistent pleas for help. The concern may be clearly focused on the real problem, may be only vaguely perceived by the parent, or it may be displaced onto the wrong person or complaint. The setting for the expression of parental concern may be during a well-child visit, at the time of a child's illness, or in an inappropriate context such as the community swimming pool. Parents generally have different expectations as to the extent to which the pediatrician will become involved in resolving their concerns. Confronted with a problem in such a poorly defined state, the pediatrician may be prompted to respond with an equally poorly focused reaction such as avoidance, unfounded reassurance, or some standard remedy.

The first task is to define the concern more fully and to determine whether the parents desire professional help. If concern has been expressed but assistance is not requested, the diagnostic process may have to be terminated at this point. It is possible that there is a sound basis for this decision; for example, the parents may have mentioned a problem that they are successfully working on and simply want to keep the pediatrician informed. An example of this situation is when a father and mother share with the physician their great distress about the child's behavior and functioning at school, but when asked by the doctor how he might help, they relate that they are already involved with appropriate consultants. It is then reported that the office visit was to complete a school physical examination form, and that their description of problems was to keep the pediatrician abreast of events.

It is possible that the pediatrician feels concern, but the parents are not taking appropriate steps and do not accept the offer for help. In this situation the physician can only make clear the reasons for the concern and describe the type of help likely to be available for management. Subsequently, the physician can observe and monitor the concern and the problem at later contacts. For example, the parents of a difficult infant insisted that their child's irritable behavior was due to milk allergy, even a month after they had on their own changed her to a milk-free diet. They felt no need for further investigations by the physician.

If the concern suggests a serious problem and the parents are unwilling to allow the pediatrician to investigate, then he or she may have to intervene on behalf of the child and consider child protection services. For example, if one learns from the parents or from another source that there is a strong possibility of child abuse or neglect, one is morally and legally obliged to take further steps.

3.2. Agreement

Before the diagnostic process can continue, there must be an agreement about whether and how the concern will be investigated. The general pediatrician's situation differs from that of the medical or mental health consultant. By the time the family appeals to specialists for help, a specific problem has usually been identified and the parents are seeking a solution. In developmental and behavioral aspects of pediatrics, the need for such an agreement is greater than in the more biological issues of medical care. For an earache or dysuria, the diagnostic problem and establishment of therapy is largely in the hands of the physician. For psychosocial issues, however, the process of evaluation and management is shared with the family. An agreement must be established as to what the family expects and what the physician will provide. In practice it is often only an implied agreement; but the greater the clarity at this point, the better the chances of effective collaboration through the diagnostic process. An example of a problem at this point was raised by a pediatric intern who was puzzled by a mother's request that he urge her son to be more faithful about saying his prayers. The clinical supervisor urged the intern to consider that there might be other problems in the parent–child relationship or in the child's behavior, but persuading children to conform to their parents' religion is not a role to which the pediatrician should agree.

The next step is to define the problem more thoroughly: what are the frequency, intensity, and duration of the symptoms; who is bothered by them and why; what management has been tried already and with what success? An initial assessment should be made at this point of the child's physical, neurological, developmental, and behavioral states, temperament, and the environmental input and interactions. These issues are all generally covered in a standard comprehensive history and physical examination.

An important diagnostic decision at this point is to determine if the child's development or physical states may be questionable or abnormal in any way.

3.3. Developmental or Physical Problem?

The question of a possible problem in these areas must be pursued in order for the diagnostic process to move forward. These issues are not more important than behavior, but are in danger of being neglected if not considered at the outset. If the practitioner knows his patient well, it may take only a moment to dispose of these matters.

The pediatrician may be capable of clarifying any uncertainty; however, referral to a medical specialist may be necessary. The investigation may uncover developmental problems such as retardation, learning disabilities, or a physical malfunction such as a neural or conductive hearing loss.

The discovery of the existence of problems and competent management strategies, however, do not obviate considerations that there may still be concerns about the child's behavior. If either the parent or the pediatrician is concerned, the investigation process should not wait until all evaluation of developmental and physical issues has been completed, but can be conducted simultaneously.

An example of the need for this comprehensive approach was presented by a child who was not paying attention well in school. She had a moderately severe conductive hearing loss due to serous otitis, but she was also inattentive before the middle-ear fluid accumulation and after it was removed.

With or without accompanying findings of a developmental or physical problem, the next diagnostic decision is whether there is evidence of a behavioral adjustment or emotional problem. Some authors classify these as separate groups. However, since emotional problems such as depression or anxiety are generally recognized by their behavioral manifestations, the term "behavioral adjustment problems" includes both groups in this discussion.

At times it is difficult to decide whether a behavioral adjustment problem is present. The issue may be clarified by defining them as disturbances in relationships with people, tasks, and oneself (Chess and Thomas, 1986). Four useful criteria of behavioral adjustment readily applied in primary child care include: (1) social competence versus undersocialization; (2) task performance versus underachievement; (3) self-assurance versus disturbance of self-relations; and (4) miscellaneous variations and deviations of feeling, thinking, and behavior.

The qualifications for the first three criteria depend on circumstances such as the age of the child. The fourth criterion describes behavior that is not normal under most circumstances, such as depression or self-destructive behavior.

In view of the unreliability of office observations and the superficiality of available behavioral adjustment questionnaires, the pediatrician must rely primarily on parental descriptions of behavior in forming judgments about behavioral adjustment. Pediatricians may shrink from this decision, feeling that a high degree of expertise is necessary. However, a few minutes of questioning using the criteria in the previous paragraph allows for at least a preliminary disposition.

The next stage in the sorting process is the determination of the severity of the behavior problem if present. The evaluation of the level as severe, moderate, or minor influences the type of intervention offered. Steps to follow if no behavior problem is found will be described shortly (Section 3.8).

3.4. Severe Behavioral Adjustment Problems

These occur when the symptoms are major, multiple, or chronic. Problems included are major antisocial behavior, school failure, major depression, psychosis, anorexia nervosa, severe obsessive-compulsiveness, overanxious disorder, phobic disorder, major conversion symptoms, and suicidal behavior. Research to date suggests a negligible role for the child's temperament in these severe problems (Chess and Thomas, 1986).

Pediatric management of these problems is seldom successful. The only appropriate course of action is prompt referral for psychotherapy. An example is the 5-year-old boy who had seemed normal on the previous visit a year before, but whose mother was now reporting deterioration of behavior with the stress of parental divorce. The child had threatened people with a knife, deliberately turned on the unlit gas stove, and showed other signs of poorly controlled and dangerous aggressiveness.

3.5. Minor Behavioral Adjustment Problems

These problems are at the other extreme and are likely to be normal variations of behavior rather than true deviations. Included here are such concerns as nail biting, thumb sucking, late toilet training, normal adolescent ambivalence toward their parents, and the capable child who gets only B's when A's could easily be achieved.

Minor problems call for minor management. Such matters can be handled relatively easily, with reassurance that the child is really behaviorally healthy. If parental concern persists despite this strategy, there is need to consider whether some extraneous factors such as the child's temperament are contributing to the worry. These other factors will be discussed later (Section 3.8).

3.6. Moderate Behavioral Adjustment Problems Related to Temperament–Environment Interactions

Between severe and minor problems there are a large number and variety of behavioral deviations presented to the pediatrician. The symptom(s) are significant but not severe. These problems range from moderate problems in social behavior such as excessive aggression toward siblings or peers or deficient school adjustment or performance, to moderate situational depression as observed with parental divorce or the death of a family member, to excessive accidents and the common "functional" physical disorders such as disturbances in eating, sleeping, elimination, and pain.

An important decision at this point is to determine if the moderate problem is related to the temperament–environment interaction. Not until this relatively advanced stage in the diagnostic process is the question raised. Some children have temperament risk factors that make them more vulnerable than others to various challenges imposed by the environment. As mentioned earlier, these risk factors embrace not only the better-known syndromes of the difficult and the slow-to-warm-up child, but also a growing list of predisposing characteristics such as high sensitivity (low sensory threshold) and low task orientation (low persistence, high distractibility, and high activity) (Carey, 1985b, 1986).

Determinations of a child's temperament can be made by carefully interviewing the parents or by a questionnaire appropriate for the child's age (Carey, 1983). Brief interviewing or office observations are likely to be misleading because of unrepresentative sampling.

Management of these problems can usually be successfully achieved by the pediatrician. Steps in the process include (1) recognition of the role of the child's temperament in the interaction; (2) alteration of parental management to decrease the stress in the interaction and to cause the secondary problem in behavior to disappear; (3) helping parents to accommodate to the child's behavioral style to reduce chances of future problems; and (4) various behavior management strategies, such as discipline, behavior modification, and psychotherapy for the child in so far as these are called for (Carey, 1985a; Chess and Thomas, 1986).

The importance of defining the child's temperament is twofold: (1) the existence of a predisposing behavioral style makes more understandable why one child and not another develops behavior problems with a given amount of environmental challenge; and (2) realistic limits are placed on the intervention effort; we hope to help the behavior problem disappear but we cannot expect by our efforts to make a difficult child become otherwise. An illustrative example is the second grade difficult girl who had previously done well in school because experienced kindergarten and first grade teachers had patiently allowed her to adjust to novel situations. With a rigid young second grade teacher the child was repeatedly frustrated, had frequent temper tantrums, deteriorated in her scholastic achievement, and was threatened with expulsion from school. Understanding the child's temperament aided the diagnostic process by explaining the magnitude and direction of her reactions and guided management plans and expectations. With another teacher her behavior and scholastic performance became quite satisfactory again.

3.7. Moderate Behavioral Adjustment Problems Related to Other Factors

These are the alternative situations when moderate degrees of behavioral deviations are not related to stress from temperament–environment interactions. These factors may be problems such as physical illness or handicaps, or an unfavorable psychosocial environment, due to parental inexperience, unrealistic expectations, personal problems, or social stresses.

Pediatric management of these problems is similar to what was mentioned in Section 3.6, but different in a major way. If temperament risk factors are not involved in the genesis of the behavior problem, the management strategy consists largely of attempts to alter the noxious environmental factors and the child's interaction with them. Other elements of behavior management may also be necessary: discipline, behavior modification, and psychotherapy for the child (Chess and Thomas, 1986). An example of this situation is the 3-year-old girl whose aggressive behavior was called to the attention of her kind, hard-working professional parents by her day-care teacher. She had been adopted as an infant. Her parents had been through several miscarriages and a previously failed effort at adoption, which was terminated by the biological mother reclaiming the child. Although she was temperamentally easy as an infant and toddler, she had become a tyrant by 3 years of age because her parents felt uncomfortable about restricting her impulses. The child needed and responded favorably to clearer, more fixed limits.

There are instances in which both temperamental risk factors in the child and unfavorable environmental elements work together to produce deviant behavior in the child. An example of this would be the difficult boy who is overwhelmed by parental divorce and begins to fail in school. His more flexible sister similarly feels unhappy but continues to function well academically.

3.8. Other Management Problems

At an earlier point the decision was made as to whether a behavior problem was present. To this point the description was of consequences of determining that there was one present. What happens next if the parents are concerned about the behavior but the criteria have not been met for a behavior adjustment problem or there is only a minor one? At this point it is appropriate to apply available temperament data to obtain more if necessary. One must decide whether temperament risk factors are present and are the cause of stress and conflict because of a "poor fit."

3.8.1. Stress from Temperament–Environment Interaction

If the child has one of the common temperament risk factors such as the difficult child or slow-to-warm-up syndromes, the parents may be feeling distress in the handling of the child, but there may be no secondary problems in behavior, development, or physical function. Some parents can deal successfully with these temperament risk factors, especially if they understand them, have good coping skills, and are well supported. Other parents experience more difficulty with the same behavior, particularly if they are inexperienced, have unrealistic expectations, or are encumbered by personal problems or social stresses.

These situations are generally within the range of pediatric counseling. Principles of handling begin with a recognition of the nature of the problem and include also a reorganization of parental management toward greater sensitivity to the meaning of behavior and more detachment in reacting to it. Parents need less criticism from professional advisors and more suggestions on specific strategies and on finding relief from the challenges experienced. Psychotherapeutic intervention is seldom needed. For details on this process, the reader is referred to the article, "The Difficult Child" (Carey, 1986) and the book for parents with the same title by Turecki and Tonner (1985).

An example of this situation is the 3-year-old girl who was referred by a fellow pediatrician for consultation. He had recommended to the parents that she needed psychotherapy for her temper tantrums, but they requested a second opinion because they could not agree. A pediatric examination and a temperament questionnaire revealed that the child did not have a real behavior problem, but rather an inflexibility to change and other challenges. Pediatric counseling rather than psychotherapy was indicated.

3.8.2. Parental Misperception of Behavior

If the clinician can detect little or no behavior problem and no temperament risk factor and yet the parents express concern about the child's behavior, what is to be done? At this point it is appropriate for the pediatrician to make at least a preliminary assessment of parental psychological and social factors to determine possible origins of their concern. We should go only far enough to establish the source of concern about the child. It is not within the pediatrician's competence to become extensively involved in these matters. The trouble may simply arise from parental misinformation about what they should expect from a child. This may be easily corrected. If parental depression, hostility, or marital discord are at the root of the misperception, these issues are best referred to those who are more skilled in managing these types of problems.

Perhaps the most common example of this type of parental concern is the situation of parental inexperience and misinformation. Parents may not understand the normal variations of behavior. An example is the parents of a 2-year-old girl who expressed dismay about how loud and vigorous she was. Their first child was an unusually pleasant, docile boy who made their more average daughter seem abnormal. A contrasting example is the mother of a normally active boy who complained that he was "hyperactive" because during the stress of marital separation his normal activity seemed excessive.

It is, of course, possible for parental concern to be aroused by a combination of temperament risk factors in the child and misperceptions of the parents.

4. Summary

The first part of this chapter briefly reviewed what is presently known about temperament. The second part presented a clinical algorithm demonstrating how knowledge of the child's temperament can play an important role in diagnosis and management.

Temperament is best defined as behavioral style or the "how" of behavior. Various dimensions of temperament have been defined, the most popular being the nine characteristics used by Thomas and Chess (1977). From these have been derived various temperament risk factors, such as the "difficult child syndrome," which predispose the child to a "poor fit" with the environment and to secondary clinical problems. Temperament can be measured using parental interviews or clinical observations, but measurement is best determined in the clinical setting primarily by questionnaire. It is derived from genetic factors, which interact with the environment, and the child's physical state. These traits show some evidence of stability but they also can change. A significant role has been demonstrated for temperament in a variety of clinical problems in physical health, development, and behavior.

The algorithm or decision tree begins with somebody's expression of concern about malfunction in the child and works its way through to various diagnostic impressions and management plans. It explains the appropriate timing and method for the use of information about the child's temperament. The child's temperament may cause parental concern whether or not there is a behavior problem.

ACKNOWLEDGMENT. I should like to thank Stella Chess, M.D., Stephen Ludwig, M.D., Sean McDevitt, Ph.D., Alexander Thomas, M.D., Stanley Turecki, M.D., and Marc Weissbluth, M.D. for their helpful comments on earlier versions of the algorithm.

References

Carey, W. B., 1983, Clinical assessment of behavioral style or temperament, in: *Developmental–Behavioral Pediatrics* (M. D. Levine, W. B. Carey, A. C. Crocker, and R. T. Gross, eds.), pp. 922–926, W. B. Saunders Company, Philadelphia, PA.

Carey, W. B., 1985a, Clinical use of temperament data in pediatrics, *J. Dev. Behav. Pediatr.* **6:**137–142.

Carey, W. B., 1985b, Interactions of temperament and clinical conditions, in: *Advances in Developmental and Behavioral Pediatrics,* Vol. 6 (M. Wolraich and D. Routh, eds.), pp. 83–115, JAI Press, Greenwich, CT.

Carey, W. B., 1986, The difficult child, *Pediatr. Rev.* **8:**39–45.

Chess, S., and Thomas, A., 1986, *Temperament in Clinical Practice,* Guilford Press, New York.

Keogh, B. K., 1982, Children's temperament and teachers' decisions, in: *Temperamental Differences in Infants and Young Children* (R. Porter and G. M. Collins, eds.), pp. 269–279, Pitman, London.

Margolis C. Z., 1983, Uses of clinical algorithms, *JAMA* **249:**627–632.
McDevitt, S. C., 1986, Continuity and discontinuity of temperament in infancy and early childhood, in: *The Study of Temperament: Changes, Continuities, and Challenges,* pp. 27–38, Erlbaum, Hillsdale, NJ.
Thomas, A., and Chess, S., 1977, *Temperament and Development.* Brunner/Mazel, New York.
Thomas, A., Chess, S., and Birch, H. G., 1968, *Temperament and Behavior Disorders in Children,* New York University Press, New York.
Turecki, S., and Tonner, L., 1985, *The Difficult Child,* Bantam Books, New York.

CHAPTER 6

Managed-Care Plans

An Update

RICHARD DONN

1. Introduction

A variety of managed-care plans have proliferated in the health care market during the past several decades. The popularity of managed-health care programs in part reflects the changes in socioeconomic times and structures, modified perspectives on health practices, and the influence of changing health insurance needs. This chapter will focus on several of the more common managed-care plans and their impact on practitioner and patient.

Although the relationship of managed-care plans and the particular needs of children and adults with developmental disabilities is not addressed specifically, physicians involved in developmental medicine must research the specific accommodations to be made to both the physician and patient. It is anticipated that broad variations will exist between the different managed-care plans available.

2. Preferred Provider Organization

The preferred provider organization (PPO) mechanism for containing health benefits cost allows the consumer a free choice of providers and maintains the fee-for-service system. PPOs are not as well-defined and understood as the health maintenance organization (HMO) system.

RICHARD DONN • Systems Development, Hackensack Medical Center, Hackensack, New Jersey 07601.

However, PPOs provide industry with a mechanism for providing their employees with a wide range and scope of providers, while controlling expenditures for health care. Lissovoy *et al.* (1986) defined PPOs as: "An arrangement in which a group of health care providers agrees to provide services to a defined group of patients at an agreed-upon-fee-for-service-rate." There are five key PPO components: (1) a provider panel composed of a limited number of physicians and hospitals; (2) negotiated fee schedules; (3) utilization review; (4) consumer choice of provider compiled with incentives to utilize PPO providers; and (5) rapid settlement of provider claims.

Lissovoy and colleagues suggest that PPOs have proliferated in response to local market conditions. PPOs flourish in market areas where (1) providers sense that competition is strong enough to encourage fee negotiation; (2) employer's health care costs have risen dramatically, encouraging the use of alternate health care delivery systems; and (3) state laws do not preclude contracting selectively. The three primary forms of sponsorship of PPOs are providers, insurers, and entrepreneurs.

2.1. Provider-Sponsored PPOs

Competition is the prime motivating force. Acording to Lissovoy *et al.* (1986), hospitals use the PPO market as a means of diversifying or entering into new markets. Physicians view PPOs as a last means of preserving the fee-for-service system. For hospitals, the matter of preserving the fee-for-service system. For hospitals, the matter of PPO organization is simpler because the intrastructure is already in place, i.e., administrative systems, billing systems, facilities and medical staff. In many cases, individual hospitals have banded together to organize regional systems of several institutions.

Physicians have more difficulty in organizing because of their reliance on office practices, and the difficulty in developing the administrative backup required to process large-volume billing and extensive user groups. Physician-sponsored PPOs are generally smaller in scope than those that are hospital sponsored. In hospital-sponsored systems, a major institution is usually the organizer and spearhead of the system. Other institutions generally participate based on similar interests and market pressures. As a rule, the hospitals utilize physicians almost exclusively from their medical staff.

According to Lissovoy *et al.* (1986), in reference to provider charges, over 50% of hospital-sponsored PPOs reimbursed participating member institutions on discounted usual charges. Per diem reimbursement was the second most-popular method. Variations in these formats are noted in some PPOs, including variable rates for special care units. All hospital-sponsored PPOs reimbursed physicians on the basis of a negotiated fee schedule.

In physician-sponsored PPOs, facilities (hospitals) were on a per diem basis and at least 30% on a discounted usual charge. Physicians were reimbursed on a negotiated fee schedule.

In regard to quality control (i.e., utilization review), 90% of hospital PPOs surveyed conducted both preadmission certification and concurrent review.

2.2. Insurer-Sponsored PPOs

Lissovoy *et al.* (1986) commented that insurer involvement in the PPO market "is a defensive move similar to the offering of administrative services only contracts that followed the trend to self-insurance among large groups." Extending the market is a matter of survival to many large-volume health-insured underwriters. Insurers bring a dimension to PPOs based on their experience in the benefits market and in negotiating with providers and payers. Typically, insurer-sponsored PPOs use a case-mix (DRG) reimbursement mechanism, paying hospitals a flat fee. Fee schedules are generally utilized for physicians.

2.3. Investor–Entrepreneurial-Sponsored PPOs

Investors act as "brokers" in the business by "networking" established provider groups for individual clients or payers. They can create a "package" for potential payers by surveying specific needs. Provider panels are almost nonexistent in this scheme since they vary from contract to contract and package to package. There are, however, some entrepreneurial PPO operations that will develop a specific package and then market that package to large self-insured groups. Insurer-sponsored PPOs predominately use a per diem basis of reimbursement to hospitals and employ a fee schedule for physicians.

3. HMOs

HMOs are distinguished from PPOs in that the purchasers pay a premium to the HMO for the provision of a full array of medical and hospital services. Anthony (1986) describes HMOs as categorized based on the type of contractual arrangement between the HMO and its physician providers. Staff model HMOs have physicians as employees. Group model HMOs are characterized by a contract between the HMO and an already established group of physicians who serve the HMO patients predominantly. Network HMOs include contracts between the HMO and several group practices and/or individual providers. Independent physician associations (IPAs) model HMOs are characterized by contracts between the HMO and IPAs whereby the physicians maintain independence in their individual practices.

The HMO can offer a wide variety of services to the payers for a fixed premium rate. In many cases the HMO shares risks with the providers or insures against such risks. Physician providers are rewarded in some cases for reduction in patient hospital days/1000 enrollees.

4. Selection of Managed-Care Plans by Physician Providers

When a physician or physicians group (as a provider) is engaged in the selection of the appropriate managed-care plan, goals should be established that guide one through the process. Goals should reflect the following:

1. Acceptable level of risk. How much risk is the provider group willing to accept? For example, risk sharing may result in a more advantageous fee schedule. Risk sharing may affect the pricing arrangement. A provider who is unwilling to work on an incentive basis or share the risk with the managed-care plan should not expect to be in a favorable negotiating position.
2. Extent of control of population. A question to be answered is: How much control does the physicians provider group wish to assert, specifically relative to utilization review, peer review, and in general the quality of care rendered?
3. Percentage of the practice's patients that would be treated under contract. A minimum of 30% of a practitioner's patients is an adequate goal to achieve. The upward limit should be established, as too extensive a mix on the high side will increase the leverage of the managed-care plan over the physician's practice.
4. Geographic market targeted by the contract. The regional boundaries of the population to be served may affect the practice structure in terms of the ability to cover patients adequately.

5. Number of hospitals networked. Similar to the geographic market targeted, the number of hospitals involved in the contract is an important variable. Networking of hospitals as established by the managed-care plan dictates the number of physicians in the system.
6. Marketing services of the group. Marketing promotional strategies is a significant variable in establishing the "identity" of the managed-care plan. This has an effect on the venture's success and ultimately the income of the practitioner.
7. Terms and conditions of contract. The terms of the contract, such as termination clauses, are important in recruiting both participating physicians and clients. The termination clause, for example, may address the ability of the practitioner to separate from the managed-care plan and possible limitations of the practitioner to contract concurrently with other plans.

5. Evaluation of the HMO Quality

Several major factors are valuable in assessing the quality of a particular managed-care plan (an HMO). The following sections explore some of them.

5.1. Access to Care

It is readily apparent that access to care will in part influence the success of HMOs in attracting subscribers. Subscribers universally insist that all providers are geographically in reasonable proximity in order to maximize health care networking. Is transportation available to subscribers? Is there a methodology established to input patients into the system? These are questions that are frequently considered significant variables in the subscribed selection of a particular managed-care plan.

5.2. The Management Structure

The integrity and competency of the management structure is a critical variable in the success of a managed-care plan. A competent management system is essential to survival of any particular plan; running the day-to-day supervision and establishing efficient and effective policies and procedures necessary to make the system "work."

5.3. Miscellaneous Factors

Continuity of care is an important consideration for almost all subscribers. Exploring the types of modalities available to ensure continuity of care is a common consideration for the subscriber before committing to a particular managed-care plan. Subscribers are also sophisticated in their knowledge of technical quality, i.e., the availability of diagnostic equipment. State-of-the-art equipment and general professional expertise, inherent in the HMO, are often inventoried by the individual who is selecting a managed-care plan. Member satisfaction is often surveyed by prospective managed-care plan subscribers. Word-of-mouth testimonials are critical in evaluating and judging the quality of care (in effect, the acceptability of the HMO viewed by the users of the service).

6. Evaluating Competitive Dimensions of Private Practice

A "practice audit" can be used periodically to determine whether a practice has a competitive edge in today's market. The audit provides the ability to evaluate the practice and to make modifications that are needed to improve a competitive stature.

Demographics

Determining patient demographics requires either an internal method of tracking statistics (preferably computerized) or the services of a professional marketer. The professional marketer generally utilizes practice records, providing the practitioner with an extensive data base including:

1. Patient demographics
   a. Place of residence of patient
   b. Economic status of patient (family income)
   c. Payer of bill (patient cash, private insurance, Medicaid, Medicare, free)
   d. Family size
   e. Referral sources (how patients get to you)
   f. Annual billing per patient per family
   g. Status of accounts receivable (by patient)
   h. Purpose of visit
   i. Number of visits per year

2. Services offered
   a. Direct patient care (types of services offered, i.e., evaluations, treatments, immunizations, etc.)
   b. Diagnostic
   c. Education (patients, PTA's)
   d. Community (i.e., schools, clinics, etc.)
   e. Emergency service coverage
3. User's attitude toward practice—methods of evaluation
   a. Patient questionnaire—results
   b. Telephone survey

4. Changes in all of the above "over time"

7. Conclusions

In summary, the following guidelines will in part serve the practitioner in the selection of a Managed Care Plan to meet their particular needs:

1. Selection of a managed-care plan requires *careful* investigation and consideration by the practitioner.
2. An analysis of the particular benefits inherent in a specific managed-care plan is essential to the selection process.
3. The practitioner should conduct a practice audit in order to assess service capability and to determine the available market; data utilized in deciding on a managed-care plan (if indeed association is desirable).
4. The practitioner should compare the assets and deficits (liabilities) of several competing managed-care plans before deciding on one or more with which to be associated.
5. Managed-care plans are increasing in popularity and often reflect the needs and posture of the market place. They should not be ignored, as they impact significantly on our health care delivery system.

The managed-care plans are an integral part of our health service. It is essential that a careful analysis of the various plans be performed, particularly for physicians involved in developmental–behavioral pediatrics. This subspecialty of pediatric medicine has unique needs and compensations. It is critical that the issues of developmental–behavioral pediatrics be reviewed within the context of financial limitations for patient and practitioner. As managed-care plans cannot be ignored, neither can the special problems of children and adults with developmental disabilities.

References

Anthony, M., 1986, Developing a network strategy, *Caring* **5**:57–61.

Lissovoy, G., Rice, T., Ermann, D., *et al.*, 1986, Preferred provider organizations: today's models and tomorrow's prospects, *Inquiry*, **23**:7–15.

CHAPTER 7

The Learning-Disabled Child

Pediatric Roles in Assessment and Management

PAUL H. DWORKIN

1. Introduction

1.1. The Concept of Specific Learning Disabilities

Any description of pediatric roles in the assessment and management of school-related learning problems must acknowledge the confusion and controversy in the field of learning disabilities. Of the many factors leading to school dysfunction, learning disabilities are the most prevalent and perplexing. The confusion surrounding this difficult problem results from the lack of any uniformly accepted definition of learning disabilities and from the divergent perspectives held by different disciplines.

1.1.1. Definition and Terminology

A wide variety of definitions and terms have been employed to describe school failure among children who are neither sensory impaired nor mentally retarded. For example, Feagans (1983) uses the term "learning disability" to describe "a heterogeneous population of

PAUL H. DWORKIN • Department of Pediatrics, Division of General Pediatrics, University of Connecticut Health Center, Farmington, Connecticut 06032.

children who display persistent school achievement problems that are not easily explained by poor intellectual abilities" (p. 487), whereas Wender (1981) broadly defines learning disabilities as "a cluster of biologically based disturbances in development that significantly impair school performance" (p. 91). Although the term "learning disabilities" or "specific learning disabilities" has retained the widest acceptance since the 1960s, a variety of other terms have been proposed, such as "minimal brain dysfunction," "dyslexia," and "perceptual handicap."

In response to the problems of varying terminology and definitions, the National Advisory Committee on Handicapped Children (1968) in a report to Congress recommended a definition of learning disabilities that includes five major components: (1) the failure to learn academic skills; (2) the absence of physical problems, poor instruction, cultural–environmental factors, sensory impairment, and mental retardation as the causes of poor school performance; (3) implied deviant central nervous system functioning; (4) a discrepancy between academic performance expected on the basis of intelligence and actual academic achievement; and (5) a disorder in one or more of the basic psychological processes involved in understanding or using language. While such a definition has not achieved uniform acceptance, it has been incorporated into such important legislation as the Education for All Handicapped Children Act (PL 94-142).

1.1.2. Disciplinary Perspectives

Various disciplines view the learning-disabled child through their own unique perspectives, which results in a maze of terminologies, proposed causes, and intervention strategies. For example, the developmentalist views deficits in various areas of development (i.e., auditory–language, visual–perceptual–motor function) as predisposing a child to specific learning problems. The neurologist considers learning disabilities to be a pathologic condition resulting from a defect within the brain, whether the consequence of maturational lag, focal maldevelopment, or defects in overall brain organization. Educators emphasize the discrepancy between academic potential and performance. Language specialists stress the relationship between impaired linguistic abilities and poor academic achievement. These divergent perspectives are not mutually incompatible. Furthermore, an appreciation of these divergent disciplinary perspectives affords the pediatric practitioner the opportunity for more successful interdisciplinary communication.

1.2. Factors Molding Pediatric Roles

Any description of pediatric roles in learning disabilities must also acknowledge that multiple factors determine the extent of a given practitioners' involvement with such problems. Certain of these factors are inherent characteristics of the field of pediatrics, while others reflect the setting within which the practitioner functions, as well as characteristics of the practitioner himself. For any particular practitioner, these factors uniquely merge to produce a particular level of involvement.

1.2.1. Discipline-Related Factors

Pediatricians have a long history of child advocacy and are committed to promoting the optimal growth and development of children. Pediatric practitioners have unique access to infants and young children and are usually able to view the child within the context of family and community. Physicians and other health care providers are generally perceived as having a broad knowledge base about childhood issues. Consequently, they are often called on to provide guidance regarding acceptable treatment approaches to learning problems.

1.2.2. Practice-Related Factors

Pediatric involvement with learning problems is, as a rule, time-consuming. Thus, such factors as mode of practice (e.g., solo or group), practice size, availability and skills of office personnel, and reimbursement policies will all influence pediatric roles. For example, the use of neurodevelopmental screening instruments may be more common among pediatric practices that employ nurse practitioners.

1.2.3. External Factors

An evolution in pediatric practice has resulted in greater pediatric involvement with learning problems. Changes in patterns of morbidity have resulted in greater pediatric responsibility for developmental issues. Legislation, such as the Education for All Handicapped Children Act, has a major effect on the way physicians address school-related problems. The availability of local resources, such as psychoeducational personnel, also impact on pediatric roles, as does the recent "explosion" of knowledge in the field of child development.

1.2.4. Practitioner-Related Factors

Numerous studies have documented the inadequacies of pediatric training in the area of learning problems (Dworkin *et al.*, 1979). Negative feelings regarding competency and training must certainly influence pediatric roles in this area. The practitioner's professional and personal attitudes and interest further influence such roles.

2. Pediatric Assessment: Beyond Basic Competency

Despite the confusion and controversy surrounding the field of learning disabilities, there undeniably exists a group of children who have remarkable difficulty with academic learning. Pediatricians are frequently confronted by parents and school systems who seek assistance in dealing with these children. Thus, despite a lack of consensus concerning the nature of learning disabilities, the pediatric practitioner must possess sufficient knowledge to participate meaningfully in the assessment and management of these children.

2.1. An Overview of Pediatric Assessment

As has already been suggested, the role of pediatric assessment for the learning-disabled student is determined by numerous factors. For the child already identified by psychoeducational evaluation to be learning disabled, the purpose of the physician's assessment is to exclude medical factors that may contribute to learning problems. In general, the yield from such assessments is quite limited. Although physical disabilities certainly do have important implications for classroom functioning, such disabilities have usually been identified earlier during routine pediatric care.

Pediatric assessment assumes a broader role when a suspicion of learning disability arises in a child with unexplained school failure. The practitioner may then initiate a search for so-called "clinical correlates" of learning disabilities. The identification of "red flags," combined with the elimination of physical or sensory factors as causes of school dysfunction, emphasizes the need for psychoeducational evaluation to either confirm or refute an impression of learning disability.

2.2. Clinical Correlates of Learning Disabilities

2.2.1. The Concept of Clinical Correlates

A wide variety of clinical correlates have been described for learning-disabled children. Mattis and co-workers (1975) noted that "almost every disorder of higher cortical functioning recognized in children has been found in greater frequency in [learning-disabled] children than in normal controls. . ." (p. 150). The prevalence of many clinical correlates among learning-disabled children is unclear, since studies have yielded contradictory findings. Furthermore, the significance of such associated findings has, in general, been misinterpreted. Certain correlates (e.g., visual–perceptual motor problems) have been inappropriately perceived as actually causing learning disabilities. However, such causality is extremely difficult to prove and many such associated findings are more likely coexisting symptoms or consequences of learning disabilities. Certain correlates, such as deficits in intersensory integration, have been interpreted as being equivalent to learning disabilities, despite the need for psychoeducational evaluation to establish a diagnosis. Despite such misconceptions, an appreciation of the frequency and significance of various associated findings among learning-disabled children is useful in both confirming the need for psychoeducational evaluation and enabling the pediatric practitioner to counsel parents and school systems about the importance of such findings.

2.2.2. The Significance of Specific Clinical Correlates

The significance of certain clinical correlates of learning disabilities have been supported by various studies. Other proposed correlates have not been consistently identified to occur more frequently among learning-disabled children than normal controls.

2.2.2a. Historical Findings. For most learning-disabled children, the medical history is not characterized by any specific findings. The prenatal history may suggest a somewhat increased incidence of unfavorable events, including prematurity. Early health problems of possible special relevance include recurrent or persistent otitis media, lead poisoning, and iron-deficiency anemia. Family history typically reveals an increased incidence of learning disabilities among family members.

2.2.2b. Minor Congenital Anomalies. The traditional physical examination of learning-disabled children is usually normal. As increased incidence of so-called minor congenital anomalies has been reported in some studies of learning-disabled children. Such findings, however, are probably less prominent in learning-disabled children than among children with attention deficit disorder. Examples of such minor anomalies include epicanthal folds, hypertelorism, low-set ears, high-arched palate, clinodactyly, and syndactyly (Waldrop *et al.,* 1968).

2.2.2c. Neurologic Abnormalities. The extent to which neurologic abnormalities are identified among learning-disabled children depends on the interpretation and significance of so-called "soft" neurologic signs or neuromaturational delay. Findings such as difficulties with rapid alternating movements (dysdiadochokinesia), mirror movements (synkinesia), and choreiform movements are more prevalent among learning-disabled children. Signs of definite neurologic abnormalities, however, are not found more commonly among children with learning disabilities. Despite the higher incidence of learning disabilities among children with documented neurologic disorders, such as cerebral palsy and epilepsy, these conditions are relatively infrequent and account for a relatively small portion of the total number of learning-disabled children. Neurophysiologic (e.g., EEG) and neuroanatomic (e.g., computerized axial tomography) studies similarly fail to consistently suggest a higher incidence of neurologic abnormalities among the learning-disabled population.

2.2.2d. Motor Abnormalities. A number of studies suggest that learning-disabled children as a group are rather awkward and clumsy (Peters *et al.,* 1975). Clumsiness may be apparent when these children are asked to perform certain motor tasks (e.g., hopping on one foot, standing on one foot, tandem gait). Developmental history may suggest delays in accomplishments such as first sitting without support or walking alone.

2.2.2e. Speech and Language Difficulties. The higher prevalence of speech and language difficulties among learning-disabled children has been documented by many studies. Examples of such difficulties include problems with auditory discrimination and auditory comprehension. Developmental history may suggest delays in speaking first words or phrases. The "typical" profile of the learning-disabled children on intelligence testing reveals a discrepancy between verbal and performance subtest scores and generally poorer functioning on the verbal sections. These findings have been cited in support of the postulate that learning disabilities are the final expression of a more general linguistic disability.

2.2.2f. Temporal–Sequential Deficits. The faulty perception and retention of temporally organized stimulus patterns of learning-disabled children have been well recognized. These children are often confused by serial commands and time relationships such as "before" and "after." The significance of these findings among learning-disabled children remains speculative. Levine and co-workers (1983) suggested that weakness in this area may be associated with "problems following directions and acquiring skill in mathematics, reading comprehension, writing, and spelling" (p. 895).

2.2.2g. Directional Disorientation and Laterality Awareness. The extent to which learning-disabled children have difficulties with right–left confusion is unclear. While various studies have revealed significant differences between learning-disabled children and controls with tasks such as "touch your right knee with your left hand," other investigations have failed to confirm these differences. In general, research suggests that directional disorientation may be associated with learning problems in a limited number of younger students.

2.2.2h. Visuoperceptual Defects. As a result of Orton's studies in the 1920s, visuoperceptual difficulties have been regarded as a common problem among learning-disabled children. Subsequent research suggested, however, that the evidence linking visuoperceptual difficulties with learning disabilities was rather weak. Findings such as difficulties with figure–ground perception may be important only in a small subgroup of learning-disabled children, particularly at younger ages.

2.2.2i. Oculomotor Deficits. The correlation between eye disorders and learning disabilities is controversial. Many studies have evaluated the prevalence of ocular disorders such as refractive errors, strabismus, amblyopia, visual field defects, and defective stereopsis among learning-disabled children. The results have revealed no increase in ocular disorders compared with children without learning problems. Furthermore, the importance of faulty eye movements in reading disability remains conjecture until validated by critical study.

2.2.2j. Deficits in Intersensory Integration. Reading is an intersensory task, requiring the ability to transform temporally distributed auditory patterns (the sounds of words) into spatially distributed visual configurations (a row of letters). Several studies suggest that learning-disabled students are less adept than achieving students at translating auditory cues (i.e., a sequence of taps) into visual patterns (i.e., dots). Results from a larger number of investigations, however, have not been consistent. Consequently, it is difficult to implicate problems with intersensory integration as a major correlate of learning disabilities. Rather, deficits in this area may be characteristic of a limited number of learning-disabled students.

2.2.2k. Deficits in Conceptual and Cognitive Thought. Disorders in higher cognitive processes (e.g., memory, attention, symbolic thought, and perception) have been identified among learning-disabled children (Longfellow and Freeman, 1977). While the definition of learning disability presumes cognitive functioning with the broad range of normal, surveys of learning-disabled children consistently suggest a slightly lower mean IQ in the range of 93–95.

2.2.2l. Mixed Dominance and Laterality Preference. The likelihood of encountering non-right-handedness and deviant hand and eye preferences among learning-disabled children is suggested by Orton's theory of disturbed cerebral hemispheric balance, with a lack of clearly established hemispheric dominance for specific functions (Orton, 1925). Some studies have supported the hypothesis that learning-disabled children tend to display a higher incidence of non-right-handedness. Other population-based surveys have failed to document any clear relationship between academic achievement and hand preference, eye preference, foot preference, or mixed hand and eye preference.

2.2.2m. Behavioral and Emotional Difficulties. Emotional or behavioral difficulties are the inevitable consequences of years of school failure. Available evidence suggests that many behavioral and emotional problems of school children, such as conduct disorders and depression, result from chronic exposure to school failure and accompanying impairments of self-esteem and self-image. Problems with attention span and activity level also characterize the learning-disabled student.

In summary, research has documented a variety of clinical correlates of learning disabilities. Such correlates include historical findings, minor congenital anomalies, neuromaturational delay, motor abnormalities, speech and language difficulties, temporal–sequential deficits, visuoperceptual deficits, deficits in conceptual and cognitive thought, and behavioral and emotional difficulties. The importance of other correlates has not been consistently confirmed, including directional disorientation and laterality awareness, oculomotor deficits, deficits in intersensory integration, mixed dominance, and laterality preference.

2.3. Guidelines for Pediatric Assessment

Certain guidelines should be kept in mind when performing a pediatric assessment of children with possible learning disabilities. First, the evaluation must consider the multiple factors that may influence school functioning. Examples of such diverse factors include the child's general health, physical status, hearing and vision, motor development, visual processing abilities, auditory–language functioning, memory skills, cognition, temperament, emotional status, learning style, school behavior, and community resources. Second, although certain aspects of an assessment have traditionally been assigned to various professionals (i.e., psychologists, educators, social workers, physicians), few factors are limited to the confines of one discipline. Factors such as a child's general health and physical status are regarded as medical issues, whereas learning style and school behavior are considered within the psychoeducational sphere. The majority of factors, however, may be viewed independently by different professionals, thereby offering the opportunity to increase the reliability of individual assessments. Pediatric assessment must therefore allow for an interchange of ideas and communication between medical and educational personnel.

2.4. One Pediatric Model

One example of a pediatric office-based approach to the child with possible learning disabilities has been described and evaluated (Dworkin *et al.*, 1981). Within this approach (Table 1), two office visits are used for assessment and one follow-up visit is scheduled to discuss findings and recommendations. During the initial visit, which requires approximately 45 min, a complete history is obtained and a physical examination including a search for minor congenital anomalies, vision screening, and

Table 1. One Pediatric Model of Assessment of the Child with Learning Disabilities

Visit one (45 min)
History
Physical examination (including search for minor congenital anomalies)
Vision screening
Hearing screening
Dispersal of questionnaires (parent, teacher)
Visit two (45 min)
Neurodevelopmental screening
Projective testing
Referral for psychoeducational testing
Follow-up visit (30 min)
Discussion of finding, recommendations, referrals

hearing screening is performed. At the conclusion of the visit, parent and teacher questionnaires are distributed. These questionnaires are designed to facilitate the collection of historical data and to provide information regarding the child's present developmental and behavioral functioning within the home and school (Levine, 1981).

A second office visit, also requiring about 45 min, is subsequently scheduled to perform neurodevelopmental screening. The Pediatric Early Elementary Examination (PEEX) and the Pediatric Evaluation of Educational Readiness (PEER) are examples of age-appropriate assessment tools used within this model (Levine *et al.,* 1980). During this visit, simple projective tests, such as the Winnicott Squiggle Game, asking the child to draw a picture of his family, and asking the child for three wishes, are performed to screen the child's emotional status. The need for referral for psychoeducational testing is determined on the basis of this assessment. Criteria for referral include the identification of "clusters" of clinical correlates suggesting the possibility of learning disabilities, general delays suggesting the possibility of cognitive impairment, or learning problems for which no apparent cause is identified.

Following this evaluation, a follow-up visit of 30–45 min is scheduled with parents and child to discuss findings and recommendations. The pediatrician also prepares a written report that includes the results of assessment, recommendations, and arrangements for follow-up. Reports are distributed to parents and to schools with the written consent of a responsible family member. The charge for pediatric assessment within this model (approximately $200) is prorated from a fee of $30 for a routine office visit, typically requiring 15 to 20 min.

2.4.1. Implementation of Recommendations

In order to evaluate the usefulness of this model of pediatric assessment, parents and school personnel were interviewed 2 to 6 months following assessment to determine implementation rates of recommendations. Overall, 66% of parent recommendations were implemented, including 72% of medical, 58% of mental health, and 64% of educational recommendations. Seventy-two percent of school recommendations were implemented. Thus, recommendations offered through this process were viewed as appropriate by parents and educators (Dworkin *et al.,* 1981).

2.4.2. Validity of Parental Descriptions

The usefulness of this model was also evaluated by a second study that assessed the validity of parental descriptions of their children's school problems. Subjects included 52 school-age children referred by their parents for pediatric assessment because of school-related problems. Parental descriptions were categorized by specific criteria into three areas of concern: developmental, attention–activity, and social–emotional. Following complete pediatric assessment, findings were similarly categorized into three problem areas. Overall, 60% of parental concerns were confirmed by assessment, including 66% of developmental, 74% of social–emotional, but only 37% of attention–activity concerns. Of findings documented by assessment, 14% had not been suggested by parental descriptions, including 22% of developmental, 15% of attention–activity, and 13% of social–emotional problems. The results suggest that pediatric assessment should not be based solely on parental descriptions of children's school problems. The results do support the usefulness of additional information, such as school data and developmental screening, to clarify children's classroom difficulties.

3. Management of Learning Disabilities: Effective or Elusive?

3.1. An Overview of Pediatric Roles in Management

The mainstay of treatment of learning disabilities is educational intervention rather than medical therapy. However, pediatric participation in the management of the learning-disabled child involves a variety of possible roles. Traditional pediatric activities include counseling and the treatment of underlying conditions, such as a seizure disorder. Other roles such as participating in the development of a child's educational program and facilitating the appropriate utilization of community resources are somewhat less traditional but also feasible (Table 2).

3.1.1. Counseling

Pediatric counseling is an important method of intervention that may serve a variety of functions. Clarification of the child's strengths and weaknesses often leads to more appropriate expectations and alleviates undue concern. Anticipatory guidance may be offered with regard to commonly occurring consequences of school dysfunction, such as loss of self-esteem and acting-out behavior. Explaining the legal rights of children and families under the Education to All Handicapped Children Act is another critical aspect of counseling. Offering scientifically based opinions about so-called "alternative" or nontraditional treatment strat-

Table 2. An Overview of Pediatric Roles in Management of the Learning-Disabled Child

Counseling
Clarification of child's strengths and weaknesses
Alleviation of undue concern
Anticipatory guidance
Explanation of legal rights of children
Critical evaluation of nontraditional strategies
Explanation of specific behavior-management techniques
Specific medical intervention
Treatment of underlying medical condition
Use of medication to promote school performance
Further investigations and referrals
Laboratory tests
Referral to subspecialists, other disciplines for consultation, treatment
Educational strategies
Participation in multidisciplinary planning of educational programs
Utilization of community resources
School system
Community-based services

egies for learning disabilities, such as dietary manipulation, is another important aspect of the counseling process. Depending on the expertise and interest of the pediatrician, specific behavioral management advice such as the use of positive reinforcement and time-out may be offered.

3.1.2. Specific Medical Intervention

The treatment of any underlying medical conditions, such as a seizure disorder, is the most traditional of pediatric roles. The prescribing and monitoring of stimulant medication for attention-deficit disorder is another example.

3.1.3. Further Investigation and Referrals

Pediatric assessment may, in fact, raise more questions than answers. For some children, specific medical concerns may suggest laboratory studies such as chromosome studies, lead testing, and anemia screening. Referrals for further investigations may be in order, including referrals for psychoeducational testing and language assessment by a speech–language pathologist. For the child with more formidable behavior problems, referral to a mental health professional is usually indicated.

3.1.4. Educational Strategies

It is highly unlikely that the pediatric practitioner will have the expertise to suggest specific educational interventions or independently select an educational program for the learning-disabled child. Nonetheless, the practitioner can participate with other professionals in the development of a child's educational plan. The physician's participation is often reassuring to the family who regard the pediatrician as an advocate for the child and as being knowledgeable about a broad range of child-related issues.

3.1.5. Utilization of Community Services and Resources

The pediatric practitioner can also serve an important role as an ombudsman, introducing children and families to important community and educational resources.

3.2. Specific Intervention Strategies

In order to meaningfully participate in the management of learning-disabled children, some knowledge of specific intervention strategies is necessary. Effective treatment of learning disabilities is elusive. Treatment strategies have been remarkable for their variability and for limited research-based information about their effectiveness (Feagans, 1983). Intervention, however, can certainly help the learning-disabled child improve classroom functioning and also foster a positive self-image and enhance self-esteem.

3.2.1. Educational Intervention

Educational intervention is the mainstay of treatment for children with learning disabilities. Intervention is provided through the process of remedial instruction. The main elements of remedial instruction include: (1) identification of the skills to be learned; (2) a statement of objectives for instruction; (3) assessment of individual skill development; (4) identification of appropriate teaching activities and material; and (5) evaluation of the results of instruction (Guthrie and Seifert, 1978). The success of remedial instruction may be promoted by using material that ensures the child's interest, enhancing confidence through early success, and providing rewards for progress.

Remedial instruction for academic delays generally consists of direct instruction of specific academic skills, rather than attempting to improve the child's functioning in select areas of development (e.g., visual processing or fine motor). Studies of the effectiveness of remedial instruction reveal short-term academic gains, as well as the need for ongoing instruction in order to ensure that such gains are maintained. The issue of whether certain remedial instruction techniques are more effective with specific types of learning disabilities is controversial. In general, studies have failed to suggest that any one remedial technique is consistently more effective. For example, when Silberberg and co-workers (1973) examined the relative effectiveness of four different remedial reading techniques (a visual–sight approach, a kinesthetic approach, an auditory–phonic approach, and a multisensory model) with 102 learning-disabled third-grade students, no single method was more satisfactory in promoting long-term gains. Even when a specific remedial technique is selected on the basis of a child's particular profile of strengths and weaknesses (e.g., "auditory" vs. "visual" learners), no clear-cut advantages are appreciated (Longfellow and Freeman, 1977). Thus, the process of diagnostic teaching should serve as the basis for identifying the most effective remedial instruction for a given child.

3.2.2. Behavior Management

3.2.2a. Behavior Modification. A variety of behavior-modification strategies have been used for learning-disabled students to promote academic achievement and to decrease undesirable classroom behaviors. Examples include conditioning through token reinforcement programs and electromyograph (EMG) feedback. These techniques have not proved to be of benefit in improving academic achievement. They are useful, however, in ameliorating undesirable classroom behaviors, such as difficulties with attention and activity.

3.2.2b. Counseling and Psychotherapy. Counseling is an important adjunctive therapy to educational intervention for the learning-disabled child. The primary goal of this therapy is to address issues of diminished self-esteem, poor self-image, anxiety, depression, and other emotional consequences of chronic exposure to school failure. In addition, counseling of parents and teachers may alter their perception of the child as being "lazy" or "unmotivated."

3.2.3. "Alternative" or Nonstandard Therapies

Effective treatment of learning disabilities is generally elusive. It is not surprising, therefore, that a variety of nonstandard therapies have been suggested for use with learning-disabled children. Nonstandard treatments are typically based on the presumed importance of certain clinical correlates among learning-disabled students. For example, neurophysiologically based treatments assume that visuoperceptual deficits, oculomotor deficits, or deficits in intersensory integration are etiologic factors in learning problems. There is no evidence, however, to justify these presumptions. It is also not surprising that these alternative approaches have not been supported by scientific study (Golden, 1980).

3.2.3a. Perceptual Training. A variety of visuoperceptual exercises involving eye movements, sequencing and spatial relationships, form perception, figure–ground perception, visual memory, and visuomotor tasks have been used in attempts to enhance the academic performance of learning-disabled children. The lack of efficacy of these exercises, as suggested by most studies, is consistent with the rather weak correlation between visuoperceptual functioning and learning disabilities.

3.2.3b. Sensory Integration Therapy. This therapy attempts to enhance academic performance by improving through vestibular, postural, and tactile stimulation the brain stem's efficiency in processing sensory input. However, studies of sensory integration therapy have yielded, at best, equivocal results. Further study is needed to resolve this issue to substantiate claims of academic success.

3.2.3c. Optometric Training. There is no higher incidence of oculomotor disorders among learning-disabled students. Similarly, there is no evidence to support the benefits of a vision-training program designed to correct "faulty" eye movements presumed to cause learning problems.

3.2.3d. Orthomolecular Approaches. There are no data to support the usefulness of megavitamins and trace minerals in the treatment of learning-disabled children. Similarly, no benefits have been documented for dietary manipulation, such as the avoidance of artificial food colors and flavors or natural salicylates.

3.2.3e. Medications. Drugs including stimulants, diazepam, antihistamines, and tricyclic antidepressants have been employed in attempts to improve the academic achievement of learning-disabled students. Students have consistently failed to document academic gains from medications. Despite their possible value in addressing coexisting attention deficits, anxiety, or depression, medication appears to be of no value in directly improving the academic performance of learning-disabled students.

4. Summary

Of the many factors leading to learning problems, learning disabilities are the most prevalent and perplexing. Divergent perspectives held by different disciplines and the lack of any uniformly accepted definition contribute to the confusion surrounding this complex problem. While assessment and treatment of the learning-disabled child are multidisciplinary tasks, pediatric roles in evaluation and intervention can be defined. For the child suspected of being learning disabled on the basis of psychoeducational assessment, pediatric evaluation consisting of a medical history, physical examination, and neurodevelopmental assessment serves to exclude medical factors that may contribute to school problems. For the child with unexplained school failure, identification of clinical correlates of learning disabilities emphasizes the need for psychoeducational referral. Clinical correlates suggested by various studies include: (1) speech and language difficulties; (2) temporal–sequential deficits; (3) directional disorientation; (4) visuoperceptual difficulties; (5) deficits in intersensory integration; (6) deficits in conceptual and cognitive thought; (7) disturbances in finger recognition; (8) motor abnormalities; (9) behavioral and emotional problems; and (10) neuromaturational delay.

Pediatric participation in the management of the learning-disabled child involves a variety of roles. Counseling includes the provision of anticipatory guidance, explanation of the legal rights of school children, alleviation of undue concerns, clarification of strengths and weaknesses, and advice regarding the efficacy of "alternative" strategies. Specific medical intervention, such as drug therapy, for underlying conditions and arranging for further investigations and referrals are also traditional pediatric roles. Participation in the development of the child's educational program and facilitating the appropriate utilization of community resources are also possible, depending on the pediatric provider's interest and expertise.

Effective treatment of learning disabilities is elusive. Educational intervention such as remedial instruction is the mainstay of treatment. Behavior management techniques such as behavior modification and counseling are important adjuncts to educational intervention. A variety of "alternative" or nonstandard therapies are not supported by scientific study. These include such neurophysiologically based treatments as perceptual training, sensory integration therapy, and optometric training and also biochemically based treatments, including megavitamin and trace mineral therapy, treatment of presumed hypoglycemia, and dietary manipulation. A variety of drugs, including stimulants, have been employed in attempts to improve academic functioning without striking benefits.

References

Dworkin, P. H., Shonkoff, J. P., Leviton, A., *et al.*, 1979, Training in developmental pediatrics. How practitioners perceive the gap, *Am. J. Dis. Child.* **133:**709–712.

Dworkin, P. H., Woodrum, D. T., Brooks, K. S., *et al.*, 1981, Pediatric-based assessment. Children with school problems, *J. Sch. Health* **51**:325–329.

Feagans, L., 1983, A current view of learning disabilities, *J. Pediatr.* **102**:487–493.

Golden, G. S., 1980, Nonstandard therapies in the developmental disabilities, *Am. J. Dis. Child.* **134**:487–491.

Guthrie, J. T., and Seifert, M., 1978, Education for children with learning disabilities, in: *Progress in Learning Disabilities,* Vol. 9 (H. R. Myklebust, ed.), Grune and Stratton, New York.

Levine, M. D., 1981, *The ANSER System,* Educators Publishing Service, Cambridge, Massachusetts.

Levine, M. D., Brooks, R., and Shonkoff, J. P., 1980, *A Pediatric Approach to Learning Disorders,* John Wiley and Sons, New York.

Levine, M. D., Meltzer, L. J., Busch, B., *et al.,* 1983, The Pediatric Early Elementary Examination: Studies of a neurodevelopmental examination for 7- to 9-year-old children, *Pediatrics* **71**:894–903.

Longfellow, C., and Freeman, E., 1977, Reading disability, in: *Children's Medical Care Needs and Treatments,* Vol. 2 (Harvard Child Health Project), pp. 225–311, Ballinger, Cambridge, Massachusetts.

Mattis, S., French, J. H., and Rapin, I., 1975, Dyslexia in children and young adults: Three independent neurological syndromes, *Dev. Med. Child. Neurol.* **17**:150–163.

National Advisory Committee on Handicapped Children, 1968, *Special Education for Handicapped Children. First Annual Report,* U.S. Department of Health, Education and Welfare, Washington, D.C.

Orton, S. T., 1925, "Word blindness" in school children, *Arch. Neurol. Psychiatry* **14**:581–615.

Peters, J. E., Romine, J. S., and Dykman, R. A., 1975, A special neurological examination of children with learning disabilities, *Dev. Med. Child. Neurol.* **17**:63–78.

Silberberg, N. E., Iverson, I. A., and Goins, J. T., 1973, Which remedial reading method works best? *J. Learn. Dis.* **6**:547–556.

Waldrop, M. F., Pederson, F. A., and Bell, R. Q., 1968, Minor physical anomalies and behavior in preschool children, *Child Dev.* **39**:391–400.

Wender, E. H., 1981, Learning disabilities in children, *Pediatr. Rev.* **3**:91–98.

CHAPTER 8

Television Viewing

Impact on Child and Adolescent Development

MARVIN I. GOTTLIEB

1. Introduction

The quantity *and* quality of television viewing are probably the single most significant experiential factors influencing the behavior, health practices, and attitudes of children and adolescents. Children spend considerably more time watching television than hours spent in school. Approximately 14,000 hours are devoted to formal educational instruction, but an average of 16,000 to 20,000 hours are allocated for watching television. Analysis of the program and commercial content during those hours devoted to television viewing is even more alarming. Children and adolescents are exposed to about 350,000 commercials, numerous acts of violence and aggression, and as many as 18,000 murders (McCowan, 1979). The combination of these factors (the extraordinary amount of time that a child is occupied in watching television, as well as the nature of the program content) strongly suggests that the electronic media has a very significant influence on child and adolescent development. Parents and professionals have become increasingly concerned that current television-viewing practices may have an *adverse impact* on the behavior and psychosocial attitudes of children and adolescents. These justifiable apprehensions are engendered by an awareness that (1) the majority of television contacts for children are unsupervised; (2) commercials and television programs may be unrealistic and inappropriate for a young and "captive" audience; and (3) the repetitive

MARVIN I. GOTTLIEB • Institute for Child Development, Hackensack Medical Center, Hackensack, New Jersey 07601; and Department of Pediatrics, University of Medicine and Dentistry of New Jersey–New Jersey Medical School, Newark, New Jersey 07103.

format of television messages and themes may in effect be a form of "electronic brain washing."

The "television experience" has created a psychoeducational paradox for child health care professionals. On the one hand, television is a most effective and valuable educational media for children with obvious potentials for expanding their knowledge base, broadening their life experiences (albeit vicariously), and enhancing the scope of cultural interactions. Unfortunately, there are several serious negative implications of television viewing relating to the unrealistic nature of various programs and commercial messages. Television may be providing the child and young viewer with a heavy diet of aggression and violence, misleading representations that promote poor health practices, and superficial, unwholesome value systems (Fosarelli, 1984). The "television experience" has meteorically evolved from a relatively inexpensive method of home entertainment to a very influential and powerful household companion with the capacity to shape patterns of behavior and life-attitudes. Health care professionals and child advocates have become increasingly concerned about the unresolved issues regarding television's impact on the impressionable audience of children and adolescents. Indeed, television has mandated new responsibilities in professional advocacy and a more specific role in helping to design television programs for children.

There is general agreement among health care professionals that numerous psychobiosocial problems may be related to inappropriate television viewing. It has been postulated that children learn from watching television and what they learn may be either beneficial or harmful (Palumbo, 1985). This chapter will focus only on several selected areas of concern: (1) the possible effects of television on promoting aggressive/violent behaviors; (2) the influence of television in promoting imitative behaviors (the "Werther effect"); (3) the role of television in initiating poor physical and mental health practices (e.g., obesity, substance abuse, and inappropriate psychosexual models); and (4) the potential negative impact of unmonitored television time on reading and learning skills. The scope and depth of this review is necessarily limited by reasonable literary restrictions. However, a relatively extensive reference list is provided for readers interested in pursuing a more comprehensive study of this important issue.

2. General Epidemiological Considerations

The current television practices of children and adolescents are generally regarded as "poor" from developmental and psychosocial perspectives. In a recent report from the American Academy of Pediatrics

Task Force on Children and Television (1984), several major adverse effects of television viewing were delineated: (1) it promotes an inclination toward violence and an apathy when violence is observed; (2) it increases consumption of high-caloric snacks and an associated prevalence of obesity; (3) it promotes passive rather than active learning; (4) it conveys a variety of unrealistic messages regarding drugs, alcohol, and tobacco (indirectly encouraging their use); and (5) it conveys an unrealistic view of problem solving or conflict resolution. Realistically, television must be regarded as *the* major source of information for most children and one of their most significant developmental influences (Zuckerman and Zuckerman, 1985).

The possible negative psychobiological and psychosocial impact of television viewing is underscored by an analysis of some of the dramatic statistics: 96% of American homes have at least one television set and over 60% have more than one. The TV set has become *the* most common and widely used household appliance.

Television seemingly has "hypnotic powers" capable of capturing and captivating a young audience, who will view whatever happens to be available at that particular moment (Gerbner, 1985). Americans generally spend more time watching television than any other activity, except possibly for sleeping. Television, as a rule, promotes physical inactivity and social isolation for the avid child viewer. It has displaced other more meaningful physical, psychological, and social activities in the life of many children, adolescents, and adults. In addition to television per se, various spin-offs of the industry (e.g., electronic games, video cartridges, satellite dishes, cable TV, etc.) are likely to further impact on the already consuming life-style of the child and adolescent (Ellis, 1983).

It appears that each year there is an escalating influence of television on all aspects of life. Television has a uniqueness shared by no other communications media and its influence on human behavior is similarly unique. The Committee on Social Issues Group for the Advancement of Psychiatry (1982) responded to the question, "What's so different about TV?"

> What's so different? The answer is plain. Television is ubiquitous and continuously accessible and, in this regard, unique. Television is viewed in almost every home, by members of every social and ethnic class and every age group, by the preliterate and the senile, by the prisoner and the school child, by the executive and the laborer. Because it is ubiquitous, television's effects, both positive and negative, are far more significant than if it affected only small numbers of people in isolated sectors. Coupled with the intensity of viewing by a substantial part of the audience and the extended periods of time over which these audiences view television, the size of the audience deepens our concern for their psychosocial health and development. (p. 7)

> Television has the largest global audience ever assembled simultaneously and regularly for any experience, including church. Well over half the people on earth are said to be directly exposed to it. Television sets now outnumber telephones (364 million compared to 360 million). Precisely because of these dimensions, television is different from any other form of communication. It is, in our opening words, unique in human experience. (p. 8)

George Cornell, reporting in the March 19, 1977 edition of the *Chicago Tribune,* described America's passion for television as the "electronic religion" because of its pervasiveness in our lives (Leary, 1979).

2.1. Quantitative Considerations

As noted previously, the television set is probably *the* most popular and most frequently utilized household appliance. Indeed, 99% of American homes with young children have at least one TV set (Murray, 1973). The incidence of possession is equaled only by its seemingly limitless hours of usage! In the United States, the average viewing time is usually more than 2 to 3 hours each day (Lyle and Hoffman, 1972). In the age category 6- to 11-year-olds, the average television-viewing time is slightly more than 24 hours per week (Nielson Report on Television, 1983). Almost a decade ago it was estimated that on any given night more than 20 million children and adolescents (2- to 17-year-olds) were watching television at 9 PM, 13 million at 10 PM, and 5.3 million at 11 PM (Hickey, 1979). The statistics for today's schedule of television viewing is probably more exaggerated. Television contact time per se appears to be increasing dramatically. In addition, there is a plethora of enticing (but time-consuming) new television devices, such as cable, videocassettes, disc, and video games (Ellis, 1983). As an example of the negative spin-off of new technologies, cable television owners watch approximately 10 hours more per week than households with only standard channel selections (Smith, 1980).

With specific reference to adolescents as a group, it is recognized that they have increased their television viewing to approximately the same level as younger children. On the average, adolescent girls watch approximately 21 hours of television each week and teenage boys about 23 hours per week (Strasburger, 1985). In an urban sample of adolescents, Lawrence *et al.* (1986) determined that they watched television approximately 147 minutes per day (17¼ hours per week) compared with their mothers who spent 136 minutes per day and their fathers 124 minutes per day. On average, the adolescents in this study watched television *with* a family member less than 50% of the time. The time that is spent viewing television with parents should not be misconstrued as true "family television." More often than not, there is very little dialogue with family members regarding the content of commercials or programs. The opportunity for family interaction during mutual television participation is available but the opportunity is usually poorly utilized.

2.2. Qualitative Considerations

The issue of excessive television viewing is dwarfed only by the potential biological and psychological problems generated by the *content* of programs and commercials. Television has been increasingly accused of having a negative impact on both the mental and physical well-being of children and adolescents (Dietz and Gortmaker, 1985; Palumbo, 1985; Zuckerman and Zuckerman, 1985). Strasburger (1985) suggested that we are involved in a "chicken-and-egg dilemma"; that is,

> . . . does television merely reflect society and its changes during the past 30 years (e.g., increasing rates of teenage sexual activity and drug use) or is television directly responsible for some of those changes? (p. 814)

Although there is an occasional disclaimer, the general concensus of professionals is that television contributes significantly to molding the behavioral and health habits of children and adolescents. Among the conclusions of the 1982 National Institute of Mental Health report on television and behavior (Rubinstein, 1983) is the challenging statement that:

> Television can no longer be considered as a casual part of daily life, as an electronic toy. Research findings have long since destroyed the illusion that television is merely innocuous entertainment. While the learning it provides is mainly incidental rather than direct and formal, it is a significant part of the total acculturation process.

3. Developmental–Behavioral Implications: Negative Effects

Thus far the discussion on the impact of television viewing by children and adolescents has been addressed within the framework of broad statistical concepts. At this point a more specific analysis of television's influence on various aspects of child/adolescent development and behavior will be reviewed briefly.

3.1. Television and Aggressive/Violent Behaviors

A major area of parental and professional concern is the potential adverse influence of television violence on the behavior of children and adolescents (Rothenberg, 1975; Eron, 1982; Huesmann *et al.*, 1983, 1984; Singer, 1985). This relationship has been studied more extensively than any other aspect of television viewing. In 1982, a major study group reporting to the Surgeon General concluded that there was a significant relationship between violence portrayed on television and aggressive behaviors in children (McGowan, 1979). Numerous reports, both in the pediatric and psychiatric literature, support the postulate of a causal relationship between the two. Television violence appears to increase the child's tolerance of real-life aggression (Drabman and Thomas, 1976). Feinbloom (1976) specifically suggested that the violence depicted on television would encourage children to (1) be more aggressive in interactive play; (2) be more willing to physically harm others; and (3) select aggression as a response in resolving conflict situations. A significant conclusion of the 1982 NIMH report (Rubinstein, 1983) was that viewing television is reflected in aggressive behaviors by children.

Signorielli *et al.* (1982) concluded that television programs for children are about six times more violent than programs for adults. Since 1967, this pattern has essentially remained stable, although cyclic increases and decreases may vary from year to year. In general, the content of television programs in the United States are more physically aggressive and violent than in other countries (Addison, 1977). It is a paradox that television programs designed for children (cartoons in particular) as a rule are more violence oriented than programs scheduled on prime time (Gerbner *et al.*, 1981). It has been estimated that an alarming 92 to 98% of all programs designed for children contain some violence, with an occurrence rate of 17 to 25 violent episodes per hour of viewing time. By any criteria, this can be regarded as an excessive television diet of aggression and violence that is directed toward a young and impressionable audience. Most professionals are apprehensive that the repetitive viewing of aggression and violence has a significant negative impact on the behavioral development of children and adolescents, but admit that some controversy persists (Fosarelli, 1984).

What are the evidences that a cause-and-effect relationship does exist between television and children's behavior? Various laboratory studies appear to support the postulate that there is a direct relationship because children imitate the violence they have recently viewed on television. Bandura *et al.* (1963) noted that 3- to 5-year-old children, who had observed a film depicting aggressive play with toys, subsequently imitated the behaviors displayed in the film. In general, the children in this study were more aggressive in their interactions. In a similar context, 5- to 7-year-old children who had viewed violent cartoons demonstrated subsequent aggressive behaviors (Steuber *et al.*, 1971). Several studies further suggested that nursery school children and 5- to 9-year-old children exhibited an imitation effect and a willingness to hurt other children after viewing violence on television (Liebert and Baron, 1972). The "copy-cat phenomenon" has similarly been observed among children who viewed television stunt performances and other daring acts. For example, the "Evel Knievel syndrome" in essence is the imitation by children and adolescents of inappropriate bicycle stunts, mimicking the motorcycle stunts performed by a professional (Wharton and Mandell, 1985). Within the context of imitation of television, it should be noted also that paradoxically children themselves may become victims of violence as a result of impressionable parents who have viewed aggressive/violent behaviors directed toward their children (Wharton and Mandell, 1985).

A few disclaimers have been reported, arguing that viewing violence on television may have a *positive* influence in lowering aggressive behaviors; in essence, a "cathartic effect" (Feshbach, 1961). The catharsis theory was repudiated in the first report to the Surgeon General and in the subsequent 10-year update (Rubinstein, 1983). Milavsky *et al.* (1982), based on a panel survey of approximately 3000 children over a 3-year period, concluded that television had no significant relationship with aggressive behaviors.

Although occasional research interpretations, such as those cited, have questioned the psychosocial influence of television violence, the cumulative evidence from multiple studies appears to support the position that a negative cause-and-effect relationship has been established. Palumbo (1985) commented more emphatically that, "Although some debate remains about these findings, most notably from network researchers, excessive viewing of violent programming can only be harmful and should be strictly monitored and limited."

3.2. Television and Youth Suicide

The potential influence of television as a factor promoting imitative suicide is a speculation based on studies of the "Werther effect."* Phil-

*Over 200 years ago, following the publication of Goethe's novel *The Sorrows of Young Werther,* it was reported that people imitated Werther's manner of death by suicide. The Werther effect postulates that a suicide publicized by the media has the potential for triggering an imitative behavior in certain vulnerable individuals.

lips (1974) reported that suicides increased shortly after a suicide had been publicized in the newspaper in both the United States and Britain during the period 1947–1968. Phillips suggested that the more publicity generated by a suicide, the larger the rise in the number of copy-cat suicides. In a subsequent report, Phillips (1979) presented new evidences that imitation and suggestion influenced social behavior. In this study, he demonstrated that automobile fatalities increased significantly following a publicized suicide. More recently, evidence has been presented that in the United States suicide has increased significantly after suicide stories received repeated television coverage on evening news programs (Bollen and Phillips, 1982). Wasserman (1984) challenged some of these findings, suggesting that on reexamination of previous postulates there was no significant rise in the national suicide rate following articles on the front page of *The New York Times*. Wasserman, however, did note that there was a rise in the national suicide rate in the month following newspaper reports of the *suicide death of a celebrity*. He suggested that suicide imitation is probably much more selective than originally suggested by Phillips. Horton and Stack (1984), from an analysis of suicide statistics, concluded that the "Werther effect" had no impact on suicide per se. The authors noted, however, that the problem of suicide can better be understood from the standpoint of an economic paradigm than from an imitation paradigm.

3.3. Television and Pediatric Health Practices

Television is the single largest resource for health-related information for the American people, and as Gerbner (1984) relates, "particularly to that vast majority who do not seek information." The average child viewer is exposed annually to approximately 25,000 commercials of which about 20% are for food products and more than 2500 are for sweets high in calories and of little nutritional value. There is some professional agreement, however, that there is potential harm resulting from the extraordinary numbers of commercials presented to children (Galst and White, 1976; Gerbner, 1984; Palumbo, 1985). Young television viewers are often unable to comprehend the selling intent of commercials (Palumbo, 1985). It is recognized that this vulnerable audience is strongly influenced by high-pressured selling techniques, often influencing family purchasing practices. Several criticisms have been directed toward various television advertisers in regard to their food promotions, because they take advantage of children by (1) misrepresenting the nutritional value of sugared cereals and candy; and (2) promoting parent–

child discussions over what products should be purchased (Fosarelli, 1984).

The content of television programs is similarly subject to criticism because frequently they depict characters "grabbing a snack on the run."

3.3.1. Substance Abuse

The portrayal of alcohol on television is equally misleading and potentially harmful. Frequently, individuals are seen to relieve their tensions, anxieties, frustrations, and conflicts by "taking a drink." Gerbner (1984) concluded that "the more television you view, the more complacent you are about eating, drinking, and safety but at the same time the more you believe in the magical power of medical science."

In a laboratory study of alcohol use on television and its effect on children's behavior, it appeared that subjects who viewed televised drinking were significantly more likely to select alcoholic beverages for adults but not children (Rychtarik *et al.,* 1983). The basis for children not selecting alcoholic drinks is perhaps a flaw in methodology, in as much as the television vignette did not show children drinking and because there are strong prohibitions against alcohol consumption by children. Nevertheless, it is generally assumed that television commercials and program content both overtly and subtly influence young viewers, particularly adolescents, in the belief that there is a "good life" associated with alcohol (Palumbo, 1985). Kotch *et al.* (1986) demonstrated that among fifth- and sixth-grade children, randomly assigned to experimental and control groups, who observed videotapes in which the principal characters consumed alcoholic drinks in the experimental but not in the control conditions, only boys who saw the film with drinking were more apt to respond that the good things associated with alcohol were more important than the bad things. The impact of television viewing on promoting alcohol consumption must be considered a potential health hazard. This hypothesis is underscored by the fact that alcohol is *the* most frequent beverage consumed on television; indeed, almost 100% of television dramas in some way involve the use of alcohol (Breed and DeFeo, 1984).

Strasburger (1985) concluded that "the extraordinary rises in teenage sexual activity and drug usage have coincided with the video explosion of the past thirty years is too provocative an occurrence to dismiss as sheer coincidence" (p. 814). He notes that "alcohol is a nearly ubiquitous drink on TV, yet the true effects of alcohol or alcoholism are rarely depicted." Alcohol as depicted on television is a social "crutch" or the quick way to resolve or relieve the tension of a crisis. The true consequences of excessive alcohol consumption are addressed relatively infrequently.

3.3.2. Obesity

Dietz and Gortmaker (1985) suggested that television is a major factor contributing to childhood obesity, because:

- Watching television reduces energy-expending activities
- Foods promoted on television are calorically dense (e.g., sugared breakfast cereals, candy, carbonated beverages)
- Nonnutritious food references occur even more frequently on prime time
- Inappropriate messages regarding food utilization are often presented in a repetitive, heavy dosage

The hypothesis implies a cause-and-effect relationship between the time spent watching television and subsequent obesity, even when controlled for confounding variables.

Fosarelli (1984) suggests that the youngest children are the most impressionable and therefore most apt to be influenced by television commercials because of their (1) inability to distinguish between fact and fiction, (2) naïveté about the sophisticated promotional techniques used in television commercials, and (3) gullibility as consumers. It is of interest that among young children the most frequently requested items at the supermarket are for cereals and candy (the edible items most frequently "pushed" on children's prime time). The American Academy of Pediatrics (1984) issued a statement emphasizing that "television viewing increases consumption of high caloric density snacks, and increases the prevalence of obesity." Lewis (1986–1987) recounts a workshop presented by Dr. W. H. Dietz in which he reported that the total number of children in the 6- to 11-year age group who are obese increased 54% and the 12- to 17-year age group has increased 30% during the past 15 to 20 years.

A pilot study of a one-week period of prime-time dramatic programs revealed that eating, drinking, or talking about food occurred on an average of nine times per hour. "Grabbing a snack" occurred in almost 40% of all eating-drinking episodes. In weekend daytime children's programs, snacks increased about 45% and traditional meals declined 24% (Gerbner *et al.,* 1981). Although obesity occurs in approximately 25 to 45% of the population, the pilot study of prime-time television programs revealed that fewer than 6% of all males and 2% of all females were obese.

3.4. Television and Reading/Learning Skills

Television when utilized appropriately is an extremely effective educational vehicle for viewers of all ages. In a monitored school and/or home environment, selected and specifically designed television materials may provide a meaningful learning experience, particularly for children and adolescents. Most professionals agree that television has unlimited potential as an adjunct to traditional teaching methods. Creative programming can provide numerous opportunities for children and adolescents to expand their knowledge base by bringing to the classroom and to the home a rich and unique assortment of learning experiences.

Serious questions, however, have been raised regarding television's influence on specific learning abilities, particularly on reading skills. This area has not been well researched and conflicting evidences have been reported. Several early studies suggested that there was no significant relationship between television viewing and academic achievement (Ridder, 1963). In a more recent investigation, it was noted that children who watched television devoted significantly less time to reading. However, when IQ and socioeconomic status were controlled, the amount of television viewing was *not* associated with reading ability (Zuckerman *et al.,* 1980). On the other hand, several adverse learning characteristics have been attributed to television viewing practices. Learning from television is a passive rather than an active process. As a rule, television detracts from meaningful educational exercises, such as reading or using active learning skills (American Academy of Pediatrics Task Force on Children and Television, 1984). Several investigations suggest that the duration of weekly television contact is inversely correlated with academic performance (Morgan and Gross, 1982; Ridley-Johnson *et al.,* 1983). Preschoolers who spent more time watching television than their age-mates did not perform as well in the first grade (Burton *et al.,* 1979). The negative impact of television on reading abilities of school-age children is generally assumed to be the result of displacement of reading time and reduced incentives to read (Hornik, 1978).

Zuckerman and Zuckerman (1985) reported that television has been blamed for children's decline in reading skills as well as fostering a pervasive apathy for education. From their review of the literature, however, they concluded that television does not appear to have a major negative influence on most children's reading skills or their classroom behaviors. It is obvious that controlled research is required if these important psychosocial issues are to be resolved.

4. Guidelines for Management of Television Practices

Television viewing for children when managed carefully (i.e., screened for program content, used as an educational tool with adult explanations and limitations as to consumer time) may become one of our most meaningful teaching adjuncts. It is readily apparent that television is a captivating media that can broaden the child's knowledge base and expand their cultural perspectives. The electronic media similarly has the potential for shaping positive values for children and adolescents.

"Controlled" television implies that adults will accept responsibility for monitoring their child's viewing, but also suggests important responsibilities for the networks.

Parents can assume a more active role in ensuring a healthy television milieu for their children by providing the following safeguards:

- Limit television viewing, allowing adequate time for exercise, homework, and other recreational activities
- Avoid using television either as a reward and/or punishment
- Join children in *family* viewing, encouraging family members to have a dialogue about content of programs and commercials
- Set a good adult example by discriminating television viewing and limiting time spent with the television set

A particular concern for parents relates to "family dialogue" when viewing television. Fosarelli (1984) suggests that appropriate discussions could focus on (1) the depiction of violence, its motives and consequences; (2) the "fantasyland" and fictional nature of television dramas; (3) the misrepresentations, inaccuracies, and glorifications of television's portrayal of characters; and (4) the high-pressured selling/promotional techniques employed in commercials. As the family becomes more conscious of these television hazards, discussions would become increasingly enlightening for children and adolescents. The net result may be the development of a more sophisticated viewing audience. It should be stressed also that television can become a focus for initiating meaningful family communication system, addressing issues that relate to family dynamics and psychosocial problems (e.g., drugs, alcohol, sex, suicide).

It has generally been assumed that it is the parent's responsibility to monitor what their kids are watching; however, the industry has equal obligations. Issues of alcoholism, substance abuse, sexual activity, obesity, violence—among other psychosocial problems—requires that the television programmers provide a selection of appropriate, accurate, and educational programs on these subjects. Meaningful facts about these issues may necessitate equal television time to counteract fictional/promotional programming. Although censorship is not advocated, wholesome television programming is urged for children and adolescents. The identification of impressionable youth with television celebrities further provides a unique opportunity for establishing positive role model identities.

There is undoubtedly a role for health care professionals as advocates in promoting more wholesome television for young viewers. Unfortunately, it appears that the vast majority of pediatric training programs do *not* provide educational opportunities for housestaff to learn the impact of television on children and/or to discuss these issues with parents (Smith *et al.,* 1986). The American Academy of Pediatrics Task Force on Children and Television (1984) has proposed several specific recommendations for parents and professionals:

- Educate pediatricians about the consequences of current television practices for children and adolescents; approaches should include well-designed curriculum for medical students, house officers, and practicing pediatricians.
- Provide adequate material for effective counseling of children, adolescents, and their families
- Support legislation that improves programming content and reduces commercials directed at children
- Provide for greater interactions with the networks (producers, writers, etc.), providing improved quality of programming and advertising
- Monitor technologies that can provide parents with opportunities to control television-viewing habits

5. Summary

Television viewing by children and adolescents has become a major biological, psychosocial, and educational concern for health care professionals. The behavioral and learning consequences of current television practices (program content, commercials, and extensive viewing time) are not well-defined by controlled research studies. Nevertheless, there have been increasing apprehensions that the electronic media has become a dominating influence in shaping the child's psychological, social, moral, and value systems. It is similarly recognized that television plays a significant role in shaping the child's and adolescent's attitudes toward a variety of health issues: alcohol use, food practices (obesity), sexual activity, drug abuse, and so forth.

The average television viewer (child and adult) is nonselective, generally watching whatever is most appealing at the moment (Gerbner, 1985). Gerbner comments that "television has become the functional equivalent of a new religion" and that "for the first time in history, children are born into a symbolic world that does not originate with parents, church or school and requires no literacy." Gerbner (1985) raised serious issues that must be addressed by parents and health care providers. On the subject of violence he commented that we should have grave concerns that television violence may convert viewers into believing in a "mean world syndrome", noting that "prime time is a time of power, that is why it has so much violence." He concludes that television fosters a negative perspective on values:

> We absorb a sense of mistrust and insecurity, a sense of living in a mean and dangerous world in which we must protect ourselves and must depend on strong people and measures for protection. If anything, it is a device that tends to put people in their place according to their status. It makes those who are lower in status feel weaker, more vulnerable and more easily controlled. (p. 826)

Gerbner further hypothesized that there is a direct cause-and-effect relationship between the amount of television exposure and expressions of insecurity, vulnerability, and dependence. Television appears to promote mechanisms that maintain and exacerbate the injustices and inequalities of our society, concluding "that is how violence really works." Strasburger (1985) eloquently summarized the cogent issues:

> For centuries, physicians have fought disease. Now pediatricians face a new morbidity: childhood accidents and violence (homicide and suicide) are the leading causes of death after 1 year of age, and sexual activity and drug use among teenagers are sources of major morbidity. This new morbidity requires a new breed of pediatrician, one that is more sensitive to cultural influences on children and adolescents, willing to do counseling with families about psychological issues, and perhaps even do "soft" (i.e., non-"bench") research. As data are gathered, perhaps every television set will one day bear the label: "Caution: Too much of inappropriate viewing may be hazardous to your health." (p. 820)

Television as currently programmed for children and adolescents presents a formidable challenge for parents and health care professionals. The advantages of wholesome programming are obvious. The concerns focus on an equally obvious recognition that: (1) television-contact time is extraordinarily high; (TV is often utilized as a babysitter, a surrogate parent); (2) television may be an even more significant factor in the life of "latchkey children"; (3) some children are more affected by television viewing than others; and (4) television may "be the main window to the world for children from low socio-economic groups" (Palumbo, 1985).

If, indeed, television practices are suspected of being "hazardous to the health of our children," it is a professional mandate that these issues be explored with well-constructed, controlled studies. Professional apathy may be reflected in television's potential to become one of the most significant epidemiological factors capable of jeopardizing the psycho-social/educational development of children and adolescents. On the other hand, television has great potential for enhancing the development and quality of life for young people.

References

Addison, F. S., 1977, TV violence and viewer aggression: A cumulation of study results 1956–1976, *Pub. Opin. Q.* **41**:314–331.

American Academy of Pediatrics Task Force on Children and Television, 1984, *Children, Adolescents and Television,* December.

Bandura, A., Ross, D., and Ross, S., 1963, Imitation of film-mediated aggressive models, *J. Abnorm. Soc. Psychl.* **66**:3–11.

Bollen, K. A., and Phillips, D. P., 1982, Imitative suicides: A national study of the effects of television news stories. *Am. Sociol. Rev.* **47**:802–809.

Breed, W., and DeFeo, J. R., 1984, Drinking and smoking on television, *J. Pub. Health Pol.* **31**:257–270.

Burton, S. G., Calonico, J. M., and McSeveney, D. R., 1979, Effects of preschool television watching on first grade children, *J. Commun.* **29**:164–170.

Committee on Social Issues Group for the Advancement of Psychiatry, Roy W. Menninger, Chairperson, 1982, *The Child and Television Drama: The Psychosocial Impact of Cumulative Viewing,* Mental Health Material Center, New York.

Dietz, W. H., and Gortmaker, S. L., 1985, Do we fatten our children at the television set? Obesity and television viewing in children and adolescents, *Pediatrics* **75**:807–812.

Drabman, R. S., and Thomas, M. H., 1976, Does watching violence on television cause apathy, *Pediatrics* **57**:329–331.

Ellis, G. J., 1983, Television's role in family interaction, *J. Fam. Issues* **4**:405–424.

Eron, L. D., 1982, Parent–child interaction, television violence, and aggression of children, *Am. Psychol.* **37**:197–211.

Feinbloom, R. I., 1976, Commentary, *Pediatrics* **57**:301–303.

Feshbach, S., 1961, The stimulating versus cathartic effects of a vicarious aggressive activity, *J. Abnorm. Soc. Psychol.* **63**:381–385.

Fosarelli, P. D., 1984, Television and children: A review, *J. Develop. Behav. Pediatr.* **5:**30–37.

Galst, J., and White, M., 1976, The unhealthy persuader: The reinforcing value of television and purchase-influencing attempts at supermarket, *Child Dev.* **47:**1089–1096.

Gerbner, G., 1984, Health, medicine, and violence on TV, *Trans. Stud. Coll. Physicians Phila.* **6:**33–40.

Gerbner, G., 1985, Children's television: A national disgrace, *Pediatr. Ann.* **14:**822–823, 826–827.

Gerbner, G., Gross, L., Morgan, M., *et al.*, 1981, Special report: Health and medicine on television, *N. Engl. J. Med.* **305:**901–904.

Hickey, N., 1979, Does America want family viewing time? *TV Guide* December, 6–12.

Hornik, R., 1978, Television access and the slowing of cognitive growth, *Am. Educ. Res. J.* **15:**1–15.

Horton, H., and Stack, S., 1984, The effect of television on national suicide rates, *J. Soc. Psychol.* **123:**141–142.

Huesmann, L. R., Eron, L. D., Klein, R., *et al.*, 1983, Mitigating the imitation of aggressive behaviors by changing children's attitudes about media violence, *J. Person. Soc. Psychol.* **44:**899–910.

Huesmann, L. R., Lagerspetz, K., and Eron, L. D., 1984, Intervening variables in the TV violence–aggression relation: Evidence from two countries, *Dev. Psychol.* **20:**746–775.

Kotch, J. B., Coulter, M. L., and Lipsitz, A., 1986, Does televised drinking influence children's attitudes toward alcohol? *Addict. Behav.* **11:**67–70.

Lawrence, F. C., Tasker, G. E., Daly, C. T., *et al.*, 1986, Adolescents' time spent viewing television, *Adolescence* **21:**431–436.

Leary, J. E., 1979, Television: The anti-wellness tool, *Health Educ.* Sept./Oct., 16–18.

Lewis, H. L., 1986–1987, Obesity: A growing problem among children ages 6 to 11, *Cardiovasc. Res. Rep.* **23:**1–2.

Liebert, R. M., and Baron, R. A., 1972, Some immediate effects of televised violence on children's behavior, *Dev. Psychol.* **6:**469–475.

Lyle, J., and Hoffman, H. R., 1972, Childrens' use of television and other media, in: *Television in Day-to-Day Life: Patterns of Use,* Vol. 4, *Television and Social Behavior* (E. A. Rubinstein, G. A. Comstock, and J. R. Murray, eds.), U.S. Government Printing Office, Washington, DC.

McCowan, D., 1979, TV: Its problems for children, *Pediatr. Nurs.* March/April, 17–19.

Milavsky, J. R., Kessler, R., Stipp, H., *et al.*, 1982, Television and aggression: Results of a panel study, in: *Television and Behavior: Ten Years of Scientific Progress and Implications for the Eighties,* Vol. 2 (D. Pearl, L. Bouthilet, and J. Lazar, eds.), U.S. Government Printing Office, Washington, DC.

Morgan, M., and Gross, L., 1982, Television and educational achievement and aspiration, in: *Television and Behavior,* Vol. 2 (D. Pearl, L. Bouthilet, and J. Logan, eds.), pp. 78–90, U.S. Dept. of Health and Human Services, Publ. No. (ADM) 82-1196, Rockville, MD.

Murray, J., 1973, Television and violence, *Am. Psychol.* **28:**472–47.

Nielson Report on Television, 1983, A. C. Nielsen Co, Northbrook, IL.

Palumbo, F. M., 1985, Television: Effects on the development of children, in: *Children are Different, Behavioral Development,* (W. K. Frankenburg, ed.) Monograph Series; No. 14, Ross Growth and Development Program, Ross Laboratories, Columbus, Ohio, pp. 1–8.

Phillips, D. B., 1974, The influence of suggestion on suicide: Substantive and theoretical implications of the Werther effect, *Am. Sociol. Rev.* **38:**340–354.

Phillips, D. B., 1979, Suicide, motor vehicle fatalities, and the mass media: Evidence toward a theory of suggestion, *Am. J. Sociol.* **84:**1150–1174.

Ridder, J., 1963, Public opinion and the relationship of TV viewing to academic achievement, *J. Educ. Res.* **57:**204–207.

Ridley-Johnson, R., Cooper, H., and Chance, J., 1983, The relation of children's television viewing to school achievement and IQ, *J. Educ. Res.* **76:**294–297.

Rothenberg, M. B., 1975, Effect of television violence on children and youth, *JAMA* **234:**1043–1046.

Rubinstein, E. A., 1983, Television and behavior. Research conclusions of the 1982 NIMH report and their policy implications, *Am. Psychol.* 820–825.

Rychtarik, R. G., Fairbank, J. A., Allen, C. M., *et al.,* 1983, Alcohol use in television programming: Effect on children's behavior, *Addict. Behav.* **8:**19–22.

Signorielli, N., Gross, L., and Morgan, M., 1982, Violence in television programs: Ten years later, in: *Television and Behavior: Ten Years of Scientific Progress and Implications for the Eighties,* Vol. 2 (D. Pearl, L. Bouthilet, and J. Lazar, eds.), U.S. Government Printing Office, Washington, DC.

Singer, D. G., 1985, Does violent television produce aggressive children? *Pediatr. Ann.* **14:**804–810.

Smith, R. D., Fosarelli, P. D., Palumbo, F., *et al.,* 1986, The impact of television on children. Current pediatric training practicies, *Am. J. Dis. Child.* **140:**78–79.

Smith, S. B., 1980, Average family viewing passes 7 hours a day, *The New New York Times,* Sept. 7, pp. 1–22.

Steuber, F., Applefeld, J., and Smith, R., 1971, Televised aggression and the interpersonal aggression of preschool children, *J. Exp. Child Psychol.* **11:**442–447.

Strasburger, V. C., 1985, Television and adolescents, *Pediatr. Ann.* **14:**814–820.

Wasserman, I. M., 1984, Imitation and suicide: A reexamination of the Werther effect, *Am. Sociol. Rev.* **49:**427–436.

Wharton, R., and Mandell, F., 1985, Violence on television and imitative behavior: Impact on parenting practices, *Pediatrics* **75:**1120–1123.

Zuckerman, D. M., and Zuckerman, B. S., 1985, Television's impact on children, *Pediatrics* **75:**233–239.

Zuckerman, D. M., Singer, D. G., and Singer, J. L., 1980, Television viewing, children's reading and related classroom behavior, *J. Commun.* **30:**166–174.

CHAPTER 9

Self-Destructive Behaviors in Children and Adolescents

Intermediary Levels of Intervention by Parents, Peers, and Pediatricians

MARVIN I. GOTTLIEB

1. Introduction

Adolescents are least likely to die of disease; however, this is the only group in the United States for whom the death rate is rising. The major causes of adolescent deaths are accidents (primarily motor vehicle related), homicide, suicide, and alcohol- and drug-associated mortalities (Shrier, 1981).

Self-destructive behaviors in various forms are not uncommon in children and adolescents. As a group these behaviors are regarded as "psychosocial emergencies." Any life-threatening behavior, regardless of age, usually requires immediate and intensive intervention by a skilled psychotherapist. As a general rule, however, it is usually parents, peers, and primary-care physicians who are the first to become aware of the child or adolescent who exhibits self-destructive behaviors and those with serious suicidal intent. Rarely does the adolescent patient or their family resolve the emotional crisis by swiftly and directly obtaining the assistance of a mental health care specialist. In most instances, the parents, peers, clergy, and pediatricians are called on to defuse the immediate life-threatening crisis and to assist in securing more expert help.

MARVIN I. GOTTLIEB • Institute for Child Development, Hackensack Medical Center, Hackensack, New Jersey 07601; and Department of Pediatrics, University of Medicine and Dentistry of New Jersey–New Jersey Medical School, Newark, New Jersey 07103.

The effectiveness of this *intermediate level of intervention* may ultimately be measured by the prevention of a child or adolescent's death by suicide. Those individuals who are the most meaningful in the life of the child or adolescent may be the first to become aware of the "signals" that suggest that there are serious psychosocial tensions confronting the potential victim. Indeed, these significant persons may be knowingly singled out by the potential victim to serve as "buffers," hoping that they will recognize the "cry for help." This great responsibility of the intermediate level of intervention, if handled inappropriately, may end in tragedy for the child or adolescent and their loved ones.

This chapter will focus on several major issues: (1) a global perspective of child/adolescent self-destructive behaviors: (2) recognition of overt and subtle warning signs of intended self-destruction; and (3) an attempt to define the roles of parents, peers, and primary-care physicians in helping seriously troubled children and adolescents. In its broadest context, seriously troubled youth may feel that the only solution to their problems is an immediate and desperate act, such as suicide. On the other hand, many more children and adolescents express their emotional turmoil and need for attention by less violent and final acts of self-destruction. Self-destruction "in the slow lane" may be acted-out through a spectrum of high-risk behaviors including alcohol and drug abuse, daring or reckless operation of motor vehicles, and inappropriate social behaviors such as running away and juvenile delinquency. Ultimately the consequences of activities designated as "self-destruction in the slow lane" may be as tragic and final as death by suicide.

It is obvious that the more acute, violent, and dramatic acts of self-destruction are suicide attempts and/or suicides. However, philosophically (and realistically) the bottom-line of substance abuse, drag racing, and similar acts may in reality represent a continuum in the spectrum of self-destruction. Regardless of the specific mode of expression, underlying factors (poor self-esteem, depression, exaggerated need for attention, etc.) may be similar for all acts of self-injury. This chapter will explore some of the epidemiological factors that contribute to precipitating self-destructive behaviors among children and adolescents.

2. The Adolescent Crisis

Children and adolescents have become increasingly exposed to numerous potentially stressful psychobiological and psychosocial hazards, which can result in highly charged anxieties, tensions, and frustrations. When coping strategies and support systems fail, or are unavailable, the child or adolescent may succumb to pressures by clinically manifesting serious depression. Over the past three decades there has been a significant improvement in the general mental health status of the population, with the exception of the adolescent age group. A variety of increasing tensions stemming from disturbed family, dynamics, peer pressures, and school and career difficulties, appear to have intensified the "adolescent crisis," perhaps serving as the precursors and precipitants for self-destructive behaviors.

The adolescent is particularly vulnerable to psychological stresses emanating from family, peer, and societal pressures. There are pressures to achieve, to determine a vocation, to establish sexual relationships, to develop independence, and to conform to the rules and regulations of society. An understanding of the epidemiological factors contributing to self-destructive behaviors is in essence an analysis of these many potential turmoils that may be experienced by the teenager during the transition from childhood to young adult. During this period of metamorphosis from child to adult, the adolescent is generally faced with a composite of confusing and anxiety-provoking organic and psychological adjustments. Adolescence is characterized by relatively rapid and dramatic physical, hormonal, cognitive, and psychological changes, which may precipitate a variety of conflicting feelings in the adolescent and the family (Shrier, 1981). The organic differentiations during adolescence are legend, including the growth spurt, primary and secondary sexual maturations, hormonal modifications, and tissue hypertrophy and atrophy. Inherent in the process of these traditional maturational physical changes are anticipated complexes of potential complications, ranging from acne to scoliosis. Any physical complication during adolescence is most often associated with exaggerated psychological and social reactions by emotionally vulnerable adolescents. Interwoven within these complex modifications in physical and sexual development are a variety of primary psychosocial adjustments (i.e., psychological issues) of adolescence. The most common psychological stressors are generally associated with resolving several basic issues: *Who am I physically? Who am I sexually? Who am I socially?*

Superimposed on this basic core of adolescent maturations and their associated complications are many significant exogenous psychostressors. For example, for many adolescents their perception of the environment is one burdened with issues (e.g., contamination of our natural resources, threats of a nuclear holocaust, etc.) that justifiably triggers depression and/or aggressive antisocial behaviors. Personal defeats, such as not being able to achieve in an increasingly competitive educational milieu and the limitations of career opportunities (in an escalating high-cost economic atmosphere) may similarly precipitate feelings of hopelessness and despair. These pychoeducational and social pressures may be further exaggerated when family support systems are unavilable and the adolescent is unable to find resources to provide coping strengths or strategies. Additional stressors serve to compound the emotional dilemmas of the "adolescent crisis," including: (1) biopsychologically complicating spin-offs of adolescent sexual practices (teenage pregnancy, AIDS); (2) powerful peer influences (experimentation with drugs and alcohol, cigarette smoking); and (3) a constant menu of media pressures (misinformation and/or misguidance from television, videotapes, and audiocassettes). The cumulative impact of these internal and external biopsychosocial tensions may render the child or adolescent vulnerable. Serious emotional confusions festering in an atmosphere of hopelessness and helplessness may dramatically culminate in acts of self-destruction. For the child and/or adolescent with poor self-concept and lack of self-confidence, these stressors are particular hazardous.

The adolescent crisis is perhaps in large measure synonymous with an admixture of weak coping strategies, feelings of futility and hopelessness, and ultimately a perceived self-destructive solution.

3. Youth Suicide

Child and adolescent suicidal behavior during the past decade has generated public and professional awareness and anxiety. The major factors responsible for this unprecedented concern are in large part the result of both an absolute and alarming increase in successful youth-suicide attempts and the phenomenon of "cluster suicides." Although we are not dealing with a new pathology in child and adolescent development, we are confronted with an escalating problem that has reached critical levels. Youth suicide has now achieved status as one of the major causes of death among adolescents, reaching what can be considered "epidemic proportions" (Brent *et al.,* 1986). Attempted suicide is one of the most common emergencies in child psychiatric practice (Pfeffer *et al.,* 1982). Hodgman (1985) comments that "episodic bursts of teenage suicide attract much attention, while suicidal symptoms in emergency departments are so common as to generate nonchalance about the ongoing pathology in the young attempter."

3.1. Epidemiological Considerations

Violent acts and self-destructive behaviors by children and adolescents were generally regarded as rare occurrences during the 1940s and

1950s. However, homicide, which now is the second leading cause of death among teenagers in the United States, showed a 300% increase in the 15- to 24-year-old age group between 1950 to 1980 (Blum, 1987a). The dramatic increasing incidence of youth suicides in the 1960s, 1970s, and 1980s justifiably alarmed the nation. Since 1950, suicide during the second decade of life in the United States has more than quadrupled, i.e., escalating from 3 per 100,000 to 12.4 per 100,000 in 1980, among 15- to 24-year-olds (Blum, 1987a)

Explanations for this changing pattern of self-destructive acts in the younger population are varied; including incriminating psychosocial stressors from family, educational, peer, and social pressures (all or combinations thereof). Regardless of any specific consideration of possible contributing factors, youth suicide and other forms of self-destruction constitute a *major* issue in the 12- to 17-year-old age group (Pediatrics Supplement, 1985; Johnson *et al.,* 1984). Suicide is a leading cause of death in this age group in the United States (AAP News, 1985), and approximately 6000 adolescents commit suicide each year. A threefold increase was reported in adolescent suicides in 1985 compared with 1980. Perhaps of even greater significance and impact is the alarming statistic that over 500,000 *suicide attempts* are reported annually. Males, because of the more aggressive methods used, generally succeed in their suicide attempt in a ratio of four to one (The University State of New York, 1984). Obviously the *reported* statistics on suicide attempts and completed suicides are extremely conservative, considering (1) the inadequacies and "cover-up" reporting of self-destructive acts; (2) the possible suicidal nature of single-vehicle accidents among adolescents; and (3) the unreported and misunderstanding of acts of aggression and violence. Many suicide attempts and successful suicides are reported as "accidental deaths," either consciously or in error. Therefore, "accidents," particularly those associated with single-vehicle fatalities, must raise suspicions regarding their cause.

Although suicide among children is rare, suicidal behavior is distressingly common. Kosky (1983) compared 20 children under 13 years of age admitted to the hospital following a suicide attempt with 50 psychiatrically ill nonsuicidal patients of approximately the same age. In general, suicidal ideation and behaviors appeared to be most frequently associated with (1) male sex; (2) experience with a personal/significant loss (e.g., parent, grandparent, sibling); (3) school difficulties and academic underachievement; (4) parental separation and divorce; (5) intrafamilial violence (child abuse); and (6) illness in the family. (Several of the high-risk factors that predispose to suicidal ideation, intent, and behavior will be explored in greater depth throughout this chapter.)

Suicide *completions* in children and adolescents are much more frequent in boys (approximately 4 : 1). Deaths usually are the result of more violent methods such as firearms and hanging. These methods are usually final acts of desperation, providing "little margin for error and minimal chance of discovery and rescue" (Greene and Keown, 1986). On the other hand, girls *attempt* suicide more frequently than boys (4 : 1). Drug overdose is the most common form of attempted suicide. As noted by Greene and Keown (1986), it is ironic that tricyclic antidepressants are the agents most commonly used in treating depression and the most commonly used for overdose. An interesting speculation and question to be resolved concerns the number of adolescents who have access to tricyclic antidepressants and may be self-medicating themselves for depression.

3.2. Depression and Suicide

It is significant that there is no universally accepted biological or psychological concept of the psychopathology of depression and suicidal behavior, particularly for adolescents. Frequently, analogies for adolescents are drawn from child and adult models. Since depression can extend throughout the life span, a single diagnostic nomenclature may be used regardless of the age of the patient. The net result may be an inappropriate or lack of identification of the adolescent with various degrees of dysphoria (Hodgman, 1985). A major reason that depression may be unrecognized in children and adolescents is that they are less likely to exhibit the "vegetative signs" of depression commonly seen in adults, such as loss of appetite, lethargy, insomnia, difficulty with concentration, and sadness (Greene and Keown, 1986).

In recent years, child psychiatrists have generally agreed that major depression is a meaningful diagnosis in children and adolescents, recognized as an affective disorder related to unipolar and bipolar illness (Humphries and Metzler, 1983; Toolan, 1981). The actual frequency of classical depression in this age group, however, has not been clearly defined. Nevertheless, the *depressive syndrome* as an identifiable entity has been established as a clinical complex, spanning all ages (Schoenback *et al.,* 1984). More recent evidence suggests that depression is increasing among children and young adolescents, with depressive symptoms increasing as children move into adolescence. It has not been confirmed, however, whether or not these children and adolescents will become chronically depressed adults (Greene and Keown, 1986).

Depressed children frequently are seen with psychosomatic complaints, lethargy, behavioral disturbances, and suicidal ideation and/or attempts. Humphries and Metzler (1983) have outlined the various diagnostic criteria for children and adolescents: depressed affect, diurnal variation, anhedonia, suicidal ideation and/or suicide attempts, poor self-esteem, pathological guilt, social withdrawal, poor school performance, psychomotor retardation, psychosomatic complaints of fatigue, sleep and appetite disturbances, and other associated symptoms. A most important clinical distinction is necessary in defining depression as a symptom and depression as a syndrome (Toolan, 1981). The differential diagnosis may be difficult to clarify, in part because of masking effects and because the syndrome may be overlooked. Renshaw (1981) noted that as a clinical entity, depression may be underestimated in children because more attention is directed to the disturbing behavior rather than the underlying cause (Table 1). Renshaw noted that "depressive equivalents" can be defined at different maturational stages from infancy through childhood to adolescence. These equivalents are manifested as physical complaints and/or behavioral disorders rather than verbalizations of "sad feelings." Renshaw cautions that masked clinical depression must be differentiated from mourning, sorrow, sadness, frustration, dejection, and other symptoms that may represent normal, transient reactions to situational stress. These normal reactions, however, are rarely sustained and lack the element of self-blame; characteristics that are significant features of severe depression.

Depression and suicide appear to be related. Estimates suggest that approximately 70% of young persons who attempt suicide have a history of significant depressive symptoms (Carlson and Cantwell, 1982). Unfortunately, as previously noted, major depressive disorder is underemphasized by clinicians and is often omitted from the initial explorations of suicide risk among children and adolescents (Fine *et al.*, 1986; Weller and Weller, 1986). In a study by Kosky *et al.* (1986), the vast majority of all cases recorded as positive for suicidal ideation were also positive for symptomatic depression, confirming the findings of Pfeffer *et al.* (1986), Carlson and Cantwell (1982), and Garfinkel and Golombek (1974).

Research studies support the hypothesis that the diagnostic criteria for major depressive disorder in children and adolescents are similar for any older age group (Puig-Antich, 1984). The DSM-III-R diagnosis of this disorder is suggested by the child or adolescent who shows evidence of one or more of the following: (1) persistent depressive mood; (2) almost complete inability to derive pleasure from the usual life activities; and/or (3) almost total loss of interest in life's activities. Puig-Antich (1984) noted that the child or adolescent generally exhibits persistent evidence of at least four of the following symptomatic clusters: (1) appe-

Table 1. Depression at Different Growth Phases[a]

Developmental stage	Clinical expression and causes	Treatment
Infancy	Anaclitic depression (genes) Results from maternal deprivation Separation from mother over 3 months Apathy and listlessness Minimal movement Poor feeding/weight loss Increased susceptibility to infection If sustained, retardation and death may occur	Reinstatement of mother Permanent mother substitute Frequent handling and fondling
Childhood	May be masked Angry outbursts School avoidance Physical complaints (i.e., abdominal pain) Whine and whimper Brooding, apathy Phobias Sleep difficulties Suicide may occur (attempts more frequent) Causes of feelings may be multiple (parental rejection, loss of a divorced parent, dealth of a family member)	Individual psychotherapy Enhance self-esteem Enhance parental attention Antidepressants of limited value
Adolescence	Extended apathy Dietary extremes (e.g., overeating or loss of appetite) Sleep disturbances (e.g., excessive or insomnia) Tearfulness Withdrawal from peer group Changes in school performance Sudden onset of stealing Initiation of substance abuse Suicide gestures, attempts, or successes—risk is high Risk of suicide very high in 15 year and older age group	Intensive psychotherapy Antidepressants not too helpful in early adolescence Medications to be administered and monitored by psychotherapist

[a]Adapted from Renshaw (1981).

tite and/or weight changes correct for normal growth; (2) sleep difficulty (insufficient to excessive); (3) psychomotor agitation or retardation; (4) loss of interest/pleasure in life's usual activities; (5) apathy; (6) fatigue; (7) thoughts of self-reproach, low self-esteem, feelings of guilt; (8) difficulty concentrating, forgetfulness; and (9) preoccupations with death, suicidal ideation, and/or behavior. When diagnosing a major depressive episode, the duration should last 14 or more days, should occur following the death of a loved one within at least 3 months, and should last more than 3 months. A major and primary challenge in the management of children and adolescents with depressive episodes is the "immediate protection against the patient's own self-destructive impulses or behaviors" (Puig-Antich, 1984).

Hodgman (1985) noted that although depression and suicide are subjects of psychobiological research, there is as yet no consistent view of these disorders. In part, research is flawed by persistent confusions between child, adolescent, and adult models of major depression and the application of a single diagnostic terminology for all ages. Confusion is often generated by the various etiological issues that relate to depression, involving genetic factors, developmental and psychological concepts, behavioral models, and sociological/environmental factors, among others. Although depression and suicide are *not* synonymous, the former coupled with self-perceived feelings of hopelessness most certainly exaggerates the risks for self-destruction.

Pfeffer *et al.* (1986), in a study of suicidal behavior in child psychiatric inpatients, outpatients, and nonpatients, concluded that there was a common denominator significant to the expression of suicidal behavior: recent and past depression, recent aggression, and preoccupation with death. In a careful evaluation of life-threatening behaviors in preschool-age children admitted to a child psychiatric setting, it was demonstrated in the suicidal group that there was a high incidence of depressed affect, morbid preoccupation with death, and thoughts of self-injury. When compared with behavior-disordered outpatient preschoolers, the inpatient group revealed significantly more morbid ideas, depressed mood, weepiness, and parental psychopathology than the suicidal and behavior-disordered outpatients (Rosenthal *et al.*, 1986). Brent *et al.* (1986), in a sample of 231 children referred for psychiatric treatment who were assessed with the National Institute of Mental Health Diagnostic Interview Schedule for Children, noted that suicidal ideation and behavior appear to be related to a broad range of psychopathology; suicidality per se is *not* related to any particular syndrome. The authors found that the various components of depression were the most significant correlates of suicidal ideation and behavior. It was noted that problems of attention, conduct, and anxiety also correlate with suicidality and that factors other than dysphoria, such as impulsivity and impaired social skills, may also contribute to suicidal behavior in children and adolescents (Brent *et al.*, 1986).

The "bottom-line" for clinicians is that the depressive syndrome must be considered in all age groups when key signs and symptoms are observed (Table 1). The clinician must recognize the significant association between depression in children and adolescents and the ultimate risk of suicidal behaviors. Urgent and appropriate professional intervention is critical.

3.3. Cluster Suicides (The Werther Effect)

Probably no single psychosocial issue during modern times has captured the awareness of public and professional interest as has the phenomenon of cluster suicides among adolescents. This devastating psychosocial behavior has focused national attention on the general problem of self-destructive behaviors among children and adolescents.

Approximately 200 years ago Goethe published a novel, *The Sorrows of Young Werther,* in which the hero committed suicide by shooting himself in the head. The book was widely circulated in Europe but ultimately banned in some countries because individuals apparently imitated the manner of Werther's suicide. The term "Werther effect" subsequently became synonymous with other descriptive designations such as copycat suicides, imitation suicide, cluster suicides, and contagious suicides (Phillips, 1974). The phenomenon of cluster suicides was most recently exemplified by the group suicide of four young people in Bergenfield, New Jersey. The Center for Disease Control in Atlanta estimates that for every successful suicide, 20 teenagers will attempt suicide (Cherskov, 1986). Teenage despair becomes evident *after* a series of teenage suicides has occurred within a school community, increasing the risk for suicide "copycats" (Cherskov, 1986).

Robbins and Conroy (1983) defined cluster suicides as a suicide attempt within a community that serves as a precipitating factor for additional self-destructive behavior. In 1974, Phillips reported that during the period 1947–1968, suicides increased immediately after a suicide story had been publicized in the newspapers. He hypothesized that the more publicity devoted to the suicide, the larger the rise in suicide attempts thereafter. Phillips concluded that the rise in suicides was due to the influence of "suggestion on suicide." Phillips (1979) extended this postulate, reporting on an analysis of the increased motor vehicle fatalities (31%) three days after a publicized suicide. He noted that the age of the drivers involved in these motor vehicle fatalities correlated significantly with the age of the person described in the suicide story and that single-car accidents increase more than any other type of vehicle accident. Bollen and Phillips (1982) and Gould and Shaffer (1986) demonstrated that television news stories correlated with a national contagion response to publicized suicides. The cumulative empirical findings of their studies revealed (1) a replication of previous reports that there is a rise in overt suicides after a publicized story of a suicide; (2) evidence that the rise occurs *after* the publication of the suicide story; and (3) the effect of publicity regarding a suicide does not extend beyond 10 days. Bollen and Phillips (1982) suggested that this study "supports the hypothesis that publicized suicides trigger imitative behavior; sometimes this behavior is overt (in the form of an explicit suicide) and sometimes covert (in the form of automobile or airplane accidents)." In a subsequent report, Phillips and Carstensen (1986) reported that teenage suicides increased more than adult suicides after stories about suicides. Cherskov (1986) pointed out that after a first suicide, school officials fear that copycats will soon follow. As noted in *Suicide Among School Age Youth* (The University of the State of New York, 1984), teachers, counselors and administrators quickly express concern that there must be other *vulnerable* students and the question is immediately raised about what can be done to prevent the possible contagious nature of the youthful suicide. Unfortunately, the report further emphasizes that "schools may bear the brunt of community criticism for not somehow preventing the suicide."

It has been suggested that adolescent cluster suicides and attempts are probably an underestimated and unreported phenomenon because (1) teenagers who attempt suicide but to not manifest physiological complications may never come to medical attention; and (2) suicide attempts are not reported to a central registry (Robbins and Conroy, 1983). There is persistent controversy, however, regarding the validity of the Werther effect, or imitative suicide behaviors. Wasserman (1984) concluded that suicidal imitation is probably much more selective than originally reported by Phillips (1974). Wasserman's study analyzed the suicide rate data with a multivariate time series model. The study controlled for seasonal effects, war, and average duration of unemployment. He found no significant association between the national suicide rate and feature articles on suicides of noncelebrities reported on the front page of *The New York Times* between 1947 and 1977. However, Wasserman did detect a significant rise in the national suicide rate occurring in the month after a celebrity commits suicide. Wasserman postulates that the basis for this phenomenon is that (1) celebrity suicides generally generate more mass media publicity; and (2) celebrities possess various social characteristics that cause individuals to identify with them.

Various disclaimers have been presented regarding the validity of the Werther effect. Horton and Stack (1984) reported "that for a properly specified model of suicide the imitation factor has no impact on suicide independent of major control variables, such as unemployment." In essence, the authors suggest that suicide can better be explained from a financial basis rather than from an imitative behavior.

Regardless of the scientific perspective assumed regarding cluster suicides, it is apparent that a growing number of communities have become victims of this devastating adolescent practice. It has been suggested that "any sort of public attention to an adolescent suicide—naming a day to commemorate the adolescent who dies, for example, or glamorizing an adolescent hero's suicide in a movie or song—can make an adolescent feel as if he'll be recognized, remembered and even admired for killing himself" (American Academy of Pediatrics News, 1985). The article further suggested that suicide may directly and indirectly be the result of peer pressure because a friend or someone an adolescent knew in school committed suicide. Similarly, it has been suggested that depressed adolescents appear to gravitate toward others who have similar emotional dysfunctions. The extended postulate further suggests that on occasion "the element or romance" may exaggerate ideation about suicide (American Academy of Pediatrics, 1985).

Delineation of various aspects of the profiles of suicide attemptors and victims perhaps may assist in understanding the nature of cluster suicides.

3.4. Myths and Misconceptions

The early recognition of the child or adolescent with suicidal intent and efforts to obtain professional assistance may be delayed, or worse, ignored, because of the prevailing myths, misconceptions, and superstitions. Unfortunately, professionals are not immune from the fables that may mask the facts about suicide. False assumptions based on popular misbeliefs about self-destructive behaviors may ultimately prove to be fatal for children and young adolescents with serious suicidal ideation. Among the more common fables are beliefs that:

- Discussions about suicide may precipitate suicidal behavior, particularly among those with prior suicidal ideation

- Individuals who talk about suicide do not commit suicide
- Suicide happens on impulse and cannot be prevented
- Suicide is inevitable in depressed individuals
- Suicide is always the act of a psychotic or mentally ill individual
- Improvement following a "suicidal crisis" means the risk is over
- Suicide happens without warning

Table 2 provides a more comprehensive list of popular myths, but more importantly it provides an explanation of the facts regarding these misperceptions (The University State of New York, 1984; Lowenstein, 1985).

Table 2. Youth Suicide: Myths versus Facts[a]

Myth	Fact
The issue of suicide has been exaggerated only because of the rare episodes of "cluster" suicides	Although overall suicide rates in the United States have remained relatively constant, in the age group 15–24 years, there has been more than a 200% increase since 1950
People who talk about suicide don't commit suicide	8 out of 10 suicide victims have given definite warnings of suicidal intent, including verbal threats
Suicide is usually a spontaneous, impulsive, "spur-of-the-moment" act and therefore cannot be avoided	Suicide is generally a result of chronic ideation with multiple clues and warning signals of the intent
Suicide represents a serious desire to die	In most instances, suicide may represent a "gamble with death"; gestures and aborted attempts may represent efforts to get attention and help
Asking an individual if they have had suicidal ideation will precipitate suicide	Suicide may be prevented by opening a dialogue that may lead to counseling and resolution of emotional distress
Suicidal individuals are mentally ill; indeed it represents the act of a psychotic person	The individual is depressed and extremely unhappy, but is not necessarily mentally ill
Once suicidal, the individual is suicidal forever	The period of crisis lasts for a limited time, but, can reoccur
Suicide is inherited	Suicide is not inherited, but suicide in the family increases the risk for other members
Intervention for a suicidal crisis with apparent improvement means the risk is over	Most suicides occur within about 3 months following signs of "improvement"
Suicide occurs most often among the rich	Suicide has no socioeconomic distribution—it is a universal happening

[a]In part adapted from Schneidman and Farberow (1961).

An important part of the intermediary level of intervention by parents, peers, and professionals is the education of both individual and community regarding what is fable and what is fact about suicide. The American Association of Suicidology (1977) cautions that many people die, who might have been saved, if a parent, peer, or professional knew the facts about suicide. The Society suggests that "if you are like most people, almost everything you have heard about suicide is false." It is recommended that a meaningful intermediary strategy is "unmasking the myths," as well as recognizing the danger signs and getting help. The American Association of Suicidology (1977) emphasizes that:

> Even if you have never thought seriously about suicide, you know how it feels to be sad. Try to magnify that feeling in your mind, add to it a sense of hopelessness—a belief that you cannot be helped and that you will never be happy again. If you can empathize with that feeling, then you can begin to understand the state of mind with which many people approach suicide—you can begin to peel away the veneer of misconception and to sense the truth that lies beneath. (p. 2)

3.5. Childhood Suicide

Suicidal tendencies among children (i.e., preadolescents) in the general population have been poorly explored. Most studies that focus on this particular age group are based on data from inpatient and outpatient psychiatric services. From this select group of children, the rates of completed suicides is relatively low (Shaffer, 1974). Nonfatal self-destructive behavior, however, is relatively common among these children (Carlson and Cantwell, 1982; Cohen-Sandler *et al.*, 1982; Pfeffer *et al.*, 1979). Nevertheless, Pfeffer (1985a) demonstrated in a study of 101 randomly selected schoolchildren, who had no history of emotional (psychiatric) symptomatology, that 12% revealed suicidal impulses. She suggests that the results of the study have several clinical implications: (1) children are capable of verbalizing suicidal tendencies; (2) there is a need for developing recognition techniques because until children were interviewed, suicidal children were not recognized as having difficulties; and (3) all suicidal fantasies and actions in children must be taken seriously.

It is recognized that in children aged 1 to 14 years, nonvehicular accidents are a leading cause of death. Finn (1986) suggests that perhaps some of these "accidents" may be classified as "suicides." In general, the incidence of suicidal behavior in children is low, possibly because (1) the National Bureau of Vital Statistics does not classify suicidal trends for children under 10 years of age, and (2) in order to avoid stigmatizing parents, children's death certificates may not reflect the self-destructive act (Brooksbank, 1985; Rosenthal and Rosenthal, 1983; Pfeffer, 1980). Self-destructive behaviors are frequently disguised and reported as "accidents" (Finn, 1986; McGuire and Ely, 1984).

It is now generally accepted that children *are* capable of suicide attempts. For some children, suicide may represent a means of escape from their distress. Finn (1986) suggests that suicidal behavior may be either an "acting out" behavior ("a cry for help") or a death wish. Regardless, most suicidal threats and/or attempts are impulsive acts. The behavioral action is utilized to force parents to pay attention to their needs. As Finn (1986) notes, "These youngsters often have histories of attention-getting behaviors ranging from minor acts to high drama. Children seldom plan suicide acts because they want to die; suicides are committed either impulsively or accidentally."

3.6. Adolescent Suicide

Suicides in the age group 15 to 19 years have more than tripled over the past 30 years, while the rates for the rest of the population have generally remained relatively stable. On the sole basis of the 5000 to 6000 annual deaths of American adolescents who commit suicide, it can be justifiably argued that such fatalities have reached "epidemic proportions" (Struner, 1986). In addition to the recognized absolute increase in youth suicide, there have been more accurate statistics because of improved reporting by medical examiners. As a rule, there is an overwhelming preponderance in successful adolescent male suicides, with firearms (33%) and hanging (18%) accounting for most of the deaths (Sturner, 1986). Females apparently have significantly higher rates of suicide ideation than males, demonstrating higher levels of emotional disturbance and lower levels of self-esteem and what was perceived as a weak or absent parental support system (Simons and Murphy, 1985). Regardless of any perspective bias regarding the relative or absolute numbers that compose the increasing incidence of youth suicide, the psychosocial issues inherent in adolescent self-destructive behaviors are overall regarded as "alarming" and a major concern to health care professionals (Eisenberg, 1980). The expanding rates of completed suicides and suicide attempts among teenagers probably represent a much more pervasive problem of depression and self-destructiveness (Smith and Crawford, 1986). The pilot study of Smith and Crawford focused on suicidal behaviors among 313 high school students in the Midwest. A shocking 62.6% of this group reported some degree of suicidal ideation or action. A suicide attempt had actually been performed by 8.4% of the group. These data suggest that suicide is a very real psychosocial issue for most high school students and "a serious concern for 1 out of 4 of these students." It is extremely difficult to be passive on this issue when it is recognized that 1 out of 8–12 high school students in this survey had actually made a suicide attempt! Based on these statistics, Smith and Crawford concluded that "we need not target our efforts solely at the seriously suicidal young person; it seems that most high school students may need our attention."

Although suicide is a relatively uncommon event among preadolescents, it is the third leading cause of death in teenagers, preceded only by accidents and homicide. Among white male youths, suicide is the second leading cause of death (Peck, 1982). During the past 20 years suicides have increased 250% among females and 300% among males, in the age group 15 to 24 years. Simons and Murphy (1985) noted that "while young people accounted for approximately 5% of all suicides in the United States in the 1960s, they account for 20% of all male suicides and 14% of all female suicides in the 1980s." Once again, these statistics must be regarded as extremely conservative and not a true reflection of the full scope of the problem (Peck, 1982). Numerous reports suggest that 25 to 50% of adolescent suicides may be "disguised," or knowingly are not reported as such. The underestimates are in part the effect of the unquestioned reliance on death certificates, which may be modified by generic citations such as "accidental death" and/or attempts to protect family survivors from the "stigmas" of an adolescent suicide (Barraclough *et al.*, 1974).

It has been hypothesized that people who commit suicide, in contrast to those who threaten or attempt suicide, come from two different populations (Peck, 1982). The suicide attempters and threateners far outnumber the group that actually committed suicides. For adolescents the ratio may be as high as 25 : 1 or 50 : 1 (Peck, 1982).

The heterogeneous factors that are involved in successful suicides, attempted suicides, and serious suicidal ideation have resulted in the design of a variety of classification systems. One schema suggests that a clinical grouping of some adolescents with serious suicidal thoughts include: (1) *depressed adolescents* (may have depressive equivalents such as psychosomatic complaints, reckless behaviors, delinquency, feelings of sadness, depression, and suicide ideation); (2) *unwanted adolescents* (perceive themselves as unnecessary to the family, may have divorced parents who fight over them, families who blame teenagers for their financial difficulties, adolescents who feel they have let the family down by school failure, delinquency, or pregnancy); (3) *adolescents with poor impulse control* (may make a fatal suicide attempt without intent on a fatal outcome, episodic violent behaviors); (4) *psychotic adolescents* (may hear voices to kill themselves); (5) *family history of suicide* (family history of suicide places adolescent at risk to attempt suicide during periods of stress); and (6) *adolescent sustaining serious trauma* (serious accidents or burns may be associated with psychosocial complications, "accidents" may in reality represent aborted suicide attempts) (American Academy of Pediatrics, 1980). Tishler (1981) outlined several of the more popular epidemiological theories of suicide: (1) the *Freudian hypothesis,* which suggests that suicidal adolescents experience loss of love, deprivation, or rejection in relation to the significant persons in their life; (2) *developmental theories,* which focus on the stresses associated with particular psychobiological stages of the life cycle, noting that adolescence is a time of physical and emotional turmoil with a tendency for impulsive overreactions to stressful situations; (3) *cognitive theories* postulate that the adolescent may have a misperception of personal immortality, characterized by a basic immaturity and incomplete intellectual development regarding the reality of death; (4) the *sociological view* of suicide conceptualizes that it is the withdrawal that causes an interruption in societal contact, followed by a sense of isolation from society; and (5) the role of *depression* and it's associated vegetative symptoms, with intensification of symptoms associated with behavioral problems related to particular stages of the adolescent's development. Peck (1982) similarly postulated that there were several subgroups composing the general category of youth suicide: (1) the very young; (2) the loner; (3) those who act out depression; (4) the psychotic suicide; (5) the crisis suicide; and (6) suicidal behavior as a form of communication (Table 3).

Gispert *et al.* (1985) reviewed the factors involved among 82 suicidal adolescents, aged 12 to 18 years. The adolescents in this survey had been admitted to an urban general hospital for evaluation of self-destructive behavior. The data revealed that most had experienced family disruption. Approximately 50% of the group were functioning poorly in school. Suicide risk correlated with current stress, but depression correlated with life-long as well as current stress. Most of the adolescents in this study were judged as being moderately depressed. In a review of the charts of 131 consecutive suicide attempts by 126 patients, Brent (1987) noted that the significant correlates of the medical lethality of suicide behavior included: (1) male sex; (2) diagnosis of affective disorder (particularly in combination with substance abuse); and (3) family history of affective disorder. In this study, demographic, social (including school function and peer/family relations), family, and environmental variables

Table 3. Categories of Youth Suicide[a]

Category	Characteristics
The very young suicide	Age group 10–14 years High incidence of learning disabilities (hyperactivity, perceptual disorders, dyslexia) Increasing frustrations Poor self-concept, loss of self-esteem Threaten and attempt suicide Extremely vulnerable period when these children lose a parent and/or have learning disorders
The loner suicide	Personality emerges age 14 and 15 years Loneliness, lack of friends, poor communication with parents and peers Parents usually normal but concerned about not being good parents Child usually learns at an early age that what he thinks of himself and what parents think are different Suicide deaths may occur with greater frequency than suicide attempts As a group do not give many clues of suicide intent Commonly diagnosed as borderline state, depressive–reactive, or "shy"
Acting-out depression suicide	Suicide ideation and attempts most common among those acting-out depression More white males in this group Behaviors are dangerous, disruptive, aggressive, violent, hostile, illegal Drug/alcohol abuse, runaways, petty crimes, assaultive behaviors Surges of depression Often come from broken homes and those in which alcohol and drugs are used
Psychotic suicide	As a group, small in number Guarded prognosis Delusions, hallucinations, and may hear messages to kill themselves Violent, bizarre behaviors Usually from single-parent families Parent(s) may be psychotic and/or alcoholic
Crisis suicide	Less than 15% of all suicidal youngsters Normal premorbid personality No history of severe emotional trauma Family usually stable

(continued)

Table 3. *(Continued)*

Category	Characteristics
	Adolescent becomes aware of sudden traumatic changes (loss of loved one, loss of status in school)
	Difficulty in concentration
	Series of classic depressive symptoms
	Typically diagnosed as reactive depression
Suicide as a form of communication	Relatively large number of threateners and attempters, rather than suicide deaths
	Suicidal when common avenues of expression of frustrated feelings are blocked
	Experience usually one of desperation and great upset
	Attempt to let other know how unhappy person feels
	Classical "cry for help"
	Frequently occurs in troubled families

[a]Adapted from Peck (1982).

were *not* reported as being significant factors. Khan (1987), from a group of 120 emotionally and behaviorally disturbed adolescents, could not identify the suicidal adolescents, based on age, sex, social class, type of peer and family relationship, academic achievement, and early loss of a parent either by divorce or death; this suggests that the variables emphasized in previous studies require validation and refinement.

Pfeffer (1985b) suggested that the factors associated with risk for suicidal behavior can be categorized into three major groups: (1) early developmental variables; (2) affective factors; and (3) family features. She emphasizes that intense states of depression and aggression are associated with suicidal risk. Pfeffer notes that, "Children and adolescents with DSM-III diagnoses of major depressive or borderline personality disorder are at especially high risk for suicidal behavior." Lowenstein (1985) reports that in the United States, 75% of all suicides are associated with depression and alocholism. Depression has an estimated lifetime mortality of approximately 15%. On the other hand, Mehrabian and Weinstein (1985) suggest that, "Contrary to the traditional view that suicide attempters are depressives, they are more likely to be neurotic or anxious types."

Gispert *et al.* (1987) had an opportunity to review the factors associated with 38 suicide repeaters and 43 nonrepeaters. They found significant differences between the two groups in the areas of: (1) school functioning; (2) life stressors; (3) suicidal intent; (4) anger; and (5) dysphoria. No significant differences, however, were found between the two groups for demographics and the nature of the attempt.

Shrier (1981) commented that the *immediate precipitant* for an adolescent suicide often seems unimportant by adult values. The underlying causes are generally complex and are often related to early childhood experiences, including: (1) parental loss through death; (2) separation from family members; (3) real or perceived emotional deprivation; and (4) feelings of alienation and hopelessness. The most commonly reported cause of suicide attempts in adolescence is rejection or separation from a boyfriend or girlfriend (the end of a teenage romance). Shrier theorized that the broken adolescent relationship may reintroduce suppressed painful feelings of a loss of love from a parent or family member. Teicher (1979) hypothesized a three-stage process that leads to social isolation and ultimately to a suicide attempt.

1. Stage 1. A long-standing history of unexpected separations from significant social interactions during the preadolescent years.
   A. *Primary factors* include death of a parent, divorce, foster placement
   B. *Secondary factors* include suicide attempts by a parent (or friend, relative), frequent family relocations
2. Stage 2. Increasing problems with advancing adolescence, including disrupted family relationships, peer pressures, and school problems. The adolescent appears unable to cope with the normal behavioral modifications of adolescence; feelings of being misunderstood and acting out behaviors to call attention to the stress (running away, rebellion, withdrawal, antisocial acts). The teenager is unable to establish meaningful and close peer relationships.
   A. *Primary factors* include increasing "loss of satisfaction and support in the three key areas of the adolescent's life—family, school, and peers"
   B. *Secondary factors* include increasing school problems and "adaptive behaviors" attempting to defuse perceived pressures
3. Stage 3. The romance is characterized by its intensity, because the adolescent feels that there is little or no time for "casual relationships." Adult figures (including parents) may have been alienated by the end of the second stage and the adolescent ac-

tively yearns for a closeness and love with a boy or girl. When the romance *fails,* "the teenager feels abandoned and totally isolated and is at risk for a suicide attempt" (Teicher, 1979).

Previous reports by Shaffer (1974, 1985) suggested that a substantial number of children and adolescents, prior to their suicides, indicated in their medical, psychiatric, and educational records that they (1) had made self-denigratory remarks; (2) felt people were against them; and (3) appeared withdrawn before their suicidal act. Shaffer believes that these are clinical features that are compatible with a diagnosis of "mood disturbance." Apparently these depressive symptoms are also common among suicide attempters. Shaffer (1985) suggests that the prevalence of depression increases with age; that is, it is less common in children and prior to puberty than in adolescence. Shaffer (1986), commenting on why suicides may be rare among children, notes that the cognitions associated with depression may require that the child have a "well-developed ability to perceive themselves, albeit in a distorted fashion, with respect to the outside world, and that this is necessary for the feelings of isolation and helplessness, which are often alleged to occur in suicidal individuals." The projected continuum of child and adolescent depression, as it is recognized in adults, has not been resolved by definitive research. The development and degradation of *self-esteem* appears to be the common denominator influencing "depression," regardless of age. Mack (1985) postulates that:

> In each stage of development after infancy the achievement of a sense of positive self-worth contributes not only to the child's sense of well-being but also to the quelling of his fears for his actual survival. In the child's eyes, his sense of self-worth is *essential* to his survival. The child who does not experience his value in the eyes of his parents will fear their abandonment and its attendant dangers to his existence. The older child and adolescent may even contemplate suicide. (p. 12)

> Most important among the immaturities of psychic organization and functioning is the poor tolerance by children of the painful affects associated with narcissistic injury and lowered self-regard. This picture of depression in childhood may be different from that of adults, characterized by hypochondriacal symptoms, accident proneness, overactivity, withdrawal from friendships (and activities), school failure, drug taking in adolescence, suicide threats or attempts, or other behaviors which are propelled by the need to avoid or escape from the emotional pain associated with diminished self-esteem. (p. 36)

Suicidal ideation is a prominent feature of depression in children and adolescents; however, the two cannot be equated in as much as some adolescent suicide attempters do not admit to feelings of depression

(Chess and Hassibi, 1986). Although there are increasing data linking suicidal behavior in adults to abnormalities of neurophysiological function, studies of these biological markers in children and adolescents have not been performed. The assumed biological basis for some adults has been demonstrated in the neuroendocrine abnormalities of cortisol secretion found with the dexamethasone suppression test in depressed adults patients. At this time, studies of biological markers for child or adolescent suicidal behaviors have not defined meaningful neurochemical indicators (Pfeffer, 1986).

Regardless of the classification schema or the primary epidemiological concept that one adopts, it is obvious that the factors associated with adolescent suicide are multivariate and relatively complex. For the clinician, the more immediate problem is the recognition of the "warning signs" of potential youth suicide and the process by which the life-threatening behavior can be averted.

3.7. Contributing Factors and Warning Signs

Children and adolescents generally verbalize their suicidal ideation and intent prior to the suicide attempt. The verbal and behavioral warning signs are often obvious, but unfortunately may be overlooked, dismissed as "just talk," or worse, they may be ignored. The significant warning signs of adolescent suicide intent can generally be grouped into four major categories: (1) symptoms of serious depression; (2) talk of suicide; (3) planning for death; and (4) previous suicide attempts (Shrier, 1981).

The *adolescent suicide* generally presents a profile that tends to be characterized by: (1) male; (2) white; (3) intelligent with academic success; (4) loners; (5) history of mental illness in the family; (6) suicidal behaviors in peers or family members; (7) previous suicide attempt; and (8) verbalized desire to die (Slaby and McGuire, 1986). The immediate precipitating event may be a broken romance, failure in school, or death of a peer or family member. In contrast, Slaby and McGuire (1986) characterize the profile of the *suicide attempter* as: (1) female; (2) drug and/or alcohol abuser; (3) disturbed parent, sibling, or peer relationships; (4) school failures; (5) involved in psychotherapy; (6) absent or unemployed fathers; and (7) depressive symptoms. Regardless of age, every suicide attempt should initiate an evaluation and "most referred for treatment" (Clayton, 1985). Clayton (1985) concluded that victims of suicide, 98 percent of whom are psychiatrically ill, come from four overlapping groups: (1) the untreated, (2) the nonpsychiatrically treated,

(3) psychiatric inpatients and outpatients, and (4) suicide attempters (sometimes emergency room patients). Prevention intervention is difficult but it seems reasonable to start with this fourth group." (p. 211).

Pfeffer (1985b) theorized that suicidal behavior is "a very complex symptom" engendered by the specific effects of underlying anger, stress, depression, and anxiety. The response to emotional strains depends on a susceptible developmental template previously fashioned by early childhood experiences and current environmental pressures such as family difficulties. Pfeffer suggests that there is a delicate balance of these various factors influencing a vulnerable individual who may in an "unstable equilibrium" exhibit a self-destructive behavior. She notes that, "Often, this shift in equilibrium occurs rapidly, so that suicidal behavior appears to have an impulsive quality."

Unfortunately there is no easy or reliable test of suicide; however, a *major* predictor is the seriousness of a previous attempt (Hodgman, 1985). Some of the warning signs for the youth at risk for suicide are summarized in Table 4.

Shrier (1981) grouped some of the warning signs that precede a suicide attempt into several major categories: (1) *symptoms of serious depression* (loss of interest in former activities; feelings of sadness, loneliness, hopelessness; loss of appetite; insomnia or hypersomnia; fatigue; sexual promiscuity; alcohol and drug abuse); (2) *talk of suicide* (preoccupations with death); (3) *planning for death* (placing "life in order";

Table 4. Warning Signs: Youth at Risk for Suicide[a]

A previous suicide attempt
Talking about suicide or suicide gestures (even in jest)
Loss of a family member or peer (particularly by suicide)
Preoccupation with themes of death
Family crises and broken home
Deep depression
Feelings of worthlessness, self-critical, poor self-esteem
Alcohol and/or drug abuse
Psychosomatic complaints
Outburst of violent or rebellious behavior
Changes in eating and/or sleep habits
Becoming socially isolated or running away
Becoming withdrawn/uncommunicative with friends or family
Difficulty concentrating
Unexplained decline in school performance
Giving away prized possessions
Getting life in order

[a]In part adapted from American Academy of Pediatrics (1985).

disposing of private and prized possessions); and (4) *previous suicide attempts* (any attempt must be taken seriously). Tishler (1982) divided suicidal risk into three broad categories based on the patients history and behaviors (Table 5). Tishler (1982) delineated these warning signs based on seriousness of risk; that is, low, medium, and high.

In essence, the *warning signs of suicide* can be grouped into several major categories: (1) verbal; (2) physical; (3) behavioral; and (4) situational signs and symptoms.

Verbalizations about suicide must be always be taken seriously. Direct statements such as, "I don't want to live anymore," or indirect comments such as "I'll show them . . . they'll be sorry when I'm gone," are definite clues of the older child's or adolescent's serious suicidal ideation. *Physical signs* are variable and may include the spin-offs of behavioral symptomatology, including appetite and weight changes (e.g., weight loss), physical fatigue from insomnia, and signs of alcohol or drug abuse. *Behavioral changes* probably constitute the largest category of signs and symptoms associated with serious suicide intent. Among the more fre-

Table 5. Major Categories of Suicide Risk[a]

Characteristic/Action	Low	Medium	High
Ambivalent feeling that act was an attempt to die	+	+/−	Clear plan for destructive act
Lethal overdose, or 20 or more pills	−	+ 15–40 pills in overdose attempt	+ 30 or more pills in overdose attempt
Cut requiring sutures, or more lethal act	−	+ Slashing requires internal and external sutures	+ Severe slashing; gunshot; hanging
Prior history of attempt	−	−	+
Statement of suicidal attempt for the future	−	−	+
High degree of perturbation or family verbalizes concern and desire for follow-up treatment	−	−	+ Severe family dysfunction; delinquency behavior; school difficulty; psychotic thinking; personal abuse

[a]Adapted from Tishler (1982).

quently encountered behavioral symptoms are the characteristic signs of depression: changes in sleeping and eating habits, withdrawal from social interactions, apathy in previously enjoyed activities, activities indicative of impending suicidal action (giving away choice possessions, increased risk activities, frequent accidents), and most significant is the history of previous suicide attempt. *Situational symptoms* are prominent, including experiences associated with loss (loss of a loved-one, loss of a pet, divorce, and critically the loss of self-esteem), problems at school, antisocial behaviors (delinquency, peer difficulties), and abuse of alcohol and/or drugs. The loss of a friend, relative, family member, or a pet may trigger the suicidal action.

The suspicion that a child or adolescent has suicidal ideation should immediately initiate the process of securing assistance for the troubled youth. This is a serious emotional and psychosocial crisis that can ill afford the luxury of time or an attitude of apathy. The prompt response to any combination of the signs and symptoms outlined may be the difference between life and death for the child or adolescent in question.

4. Self-Destructive Behaviors: "The Slow Lane"

Blum (1987a) grouped contemporary threats to adolescent health in the United States into two major categories: (1) *mortalities of youth* (accidental injuries, homicide/assault, and suicide), and (2) *morbidities of youth* (teenage pregnancy, alcohol abuse, tobacco use, drug abuse, adolescent physical and sexual abuse, and chronic illness and disabilities). The latter category partially comprises behaviors that can be perceived as self-destructive activities, but at a much slower pace than suicide. Indeed, it is generally recognized that several of the major morbidities (alcohol abuse and drug abuse) may directly and indirectly contribute to accidental injuries, homicide, and suicide, which make up the major mortalities of youth. It should again be noted that despite the dramatic reduction in deaths caused by communicable diseases, the absolute mortality rate has *not* been reduced because of the rise in violent death among adolescents.

Up to this point, this chapter has focused primarily on the more obvious and aggressive acts of self-destruction among children and adolescents; that is, suicide attempts or suicide by gunshot, hanging, slashing of wrists, overdose of pills, and single-vehicle (automobile, motorcycle) "accidents." It is not surprising that these more violent behaviors characteristically generate parent, peer, and professional concerns and anxieties. On the other hand, the more "subtle" self-destructive behaviors (drug abuse, alcohol abuse, accident-proneness, reckless/impulsive acts, and delinquency) may not cause the societal apprehensions that they should. Often these behaviors are misperceived as passing phases in adolescent development, may be overlooked by parents and professionals as significant psychopathologies, or worse, they are ignored as meaningful symptomatic clues. The "subtle" but inappropriate psychosocial activities represent an attempt at self-injury and self-degradation, albeit in "slow motion." In reality, however, they may represent latent but significant precursors for more violent acts of self-destruction by children and teenagers. Indeed, alcohol and/or drugs have been involved in approximately 50% of adolescent suicides. Several of the major morbidities of adolescence are discussed in more detail because of their overall impact as significant self-destructive behaviors (Strasburger, 1985).

4.1. Drug and Alcohol Abuse

Substance abuse (marijuana, cocaine, crack, and other drugs) have traditionally constituted a major public health problem (Table 6). However, the more widespread and insidious abuse of alcohol (a legal drug) is perhaps the more serious drug problem, regardless of age (Macdonald, 1986).

It has been estimated that approximately 10% of children aged 12 to 13 years are current drinkers (defined as having consumed alcohol within the past month). By the time they are high school seniors, two thirds are current drinkers. Approximately 90% of students have tried alcohol by the time they are high school seniors. The peer and media pressure to drink alcoholic products is pervasive throughout all age

Table 6. Approximate Incidence of Substance Abuse among Teenagers 12 to 17 Years of Age (1975–1983)[a]

Substance abused	Number experimented (in millions)	Percent of 12–17 population	Number daily users (in millions)	Percent of 12–17 population
Cigarette	16.3	71.0	4.8	21.0
Alcohol	21.4	93.0	1.2	5.5
Marijuana	13.1	57.0	1.2	5.5
Stimulants	8.0	35.0	—	—
Cocaine	3.7	16.0	—	—

[a]Adapted from Johnson *et al.* (1984).

groups and drinking has been reported as early as fourth grade. MacDonald (1986) emphasizes that *beer* is the usual alcoholic beverage consumed by children and adolescents. Beer, he comments, "is closely linked through advertising to social and recreational activities that are especially appealing to adolescents." MacDonald suggests that there is environmental pressures placed on teenagers in this regard, noting that:

> Each year $1.23 billion is spent to advertise beer, and the average teenager is exposed to an estimated 1000 ads touting alcoholic beverages. It is unlikely that teenagers will miss the message that drinking is "in" and that "sophisticated" adults drink. (p. 50)

Various investigators suggest that alcohol use at an early age is the "gateway" to increased serious drinking problems, smoking, and to significant experimentation or abuse of marijuana and other drugs. Similarly, a variety of psychological and social complications of alcohol misuse such as high-risk behaviors (sexual promiscuity, reckless driving, antisocial activities) are commonly encountered among adolescents who drink. The gravity of the problem is further highlighted by data indicating that one in seven 12th-graders report drinking to inebriation on at least a weekly basis (Blum, 1987a). Intoxication among 10th grade students, during the school year, is similarly a relatively common occurrence, approximately 40%.

Several high-risk factors have been associated with the potential for teenage alcohol abuse: a family history of alcoholism; inconsistent parental discipline; peers/friends who regularly drink or use drugs; negative attitudes about school and poor academic performance; antisocial behaviors; weak or absent family, school, and church support systems; and low self-esteem (Macdonald, 1986). Adolescents who abuse alcohol appear to manifest particular characteristics that may distinguish them from their nondrinking peers (Blum, 1987b), including increased tolerance for social inappropriateness of deviance, less interest in religious activities, relative indifference to school performance, greater family tolerance for alcohol and substance abuse, and if they are male.

A brief comment regarding marijuana use by children and adolescents: The ready availability and apathy regarding its abuse, in all age groups, strikes a similarity with the problems encountered with alcohol abuse. It has been estimated that the abuse of marijuana is widespread, involving the daily *intoxication* by approximately 120,000 American high school seniors (Schwartz *et al.*, 1987). Despite a decline in peak usage of 10.8% in 1978 to about 5% in 1985, marijuana abuse must be regarded as a relatively *common* practice among adolescents. The average age of first use is between 13 and 14 years. In a comparable situation with alcohol abuse, a significant number of one-time users (about 10%) will progress to daily use of marijuana. It is of interest that among adolescent marijuana users, there is a significant number of parents who are heavy drinkers or alcoholics. Similarly, without early intervention, marijuana abusers are likely to progress or do progress to other forms of drug abuse. Both alcohol and drug abusers are characterized by experiencing difficulty in school; that is, academic underachievement and a high incidence of failure to graduate from high school (Friedman *et al.*, 1985). Schwartz *et al.* (1987), in a study of 35 adolescents who became dependent on marijuana and were placed in an adolescent treatment facility, serious behavioral, psychosocial, and academic problems began or worsened as marijuana use escalated. As in the case with child and adolescent alcohol abusers, parents in this study were notably late in detecting the dependency on marijuana. In several cases the diagnosis was overlooked by mental health professionals.

A detailed compendium of the clinical manifestations, emergency problems, and rehabilitation strategies for adolescent drug abusers is beyond the scope of this chapter. A variety of texts are available to serve this function (Schuckit, 1984). This is not to deemphasize the need for parents and professionals to be cognizant of the spectrum of "street drugs" available for youth experimentation and use (e.g., CNS depressants, stimulants, cannabinols, PCP, opiates, hallucinogens, and crack—to mention a few). Needless to say, the recognition and provision of professional assistance for child or adolescent substance abusers is a life-saving intervention.

4.2. Inappropriate Adolescent Behaviors

Encompassed within the broad, generic classification of inappropriate adolescent behaviors are several psychosocial activities, though not life-threatening, that can profoundly influence the quality of an adolescent's life. Among these adolescent behavioral morbidities are teenage pregnancy, juvenile delinquency, running away, and other significant antisocial behaviors.

4.2.1. Teenage Pregnancy

In 1983, there were slightly more than one million adolescent pregnancies reported in the age group 15 to 19 years (Blum, 1987a) Of these adolescent pregnancies approximately 47.9% were carried to term, 38% ended in abortions, and 13.4% ended as miscarriages. Although there has been a decline in the birth and abortion rate among adolescents during the past 5 years, this decrease in incidence is slower than for women in other age groups. The American Academy of Pediatrics (1979) suggests that teenage pregnancy has reached "epidemic" proportions, reflecting poor sex education, promiscuity, and peer pressures. Regardless of these depressing and alarming statistics, *why is teenage pregnancy included in a chapter whose theme is self-destructive behaviors?*

The profound health implications of adolescent pregnancy qualifies the topic for inclusion in this review. The two major adverse health consequences of teenage pregnancy are (1) preeclampsia and (2) an excessive number of low-birthweight infants (American Academy of Pediatrics, 1979). The adolescent mother, however, is confronted with other major psychosocial issues: (1) she is usually forced to interrupt schooling; (2) she is generally economically dependent; and (3) most often she is deserted by the father. To further complicate the issue, there have been reports that teenage pregnancies may be associated with increased risks for abnormalities of child development, handicapped children, and children with depressed IQ scores. In addition, child abuse and neglect and delinquent behavior have been reported among adolescent mothers (American Academy of Pediatrics, 1979).

4.2.2. Juvenile Delinquency

Delinquency encompasses a heterogeneous group of acts that are prohibited by criminal law, ranging through a variety of offenses, e.g., theft, drug use, vandalism, and various kinds of heterosexual and homosexual acts. In the United States, status offenses involving drinking alcohol and violating curfew are also included (Farrington, 1987). In 1983, approximately 30% of all persons arrested in the United States for index offenses were under 18 years of age. The prevalence of serious delinquency appears to vary markedly with age and gender, peaking at ages 15 to 17 years and thereafter decreasing in both males and females (Farrington, 1987). Court statistics indicate that 3% of American children aged 10 to 17 years will appear in Juvenile Court for offenses other than traffic violations. (Statistics are based on only those delinquents who are apprehended!) The youthful offender generally averages age 13.5 years, with a distinct male predominance. Since the 1940s, the arrests of youthful offenders have increased at a much more rapid rate than that of adult offenders. These statistics are dramatically exaggerated by the extremely high incidence of recidivism for incarcerated juvenile delinquents. Regardless of the absolute incidence/prevalence of delinquency in adolescence, the psychosocial disorder "qualifies as one of childhood's most tragic developmental–behavioral outcomes" (Levine *et al.*, 1985).

A variety of risk factors have been associated with delinquent and antisocial behaviors: learning disabilities and failing subject in school (Novy and Donohue, 1985; Zinkus and Gottlieb, 1978); selected health problems such as vision, hearing, speech, neurological, prenatal and perinatal complications (Penner, 1982); pervasive and serious developmental disorders (Hollander and Turner, 1985); skill deficits (Dishion *et al.*, 1984); and borderline IQ's, i.e., scores below 85 (Hollander and Turner, 1985). Levine *et al.* (1985) concluded that there are "multiple delinquency-predisposing stresses (so-called risk factor complexes)," including (1) socioeconomic deprivation; (2) perinatal health stress; (3) illnesses; (4) chronic disorders of behavior; (5) family discontinuity and lack of family supports; (6) poor school performance; and (7) "neurodevelopmental disability interfering with learning and social adjustment." Cluster analysis of over 30 risk factors identified three subgroups that accounted for 70% of the juvenile delinquents (Table 7). Roff (1986) identified a high-risk group characterized by aggressive behavior associated with peer rejection, predelinquent behavior, and family disturbance or criminality producing increased risk.

The ultimate consequences of juvenile delinquency, as a form of self-destructive behavior (albeit "in the slow lane"), are associated with

Table 7. Cluster Analysis of 31 Specific Findings (High-Risk Factors) Associated with Juvenile Delinquency[a]

Group one
Lowest mean risk scores
Over one third had language delays and difficulties with mathematics
Relatively few medical problems and developmental delays
Group two
Most severely involved in all areas
Severe educational delays
Numerous neurodevelopmental findings
Sequencing problems
Language impairments
Highest prevalence of reading disorders and attention deficits
Commonly associated with chronic anxiety and depression
Group three
Highest number of medical risks
90% had serious perinatal problems
100% had been in serious accidents and had head trauma requiring medical attention
Group with most findings on physical examination
Most weaknesses in visuoperceptual function
30% had history of recurrent otitis media

[a] Adapted from Levine *et al.* (1985).

numerous ominous psychosocial connotations: (1) the potential for repetition of antisocial behaviors resulting in chronic incarcerations; (2) repeated episodes of physical and sexual exploitation; and (3) a life-style characterized by aggression, violence, and homicide (as a perpetrator or victim).

4.2.3. Teenage Runaways

The teenage runaway requires little or no formal discussion as it relates to self-destruction. The varied disastrous complications are legend, including a propensity for drug abuse, prostitution, AIDS, physical violence, homicide, and suicide. Many of the epidemiological factors associated with suicide, depression, teenage pregnancy, delinquency, and other child or adolescent psychosocial risks are operant as causes of runaway behaviors.

5. Intermediary Levels of Intervention

Serious ideation by a child or adolescent contemplating an act of self-destruction, or an attempt per se, demands the immediate expertise of a skilled psychotherapist. Securing this urgently needed therapeutic resource mandates new and critical skills for parents, peers, and primary-health care providers. Inability or undue delay in establishing an effective bridge between the potential victim and a skilled therapist may literally be a life-and-death issue. Clayton (1985) suggests that prevention of suicide "must start with the education of the nonpsychiatric physician, counsellors, clergymen, policemen, and the public."

5.1. Role of Parents

As a general rule, parents must ultimately assume the responsibility of establishing contact between their seriously troubled child or adolescent and a psychotherapist. This mandate in "intermediate intervention" can only be successfully accomplished if the parents (1) are able to recognize both the obvious and subtle warning signs of suicidal ideation and intent; (2) are receptive to sharing and acting on the observations and concerns of others, such as teachers and peers (even if the parents themselves have not recognized self-destructive behaviors); (3) can respond to the pychosocial crisis with a caring and understanding attitude and thereby develop meaningful communication with their troubled child; (4) are familiar with community resources that can provide the critically needed expert psychotherapy (or can make the necessary inquiries to locate these resources); and (5) most importantly, can suppress their own feelings of ambivalence, denial, guilt, and fears of social stigmatization, diverting their energies to promptly securing professional assistance. The key to a successful outcome may depend on the parent's ability to promptly recognize the danger signals of self-destructive behaviors and to respond quickly to the emergency—procrastination may prove to be fatal. Delays in securing needed professional help may be engendered by false assumptions such as, "Now that we are talking about the problems, everything will be OK," "We can work it out by ourselves," and other life-threatening cliches. Children and adolescents who present warning signs of suicide require immediate professional intervention. Effective psycho-therapy *cannot* be rendered by even the most sensitive and/or caring parents. In attempting to secure professional help, parents may turn to their primary-care physicians, their clergyman, crisis intervention centers, hospital emergency rooms, or other medical agencies for guidance.

Although the urgency of the moment can be readily appreciated, parents may have an equally significant role in *prevention* of child and adolescent suicides. Recent research appears to have identified some of the family pathologies that serve as precursors for self-destructive behaviors in teenagers. The link between adolescents who have experienced abuse (physical, sexual, and emotional), severe maladjustment problems, low self-esteem, anxiety, aggressive behaviors, alcohol abuse, difficulties in social adjustment, school difficulties, and suicidal tendencies have been reported (Galambos and Dixon, 1984; Garbarino and Gilliam, 1980; Garbarino, 1978). Yesavage and Widrow (1985), in a study of 45 male inpatients with major depressive episodes, noted that 44% of the variance for inpatient self-destructive acts could be accounted for by a combination of factors: (1) history of severe childhood discipline by father and mild discipline by mother; and (2) parental conflict frequently involving alcohol. It was noted that losses during childhood were of less importance than the cited measures of family instability. A pilot study to test if exposure to child abuse or neglect was associated with suicidal behavior in adolescence revealed that for both sexes prior contact with the Department of Social Services (Massachusetts) was three to six times more likely for probands than for comparison subjects. Results suggested that the higher frequency of contact with the Department of Social Services among the suicidal proband is a marker for a greater burden of disadvantage or adversive incidences experienced by these children and adolescents. In essence the study revealed that prior contact with this agency was a marker for adolescent suicidal behaviors (Deykin *et al.*, 1985). In an earlier analysis of a limited number of cases, Pfeffer (1981b) suggested that the family system of psychiatrically hospitalized suicidal latency-age children can be characterized as "functioning with intense ambivalence, rigid patterns of interaction, poor identity as a family unit due to lack of differentiation of generational boundaries, regressions to state of collective primitive ego functioning, levels of helplessness, low self-esteem and depression, and threats by any attempt for family differentiation or member individuation." Pfeffer postulates that the child with suicidal ideation and behavior has been placed in the role of providing gratification to a parent, of being "an omnipotent protector" for the parent who is distressed, and of "accepting the displaced parental hostility derived from parental unresolved infantile conflicts." It was concluded that the child with suicidal behavior may act-out almost as a desperate and last-resort measure, in order to remove their negative self-perceptions and poor self-esteem from their consciousness.

Regardless of the perspective, preventive or therapeutic, parents generally are the first to detect behavioral deviations that suggest suicidal ideation and intent. Their primary role is to secure the necessary assistance in a timely fashion.

5.2. Role of Peers

The "peer group" is perhaps one of the most significant psychosocial influences in the life of the child and adolescent; ranging from anxiety-provoking peer interactions to friends with whom the most intimate of secrets are shared. Needless to say, this relationship is unique, particularly among adolescents, and has direct implications in the problem of self-destructive behaviors. It is recognized that frequently adolescents first verbalize and act-out suicidal intent with their peer group, rather than with family members or teachers. The response of peers to these messages from their troubled friends or classmates is usually fashioned by the code of "keeping a secret." "Betraying a confidence" is generally regarded as a psychological and social taboo among teenagers! Several years ago, in response to the increasing incidence of youth suicide, a task force was organized by the Union of American Hebrew Congregations (UAHC) (Break the Silence, 1985). This task force on youth suicide focused on the role of peers in this complex, devastating psychosocial issue. In addition to designing, distributing, and making available theme-related materials, the task force of the UAHC developed a specific campaign directed at the peer group, the theme of which was to "Break the Silence." The materials that were prepared focused on the fact that the child and adolescent with serious suicidal ideation (to paraphrase from their poster), "won't tell a parent or a teacher, but a peer, a friend. If someone tells you a secret—that they are thinking of committing suicide—you can help. Listen to them. Show your care and support. But most important, tell someone. Break the silence. Break the secret. You may risk a friendship, but you may save a life." The posters and handouts emphatically underscored the message that most who commit suicide actually tell someone about their intent, but the message is often suppressed. In addition, the UAHC sponsored an excellent book, *When Living Hurts,* by the noted author/educator, Dr. Sol Gordon. The book, designed and written in the "language" for teenagers and young adults, addresses a variety of associated issues. Of particular importance to this review are the chapters entitled "If someone you know is feeling really bad or is suicidal. It could also be yourself" (pp. 5–29), and "Help. What to do when you are feeling bad. On how to help a friend who is feeling sad, depressed, bored, or lonely" (pp. 30–60).

The role of peers and their responsibility in preventing youth suicide cannot be emphasized too emphatically. This is a life-saving issue that should be popularized at home in family discussions, at school, from the pulpit, and by the media.

5.3. Role of Primary-Care Physicians

There are four basic principles in the medical management of the potentially suicidal adolescent: (1) *be available* (as a rule most suicidal adolescents feel lonely, isolated, unwanted, anticipate rejection, and often test others "to see if they really care"); (2) *don't be afraid to talk about suicide* (skill is necessary in communicating with the adolescent contemplating suicide; avoid acting shocked, don't moralize, and don't be critical; verbalize a caring attitude); (3) *referral to a psychiatrist* (a critical decision must be made as to whether the adolescent in question will require short-term crisis intervention counseling from the pediatrician *or* intensive long-term individual, group, and/or family therapy from a psychiatrist); and (4) *antidepressant medication* (these drugs are generally not of benefit, particularly when the adolescent is attempting to minimize feelings of depression by acting-out with promiscuous sex and/or drug and alcohol abuse. These principles, as outlined by Shrier (1981), focus on the interventions that can be provided by medical professionals; however, important intermediary levels of intervention must also be initiated by parents and peers.

It is universally agreed that definitive psychotherapy for the child or adolescent with suicidal intent (or who has made an attempt) demands an expertise beyond the scope of general pediatric practice. Smith and Bope (1986), however, recognize the role served by primary care physicians in establishing this definitive therapeutic relationship:

> Evaluation of the suicidal patient involves careful consideration of risk factors, including attention to subtle clues from history, and mental health examination. The most urgent decision for the physician to make is whether or not to insist on hospitalization. (p. 199)

The authors noted that adolescents who threaten suicide present a somewhat unique situation; that is, the emotional lability of an adolescent generally results in more "explosive reactions to a disappointment or loss that would be managed more successfully by an adult."

Unfortunately, pediatricians often lack involvement with suicidal adolescents because there is (1) a lack of clinical contact with the suicidal adolescent; (2) an unwillingness by adolescents and their families to seek the pediatrician's assistance; and (3) a lack of training and expertise by primary-care physicians in suicide intervention (Hergenroeder *et al.*, 1986). Hergenroeder *et al.* recommend narrowing the gulf between primary-health-care providers and the suicidal adolescent, suggesting that residency training programs should make this a priority in the curriculum.

It is important to recognize that the primary-care physician (as with parents and peers) must be able to recognize the warning signals and must be prepared to act accordingly. A genuine and caring attitude—perhaps simply stating, "I care about you"—may be the trigger that defuses a volatile life-threatening situation.

Communicating concern for the child and adolescent during this period of emotional turmoil and stress may be the first positive signal that the patient receives. Assessing the severity and depth of the suicide warning signals, exploration of underlying feelings, and demonstrating a willingness to listen (rather than to preach good mental health practices) are the initial responsibilities and intervention strategies for the physician. Securing expert counseling services for the child or adolescent, and most often for the entire family, is similarly a professional communication challenge (Pfeffer, 1980). Effectively facilitating the patient's transfer from the primary-care office setting to either the hospital or psychotherapist's office demands that patient and family have the trust and confidence in the physician to ensure compliance.

6. The Survivors

This chapter does not present a comprehensive discussion of the grieving process of family members in the tragic aftermath of a youth suicide. The death of a child, particularly an adolescent, entails a special form of grieving for parents and siblings (Dunne *et al.*, 1987; Hauser, 1987). The differences, frictions, and dynamics of adolescent–family relationships may serve to magnify the feelings of guilt, converting the normal grieving process into a pathological state (McIntosh, 1987; Ojanlatva, 1987; Rando, 1986; McIntosh and Eldridge, 1984). Unfortunately, grief counseling is *not* an integral component of many medical students and/or pediatric residency programs (Behnke *et al.*, 1984; Schowalter, 1970). In essence, the professional support for grieving members of the family may simply be lacking.

Hauser (1987) defines *bereavement* as the cumulative physiological, psychological, behavioral, and social responses exhibited by an individual following the death of a significant person in their life. Bereavement has two major components: grief and mourning. Grief is defined as the feelings and emotional responses related to bereavement. Mourning is related to the social customs and rituals that help the bereaved person grieve. Suicide engenders various types of *unresolved grief:* "denial," "chronic mourning," and "euphoria" (the least common variant). Unresolved grief is characterized by an unstable response that usually gives way to intense grief and appears to be based on gross reality distortions. Hauser (1987) outlined a variety of reasons why death by suicide can result in unresolved grief:

- Death by suicide is usually sudden and unexpected
- Death by suicide is generally violent
- Suicide creates guilt in the survivors
- Suicide often occurs in systems already experiencing stress (e.g., disturbed family relationships)
- Death by suicide can compromise the usual mourning rituals
- Suicide may lead to harmful expressions of unconscious anger and ultimately to distorted communication patterns
- Some of the usual social supports may be withdrawn following death by suicide

McIntosh (1987) notes that guilt is a prominent grief reaction of parents to the death of a child. It appears that guilt may be intensified among parents and is of longer duration. In essence, the death of a child by suicide questions the credibility of the parents; that is, the stigmatization as "bad parents." In some instances parents may feel that "poor parenting" was responsible for the suicide, generating abnormal fears about the welfare of surviving siblings. Disturbances in social interactions and marital discord may follow in the wake of the tragedy of a child's death by suicide. In addition to abnormal grief patterns in the parents, siblings may have similarly altered bereavement responses. The responses by friends of the family, by the child's peers, and by relatives may be awkward, inappropriate, and unknowingly pain provoking. At best, death of a child by suicide is an extremely traumatic experience to all concerned.

7. Summary

Self-destructive behaviors in children and adolescents have been reviewed in a broad framework, ranging from teenage runaways to youth suicide. Particular focus was directed toward the need for recognition of warning signs, replacing facts for myths, and acting judiciously in securing professional psychotherapy services. The role of parents, peers, and primary-care physicians was delineated, ranging from providing a bridge between the troubled youth and a counseling resource to providing a caring attitude and meaningful support system. The need for additional research in the epidemiology and prevention of self-destructive behaviors is readily appreciated.

References

American Academy of Pediatrics, 1985, *Surviving: Coping with Adolescent Depression and Suicide,* American Academy of Pediatrics, Elk Grove, IL.

American Academy of Pediatrics, 1979, Committee on Adolescence, Statement on teenage pregnancy, *Pediatrics* **63:**795–797.

American Academy of Pediatrics, 1980, Committee on Adolescence, Teenage suicide, *Pediatrics* **66:**144–146.

American Academy of Pediatrics News, 1985, Teen suicide, August, pp. 4–8.

American Association of Suicidology and Merck Sharp & Dohme, 1977, Suicide and how to prevent it, in: *Merck Services,* 6th printing, pp. 1–8, West Point, PA.

Barraclough, B. M., Bunch, J., Nelson, B., *et al.,* 1974, A hundred cases of suicide, *Br. J. Psychiatry* **125:**355–373.

Behnke, M., Setzer, E., and Mehta, P., 1984, Death counseling and psychosocial support by physicians concerning dying children, *J. Med. Educ.* **59:**906–908.

Blum, R., 1987a, Contemporary threats to adolescent health in the United States, *JAMA* **257:**3390–3395.

Blum, R., 1987b, Diagnostic and treatment issues in adolescent substance abuse, *Pediatr. Clin. North Am.* **34:**523–537.

Bollen, K. A., and Phillips, D. P., 1982, Imitative suicide: A national study of the effects of television news stories, *Am. Sociol. Rev.* **47:**802–809.

Break the Silence, 1985, Task Force on Youth Suicide Union of America Hebrew Congregations, 838 Fifth Avenue, New York 10021.

Brent, D. A., 1987, Correlates of the medical lethality of suicide attempts in children and adolescents, *J. Am. Acad. Child Psychiatry* **26:**87–89.

Brent, D. A., Kalas, R., Edelbrock, C., *et al.,* 1986, Psychopathology and its relationship to suicidal ideation in childhood and adolescence, *J. Am. Acad. Child Psychiatry* **25:**566–673.

Brooksbank, D. J., 1985, Suicide and parasuicide in childhood and early adolescence, *Br. J. Psychiatry* **146:**459–463.

Carlson, G., and Cantwell, D., 1982, Suicidal behavior and depression in children and adolescents, *J. Am. Acad. Child Psychiatry* **21:**361–368.

Cherskov, M., 1986, Hospitals join in the battle to stop teen suicides, *Hospitals* June 5, pp. 98,100.

Chess, S., and Hassibi, M. (eds.), 1986, *Principles and Practice of Child Psychiatry,* 2nd ed., Plenum Press, New York.

Clayton, P. J., 1985, Suicide, *Psychiatry Clin. North Am.* **8:**203–214.

Cohen-Sandler, R., Berman, A. L., and King, R. A., 1982, Life stress and symptomatology: Determinants of suicidal behavior in children, *J. Am. Acad. Child Psychiatry* **21:**178–187.

Deykin, E. Y., Alpert, J. J., and McNamarra, J. J., 1985, A pilot study of the effect of exposure to child abuse or neglect on adolescent suicidal behavior, *Am. J. Psychiatry* **142:**1299–1303.

Dishion, T. J., Loeber, R., Stouthamer-Loeber, M., *et al.,* 1984, Skill deficits and male adolescent delinquency, *J. Abnorm. Child Psychol.* **12:**37–54.

Dunne, E. J., McIntosh, J. L., and Dunne-Maxim, K. (eds.), 1987, *Suicide and Its Aftermath, Understanding and Counseling the Survivors,* W. W. Norton and Co., New York.

Eisenberg, L., 1980, Special article: Adolescent suicide: On taking arms against a sea of troubles, *Pediatrics Special Article* 315–320.

Farrington, D. P., 1987, Epidemiology, in: *Handbook of Juvenile Delinquency* (H. C. Quay, ed.), pp. 33–61, John Wiley & Sons, New York.

Fine, P., McIntire, M. S., and Fain, P. R., 1986, Early indicators of self-destruction in childhood and adolescence: A survey of pediatricians and psychiatrists, *Pediatrics* **77:**557–568.

Finn, P. A., 1986, Self-destructive behavior in school-age children: A hidden problem? *Pediatr. Nurs.* **12:**198–199.

Friedman, A. S., Glickman, N., and Utada, A., 1985, Does drug and alcohol use lead to failure to graduate from high school? *J. Drug Educ.* **15:**353–364.

Galambos, N. L., and Dixon, R. A., 1984, Adolescent abuse and the development of personal sense of control, *Child Abuse Neglect* **8:**285–293.

Garbarino, J., 1978, Child abuse and juvenile delinquency: The developmental impact of isolation, in: *Exploring the Relationship between Child Abuse and Delinquency* (R. J. Hunner and Y. Elder-Walker, eds.), pp. 115–127, Allanheld Osman & Co., Montclair, N.J.

Garbarino, J., and Gilliam, G., 1980, *Understanding Abusive Families*, Lexington Books, Lexington, MA.

Garfinkel, B. D. and Golombek, H., 1974, Suicide and depression in childhood and adolescence, *Canad. Med. Assoc. J.* **110:**1278–1281.

Gispert, M., Wheeler, K., Marsh, L., *et al.*, 1985, Suicidal adolescents: Factors in evaluation, *Adolescence* **20:**753–762.

Gispert, M., Davis, M. S., Marsh, L., *et al.*, 1987, Predictive factors in repeated suicide attempts by adolescents, *Hosp. Commun. Psychiatry* **38:**390–393.

Gordon, S. (ed.), 1985, *When Living Hurts*, Union of Hebrew Congregations, New York.

Gould, M. S., and Shaffer, D., 1986, The impact of suicide in television movies: Evidence of imitation, *N. Engl. J. Med.* **315:**690–694.

Greene, J. W., and Keown, M., 1986, Depression and suicide in children and adolescents, *Compr. Ther.* **12:**38–43.

Hauser, M. J., 1987, Special aspects of grief after a suicide, in: *Suicide and Its Aftermath* (E. J. Dunne, J. L. McIntosh, and K. Dunne-Maxim, eds.), pp. 57–70, W. W. Norton and Company, New York.

Hergenroeder, A. C., Kastner, L., Farrow, J. A., *et al.*, 1986, The pediatricians role in adolescent suicide, *Pediatr. Ann.* **15:**790–798.

Hodgman, C. H., 1985, Review article: Recent findings in adolescent depression and suicide. *J. Dev. Behav. Pediatr.* **6:**162–170.

Hollander, H. E., and Turner, F. D., 1985, Characteristics of incarcerated delinquents: Relationship between developmental disorders, environmental and family factors, and patterns of offense and recidism, *J. Am. Acad. Child Psychiatry* **24:**221–226.

Horton, H., and Stack, S., 1984, The effect of television on national suicide rates, *J. Soc. Psychol.* **123:**141–142.

Humphries, L. L., and Metzler, E. E., 1983, Diagnosis of depression in childhood and adolescence, *J. Ky. Med. Assoc.* September, pp. 693–696.

Johnston, L. D., Bachman, J. G., and O'Malley, P. M., 1984, *Drugs and American High School Students, 1975–1983*, National Institute on Drug Abuse, Washington, D.C., pp. 1–492.

Khan, A. U., 1987, Heterogeneity of suicidal adolescents, *J. Am. Acad. Child Adoles. Psychiatry* **26:**92–96.

Kosky, R., 1983, Childhood suicidal behavior, *J. Child Psychol. Psychiatry* **24:**457–468.

Kosky, R., Silburn, S., and Zubrick, S., 1986, Symptomatic depression and suicidal ideation. A comparative study with 628 children, *J. Nerv. Ment. Dis.* **174:**523–528.

Levine, M. D., Karniski, W. M., Palfrey, J. S., *et al.*, 1985, A study of risk factor complexes in early adolescent delinquency, *Am. J. Dis. Child.* **139:**50–56.

Lowenstein, S. R., 1985, Suicidal behavior: Recognition and intervention, *Hosp. Prac.* October 30, pp. 52–55, 58–68, 71.

Macdonald, D. I., 1986, How you can help prevent teenage alcoholism, *Contemp. Pediatr.* **3:**50–52, 55–58, 64–72.

Mack, J. E., 1985, Self-esteem and its development: An overview, in: *The Development and Sustenance of Self-Esteem in Childhood* (J. E. Mack and S. L. Ablon, eds.), pp. 1–41, International Universities Press, Inc., New York.

McGuire, D. J., and Ely, M., 1984, Childhood suicide, *Child Welfare* 63:17–26.

McIntosh, J. L., 1987, Survivor family relationships: Literature review, in: *Suicide and Its Aftermath* K. Dunne-Maxum, (ed.), pp. 73–84, W. W. Norton & Company, New York.

McIntosh, N., and Eldridge, C., 1984, Neonatal death. The neglected side of neonatal death, *Arch. Dis. Child.* **59:**585–587.

Mehrabian, A., and Weinstein, L., 1985, Temperament characteristics of suicide attempters, *J. Consult. Clin. Psychol.* **53:**544–546.

Novy, D. M., and Donohue, S., 1985, The relationship between adolescent life stress events and delinquent conduct including conduct indicating a need for supervision, *Adolescence* **20:**313–321.

Ojanlatva, A., Hammer, A. M., and Mohr, M. G., 1987, The ultimate rejection: Helping the survivors of teen suicide victims, *J. School Health* **57:**181–182.

Peck, M., 1982, Youth suicide, *Death Educ.* **6:**29–47.

Pediatrics Supplement, 1985, Sex, drugs, rock n' roll—Understanding common teenage behavior, *Pediatrics* **75:**659–712.

Penner, M. J., 1982, The role of selected health problems in the causation of juvenile delinquency, *Adolescence* **17:**347–368.

Pfeffer, C. R., 1980, Unanswered questions about childhood suicidal behavior: Perspectives for the practicing physician, *J. Dev. Behav. Pediatr.* **1:**11–14.

Pfeffer, C. R., 1981a, Suicidal behavior of children: A review with implications for research and practice, *Am. J. Psychiatry* **138:**154–159.

Pfeffer, C. R., 1981b, The family system of suicidal children, *Am. J. Psychother.* **35:**330–341.

Pfeffer, C. R., 1985a, Suicidal fantasies in normal children, *J. Nerv. Ment. Dis.* **173:**78–84.

Pfeffer, C. R., 1985b, Self-destructive behavior in children and adolescents, *Psychiatr. Clin. N. Am.* **8:**215–226.

Pfeffer, C. R. (ed.), 1986, *The Suicidal Child,* p. 77, The Guiford Press, New York.

Pfeffer, C. R., Conte, H. R., Plutchik, R., *et al.*, 1979, Suicidal behavior in latency-age children: An empirical study, *J. Am. Acad. Child Psychiatry* **18:**679–692.

Pfeffer, C. R., Solomon, G., Plutchik, R., *et al.*, 1982, Suicidal behavior in latency-age psychiatric inpatients: A replication and cross validation, *J. Am. Acad. Child Psychiatry* **21:**564–569.

Pfeffer, C. R., Plutchip, R., Mizruchi, M. S., *et al.*, 1986, Suicide behavior in child psychiatric inpatients and outpatients and nonpatients, *Am. J. Psychiatry* **143:**733–738.

Phillips, D. P., 1974, The influence of suggestion on suicide: Substantive and theoretical implications of the Werther effect, *Am. Sociol. Rev.* **39:**340–354.

Phillips, D. P., 1979, Suicide, motor vehicle fatalities, and the mass media: Evidence toward a theory of suggestion, *Am. J. Sociol.* **84:**1150–1174.

Phillips, D. P., and Carstensen, L. L., 1986, Clustering of teenage suicides after television news stories about suicide. *N. Engl. J. Med.* **315:**685–689.

Puig-Antich, J., 1984, Clinical and treatment aspects of depression in childhood and adolescence, *Pediatr. Ann.* **13:**37–40, 44–45.

Rando, T. A. (ed.), 1986, *Parental Loss of A Child,* Research Press Co., Champaign, IL.

Renshaw, D. C., 1981, Suicide in children, *Am. Fam. Physician* **24:**123–127.

Robbins, D., and Conroy, R. C., 1983, A cluster of adolescent suicide attempts: Is suicide contagious? *J. Adolesc. Health Care* **3:**253–255.

Roff, J. D., 1986, Identification of boys at high risk for delinquency, *Psychol.* **Rep. 58:**615–618.

Rosenthal, P., and Rosenthal, S., 1983, Suicide among preschoolers. Fact or fallacy? *Child. Today* **12:**21–24.

Rosenthal, P. A., Rosenthal, S., Doherty, M. B., *et al.*, 1986, Suicidal thoughts and behaviors in depressed hospitalized preschoolers, *Am. J. Psychother.* **60:**201–213.

Schoenback, V., Garrison, C., and Kaplan, B., 1984, Epidemiology of adolescent depression, *Public Health Rev.* **12:**159–189.

Schowalter, J. E., 1970, Death and the pediatric house officer, *J. Pediatr.* **76:**706–710.

Schuckit, M. A. (ed.), 1984, *Drug and Alcohol Abuse: A Clinical Guide to Diagnosis and Treatment,* 2nd ed., Plenum Press, New York.

Schwartz, R. H., Hoffman, N. G., and Jones, R., 1987, Behavioral, psychosocial and academic correlates of marijuana usage in adolescents, *Clin. Pediatr.* **26:**264–270.

Shaffer, D., 1974, Suicide in childhood and early adolescence. *J. Child Psychol. Psychiatry* **15:**275–291.

Shaffer, D., 1985, Depression and suicide in children and adolescents, in: *Child and Adolescent Psychiatry: Modern Approaches* (M. Rutter and L. Hersov, eds.), pp. 275–291, 2nd ed., Blackwell Scientific Publications, Oxford.

Shaffer, D., 1986, Developmental factors in child and adolescent suicide, in: *Depression in Young People* (M. Rutter, C. E. Izard, and P. B. Read, eds.), pp. 383–396, The Guilford Press, New York.

Shneidman, E. S., and Farbernow, N. L., 1961, *Some Facts about Suicide,* PHS Publication No. 852, U.S. Government Printing Office, Washington, D.C.

Shrier, D. K., 1981, Teenage suicide, *J. Dev. Behav. Pediatr.* **2:**155–159.

Simons, R. L., and Murphy, P. I., 1985, Sex differences in the causes of adolescent suicide ideation, *J. Youth Adolesc.* **14:**423–434.

Slaby, A. E., and McGuire, P. L., 1986, Prevention of child and adolescent suicide, *Psychiatry Lett.* **4:**65–74.

Smith, Jr., C. W., and Bope, E. T., 1986, The suicidal patient. The primary care physician's role in evaluation and treatment, *Postgrad. Med.* **79:**195–202.

Smith, K., and Crawford, S., 1986, Suicidal behavior among "normal" high school students, *Suicide Life Threat. Behav.* **16:**313–325.

Strasburger, V. C., 1985, Sex, drugs, rock 'n' roll: Are solutions possible? A commentary, *Pediatrics* (Suppl.) 704–712.

Sturner, W. Q., 1986, Adolescent suicide fatalities, *R.I. Med. J.* **69:**471–474.

Teicher, J., 1979, Suicide and suicide attempts, in: *Basic Handbook of Child Psychiatry,* Vol. 2 (J. D. Noshpitz, ed.), Basic Books, New York.

Tishler, C. L., 1981, Adolescent suicide: Prevention, practice, and treatment, in: *Feelings and Their Medical Significance,* Vol. 23, Part 1, pp. 23–26, Ross Laboratories, Columbus, Ohio.

Tishler, C. L., 1982, Adolescent suicide: Prevention practice and treatment, *Feelings and Their Medical Significance* Vol. 24, Part 2, pp. 1–4, Ross Laboratories, Columbus, Ohio.

Toolan, J. M., 1981, Depression and suicide in children: An overview, *Am. J. Psychother.* **35:**311–322.

The University of the State of New York, 1984, *Suicide among School Age Youth,* p. 1, The State Education Department, Office of General Education, Albany, NY.

Wasserman, I. M., 1984, Imitation and suicide: A re-examination of the Werther effect, *Am. Sociol. Rev.* **49:**427–434.

Weller, E. B., and Weller, R. A., 1986, Clinical aspects of childhood depression, *Pediatr. Ann.* **15:**843–847.

Yesavage, J. A., and Widrow, L., 1985, Early parental discipline and adult self-destructive acts, *J. Nerv. Ment. Dis.* **173:**74–77.

Zinkus, P. W., and Gottlieb, M. I., 1978, Learning disabilities and juvenile delinquency, *Clin. Pediatr.* **17:**775–780.

CHAPTER 10

Developmental–Behavioral Pediatrics

Past, Present, and Future

MORRIS GREEN

1. A Time of Change

Our society is undergoing rapid change. Most mothers now work outside the home. By 1990, one fourth of the children in the United States will spend part or all of their lives in one-parent families. Divorce, separation, and remarriage have become common events in the experience of children. Grandparents and other relatives are less available to provide support for young parents. Except for low-income families, in which a number of pediatric diseases regretfully continue to be overrepresented, children in the United States are physically healthier than they were in the past. The numerous infectious and nutritional problems that formerly occupied so much of the pediatrician's time do so remarkably less often today. Currently, the problems of children are more likely to be of a developmental, behavioral, social, or educational nature. Chronic illness, family crises, and health-damaging behaviors loom larger on the pediatric horizon, while our patients come from more diverse ethnic and cultural backgrounds than they did a few years ago.

In order to remain responsive to the child health needs of the times, pediatric practice must give increased attention to the psychosocial and developmental aspects of child and family life. Some practitioners, busy and reasonably satisfied with the way things are now, believe that no

MORRIS GREEN • Department of Pediatrics, Indiana University School of Medicine, and James Whitcomb Riley Hospital for Children, Indianapolis, Indiana 46223.

change in their practice is needed; others readily admit that the behavioral aspects of pediatrics holds no interest for them. A significant number, however, share the concern that their present style of practice does not allow them to be sufficiently aware of important family stresses and problems. Recognizing that behavioral, developmental, and learning problems are important parts of the new pediatric agenda, most pediatricians want to master the changes and realize their new opportunities. While some have had the training and experience required to provide such care, those who completed their residencies before the relatively recent special emphasis on the psychosocial aspects of pediatrics need additional preparation.

A generation ago, pediatric education in the "psychobiological" or "biobehavioral"—adjectives that I find more precise than "behavioral"—aspects of pediatrics was provided by child psychiatrists or by a small number of pediatricians with additional training in child psychiatry. Some of the latter retained their pediatric identities while others functioned as child psychiatrists or were perceived as such. As the psychobiological aspects of general pediatrics evolved, its data base increasingly came from such behavioral and social sciences as child development, psychology, sociology, cultural anthropology, and epidemiology. Later, as young pediatric academicians with a special interest and research competence in the field appeared, biobehavioral pediatrics assumed more responsibility for its own destiny, a future that will likely be further strengthened as a result of the current biologic revolution, especially in neurobiology, psychoimmunology, neuroendocrinology, genetics, and psychopharmacology.

The ability to integrate behavioral and developmental considerations into the care of all patients requires extensive training, experience, and a recognition that the behavioral and psychosocial aspects of child health are central to general pediatrics. Learning which problems they can manage themselves, which are best cared for collaboratively, and which should be referred to other mental health professionals is an educational process that cannot be much truncated. Psychobiological pediatrics is a highly complex aspect of child health care, one that involves not only cognitive material but also feelings—those of the physician as well as the patient. The medical student or pediatric resident can read and be lectured to about the biobehavioral aspects of pediatrics, observe optimal practice, have a notion as to what pediatricians do, and manage some patients with behavioral symptoms and problems reasonably well, but it takes long study, experience, and direct responsibility for the care of several hundred patients over many years to gain the maturity, judgment, observational competence, understanding, sense of empathy, and data base necessary to become highly competent in this area of pediatric care. Such broad competency is not acquired in a straight-line fashion; rather, it depends heavily on the individual resident's personality, life experiences, capacity, and goals.

Table 1 lists the subject matter that constitutes the scientific data base for the psychobiological aspects of pediatrics. The diagnostic and therapeutic skills of the pediatrician with a special interest in behavior and development are listed in Table 2. Utilizing referral to mental health professionals when appropriate, the well-prepared pediatrician may manage pediatric psychobiological disorders such as failure to thrive, rumination, developmental delay, breath-holding spells, temper tantrums, pica, sleep disorders, separation difficulties, phobias, conduct disorders, hyperactivity, attention deficit disorder, stealing, tics, school avoidance, school underachievement, anorexia nervosa, conversion reactions, substance abuse, enuresis, somatic complaints such as abdominal pain, headaches, fatigue and chest pain, hypochondriasis, the psychological aspects of long-term illness and handicap, depression, pregnancy, and other issues of sexuality.

The pediatrician also needs diagnostic skills that lead to referral to mental health professionals of children and adolescents with disorders such as autism, failure of maternal attachment, atypical behavior disorder, schizoid disorder, delinquency, persistent phobias, gender identity

Table 1. The Scientific Data Base

Normal growth and development
Adaptive and pathological psychosocial development
The nature of parent–child and family relationships
The relation of child care and parenting practices to families of various ethnic and cultural backgrounds
The reactions of children of various ages to illness and death
Family dynamics
The signs and symptoms of psychiatric and neurologic disorders (IDC-9 and DSM-III), particularly the psychosocial and psychosomatic disorders frequently encountered by pediatricians
Patient compliance
Psychopathology and symptom formation
The nature and significance of psychological tests to assess status, aptitude, and achievement
Developmental neurology
Opportunities for preventive intervention in primary care and at-risk families
The principles of the psychotherapeutic role of the pediatrician
The social psychology of education for healthy life-styles
Psychoneuroendocrinology
Psychopharmacology

Table 2. Pediatric Functions

The pediatric interview for data collection and psychotherapeutic purposes
A working understanding of developmental processes in childhood
Perceptivity of mental status as well as physical findings
Recognition of anxiety, depression, anger, and other feelings in parents
Developmental assessment
Use of the physical examination for reassurance and to promote the physician's relationship with the child
Achievement of a psychotherapeutic relationship with the child and parents
Counseling of families
Preparation of children for hospitalization and surgery
Recognition of the need for and skill in making an effective referral for psychiatric consultation or treatment
The ability to identify psychosocial strengths, vulnerabilities, and invulnerabilities of children and parents
Organization of parents' groups
Utilization of community resources, including those concerned with increasing parenting skills

disorders, chronic depression, child custody, placement away from home, and parental mental illness.

Although much of the content and skills of biobehavioral pediatrics can be introduced during a 3-year residency program, continuing education is as important as that for the biomedical aspects of pediatrics, perhaps even more so. Therefore, practitioners need ready access to several effective, relevant and convenient educational options, including direct supervision, courses, demonstrations, study groups, mini-fellowships, videotapes, audiotapes, seminars, books, articles, and consultations with a more experienced clinician.

Most residents choose pediatrics because they like children and want to help those who are sick. They are probably attracted initially more by the diseases of children, inpatient pediatrics, and organ-subspecialty care than by health promotion, prevention, or the behavioral and developmental aspects of child health. With further maturation and experience, they generally come to recognize and understand more fully the importance of the latter. Since they are so intertwined, competency in the biomedical aspects of child health is essential for effectiveness with the psychosocial dimensions of pediatrics. Such biologic front-loading is thus supportive rather than competitive.

This professional evolution may, however, be quickened by opportunities to work regularly with master clinicians who elegantly demonstrate in hospital, ambulatory, and office settings that skilled attention to the behavioral and developmental aspects of care can influence child and family health in a rewarding fashion. Discussions about disease,

disease processes, and treatment appropriately continue to rank highly in the interest and concern of pediatric residents, and they may be more apt to identify with teachers who are well-informed in the biomedical areas of pediatrics in addition to their special competency in the behavioral and developmental spheres.

The effectiveness of such teachers is reinforced when they are highly visible and promptly available to assist the house officer in both ordinary and difficult situations. While over time the resident or practitioner independently learns many of the basic biobehavioral pediatric skills and facts, ready access to informed supervision accelerates the process. These aspects of pediatric education are best learned when they are considered to be part of a resident's day-to-day training and experience in a variety of clinical settings; otherwise, they may be considered special or different rather than regular.

This learning process is enhanced by a departmental and hospital culture that includes attention to humanistic as well as scientific care. The former includes the establishment of constructive physician–patient relationships; pediatric interviewing that attends thoughtfully and simultaneously to the biomedical, the psychosocial, and the emotional; expertise in behavioral observation; communication skills; a data base that spans both the psychosocial and the biomedical; a scientific interest in human behavior; a focus on a child's and family's current and potential strengths as well as their vulnerabilities and problems; the encouragement of self-responsibility for health; the ability of the physician to recognize, understand, and be comfortable in dealing with his or her own as well as a patient's feelings; and the practice of interdisciplinary care. Personal qualities of the pediatrician such as graciousness, personal warmth, courtesy, and empathy contribute to psychological effectiveness. These and other characteristics of the master pediatric clinician are listed in Table 3.

The physician's ability to get a child to like, trust, and admire him and to be comfortable and friendly, to relate in a strongly positive fashion, and to identify with and assume, at least to some extent, the physician's ideas and attitudes toward health and his view of the child's symptoms and life situations offers a special therapeutic relationship. The doctor's supportive interest in carefully identifying the patient's successes, strengths, and resources in addition to his weaknesses, worries, feelings, puzzlements, and vulnerabilities helps establish a health-promoting bond among physician, parent, and child, contributes to the child's self-esteem, fosters his ability to assume an active role in the resolution or amelioration of his problem, and promotes the development of new capabilities.

Seasoned master clinicians who provide care that incorporates the

Table 3. Characteristics of a Master Clinician

Highly secure as to own medical competency
Projects personal warmth and empathy without being engulfed
Makes a long-term commitment to patients and their families—a kind of medical tenure in sickness and in health
Recognizes, understands, and is reasonably comfortable in dealing appropriately with feelings of anxiety, fear, depression, loss, denial, shame, suspicion, anger, and guilt in patients and families
Is aware of own personal reactions—anxiety, depression, anger, guilt, frustration, and feeling of failure; avoids the tendency to depersonalize patients and their families
Promotes parental participation
Has coping strategies for dealing with personal discomfort
Has the ability to deal with uncertainty
Identifies parents' and child's strengths as well as their vulnerabilities and problems
Gives the parents and child the feeling that they are understood
Establishment of constructive physician–patient relationship
Interviewing that attends thoughtfully and simultaneously to the biomedical, psychosocial, and affective
Expertise in behavioral observations
Communication skills
Psychosocial and biomedical data base
Focus on strengths as well as vulnerabilities and problems
Encourgement of self-responsibility for health
Shares the care of children with other professionals and seeks best services available
Believes own life, personal and professional, is highly meaningful
Is interested in persons and personal care as well as disease
Has well-developed professional linkages and secure personal support systems
Gracious, courteous, mature, trustworthy, and responsive
Able to have child identify with physician's attitude toward health
Is able to *care* for others

best of our scientific and humanistic traditions and who are admired for their clinical skill, scientific credibility, and scholarship serve as powerful role models for pediatric trainees. Since training in biobehavioral pediatrics involves feelings as well as facts, the faculty must provide considerable personal supervision, be physically available, and spend the time necessary to know, listen to, and advise the trainees. This kind of mentor relationship is crucially important.

2. Fashioning a New Identity

Apart from the extensive and complex scientific roots required to sustain its growth, biobehavioral pediatrics needs a clearer identity, one that signifies a distinctive body of knowledge. There comes a seminal time in the development of any academic field when one or more unifying themes emerge. By illuminating the interrelationships that exist and catalyzing new ways of thinking, such insights form the infrastructure on which conceptual advances and a larger body of knowledge are constructed. The scientific credibility, coherence, vitality, and growth of any discipline requires a theoretical base that serves to explain events, order observations, and generate new hypotheses for empirical research. Such constructs inform both the clinician and the investigator.

The current theoretical background for biobehavioral pediatrics is eclectic, derived from psychiatry and the behavioral and social sciences. Although the recombinant product of these disciplines and general pediatrics has been useful, what has been a diffuse process now requires more of a focus and individuation anchored by an integrative concept that encompasses the following:

1. Biological and behavioral considerations
2. The child, the family, and the ecology of the child and family
3. The interactions between the child, the family, and the environment
4. Facts and feelings
5. Individuals and populations
6. Patient care, teaching, and research
7. The patient and the physician
8. Prevention, health promotion, and treatment
9. Past and present pediatric practice
10. Pediatrics and other disciplines

3. Pediatrics and Adaptation

Adaptation is part of an established pediatric tradition. It is, after all, the daily role of the pediatrician to enhance a child's capacity to adapt to a variety of biological stressors, e.g., the administration of antibiotics to an infant with bacteremia helps the baby successfully cope with and overcome a possibly fatal stressor. Measles immunization offers a prospective adaptation to the measles virus, a potentially deleterious biologic insult. Insulin contributes to a child's immediate adaptation to the physiologic derangements caused by juvenile diabetes. In terms of psychosocial and developmental adaptation, parents and children experience both expected and unexpected transitions that test their coping repertoires. Pediatric services that help children and families master psychosocial stressors may well, in the future, be valued by society as much as those of a biomedical and procedural nature.

Pediatricians may help parents and children cope with a wide range of those psychosocial and developmental stressors that are increasingly part of our lives. Table 4 lists some of the stressors encountered by school-age children and adolescents. Adaptation may be (1) *prospective,* e.g., preparation of a family for an adoption, for an infant's emerging autonomy, for a child's entrance to school, for hospitalization, for surgery, for the changes initiated by puberty, or for the remarriage of a parent; (2) *concurrent,* e.g., coping with an infant with a difficult temperament, the birth of a baby with a handicap, separation, divorce, death, unemployment, suicide, homicide, accidents, sexual assault, serious illness, hospitalization, and the mother going to work outside the home; or (3) *rehabilitative,* e.g., managing the disorders and symptoms that result from maladaptation. Pediatricians are in an advantageous position to promote adaptive outcomes, prevent maladaptive sequelae, intervene early, or treat the symptoms that ensue from faulty adaptation.

Fostering constructive biomedical and psychosocial adaptive outcomes, helping introduce protective factors, and contributing to a child's or parent's coping strategies in relation to a wide range of developmental and life changes, events, and stressors is an important pediatric goal. Positive parental adaptive outcomes include self-confidence, self-esteem, and autonomy; enjoyment of parenthood; adequate family communication; maintenance of social supports; understanding child development; nurturant parent–child interactions; a good marital relationship; and comfort in seeking help for current problems and major stressors.

Positive adaptive outcomes in children include the ability to communicate well, express feelings, relate positively to others, and develop trusting relationships. Other strengths are physical fitness, personal achievement, a constructive assessment of personal capacities, good grooming, self-responsibility for health, high self-esteem, and the security of being cared for and loved.

4. The Adaptation of the Pediatrician

It is a commonsensical inference that physicians whose own psychological needs are being met may be more likely to be responsive to the psychosocial aspects of child and family health than would otherwise be the case. Some of the major professional stressors for which pediatric trainees can be prospectively prepared include caring for a critically ill or dying child; helping anxious patients and families; dealing productively with hostile, challenging, or threatening parents; making a diagnostic or therapeutic mistake; caring for a physically or sexually abused

Table 4. Stressors for School-Age Children and Adolescents

- Separation experiences that represent a major life change
  - The death or the anticipated death of a significant person—a parent, sibling, grandparent, friend, or pet
  - Parental separation, divorce, anticipated divorce, or desertion
  - Work or social commitments that limit parents' physical or psychological availability to the child
  - The child's fear of his own premature death because of the presence or the history (vulnerable child syndrome) of a life-threatening illness
  - Move of family or close friend
  - The child placed outside his family
  - An older sibling's marriage, entrance to college, military service
  - Secret fears about parents or siblings dying or having a fatal accident
- The family
  - Family illness
    - Organic illness of parents, grandparents or siblings
    - Sibling with long-term handicap
    - Emotional illness of parents, e.g., depression, affective disorder, schizophrenia, or anxiety
    - Alcoholism
    - Parental hypochondriasis
  - Marital discord
  - Family violence
  - Family criminality
  - Remarriage
  - Lack of family communication
  - Addition of another adult to the household
  - Social isolation of family
  - Parental unemployment, economic distress, poverty
  - Lack of mutuality in parent-child interactions
- The child
  - Inability to make and keep friends; lack of social skills
  - School and learning problems
  - Difficulty handling anger
  - Pressure for scholastic, athletic, or artistic performance; an "overachieving" child's fear of impending failure in academic or other competitive activity
  - Long-term illness or handicap
  - Hospitalization or surgery
  - Depression
  - Concerns about sexuality
  - Peer pressures
  - Being different: short, tall, overweight, ethnic or racial differences, physically handicapped, retarded, lack of social skills
  - Peer pressures: drugs, alcohol, sex, antisocial acts
  - Developmental transitions
  - Lack of community resources and future opportunities: educational, vocational, and social
  - Physical and sexual abuse
  - Overwhelming stressors
    - Witness to violence: homicide, suicide, war, accidents, rape, assault, terrorism
    - Natural disasters: tornados, hurricanes, fires, earthquakes, floods
    - Kidnapping, hostage

child; and working with multiproblem families. In addition to such professional stressors, physicians are commonly confronted with one or several additional personal stressors such as the death of a significant person, marital problems, divorce, the birth of a child with a handicap, and the competitive demands of being a physician, a spouse, and a parent.

In addition to introducing protective and stress-modifying practices into a training program or practice, residents and practitioners need to believe that their work is meaningful, have the capacity to define and persist in achieving their goals, and develop collegial working alliances with other disciplines. Other characteristics that contribute to mastery of stressful experiences include a willingness to turn to other persons in times of stress, the maturity to ask for help with comfort, the capability to use time efficiently, and the resiliency to withstand professional stressors. A continuing relationship with one or more mentors, skills in conflict resolution, recognition that physicians as well as patients have emotional needs, comfort in tending to personal and family needs, and high self-esteem are other strengths.

5. The Need for New Pediatric Ambulatory Care Models

The model of pediatric office practice fashioned originally in response to the nutritional and infectious disorders of infants, though appropriate in the past, does not meet present-day needs, especially in relation to behavior and development. Pediatric visits that are almost exclusively biomedical or disease oriented, advice that is largely directive, and a predominant focus on infants and toddlers rather than on the whole of childhood and adolescence does not fit well with today's child and family health agenda. The present challenge is to fashion and institutionalize new models of pediatric care that provide attention to the developmental and behavioral aspects of child health. These are time-intensive services.

Today, many pediatric practitioners wish to develop secondary or tertiary as well as general pediatric care competencies, including those concerned with the behavioral and developmental aspects of child health. Just as has been traditional for hospital services, three levels of care can be defined for ambulatory care based on (1) the length of time and the number of visits required; (2) the specialized training, experience, and competence needed; (3) the complexity of the problem; and (4) whether the pediatrician works alone or with others.

Level 1 *general pediatric care,* which may be defined as that delivered in the office by the pediatrician and the nurse or the developmental associate discussed below, encompasses health promotion, continuity care visits of children with long-term handicaps or illness, and the management of episodic disease or minor trauma. Anticipatory guidance (prospective adaptation), which constitutes a large part of pediatric health supervision, promotes the ability of parents and children to cope with expected developmental transitions. In view of the current expectation of parents for increased autonomy, self-help, and personal sufficiency, anticipatory "guidance" may be an outdated term except in the case of young or inexperienced mothers or other highly dependent parents. The promotion of parent and child adaptation offers an active rather than a passive role and an internal locus of control. The American Academy of Pediatrics publication, *Guidelines for Health Supervision,* contains health supervision packages that integrate the biomedical and psychosocial aspects of pediatric care for each scheduled visit from the prenatal period through adolescence.

Since the chief justification today for health supervision and promotion visits is the attention given to child development and behavior and to personalized teaching by the pediatrician, most of the other aspects of patient education should be addressed through alternative approaches that convey and reinforce authoritative, easily understood and relevant information and that encourage parents and children to be active on behalf of their own health.

Preparatory home study through the use of pamphlets, books, hand-outs, newsletters, and videotapes or audiocasettes by the parent and the child prior to the scheduled health supervision visit would allow the pediatrician to respond more fully to the parent's and child's questions and self-identified needs. Considerable time is available cumulatively over several visits to give appropriate attention to developmental and behavioral considerations, especially if fewer but longer level 1 sessions are scheduled. Other effective strategies include self-administered screening behavioral and developmental questionnaires and group sessions for parents and children.

As child developmental and behavioral issues receive a larger emphasis in health supervision visits, the contribution of the pediatric nurse may be supplemented by that of a possible new professional, the child development associate, who would be especially prepared in areas of child development, behavior, and parent education. If many of the questions and problems identified by the parent or child were answered by the pediatric nurse or the proposed child development associate, the pediatrician could concentrate on increasing the effectiveness of the visit.

Effective health promotion that includes attention to behavior and development must be personalized. The health promotion interview should be largely nondirective, cued to what the patient says, and include open-ended questions that help the parent or child share what is on their minds as well as direct questions about common developmental processes such as sleep or toilet training. When complemented by other educational and screening strategies, the interview serves to identify most of the behavioral and developmental issues that the parent or child are aware of and ready to explore. Those issues that can be addressed through information, clarification, advice, or reassurance are easily managed during level 1 care.

Well-functioning families usually need only this level of care, whereas dysfunctional ones require level 2 or 3 appointments. The pediatrician cannot expect to change patient behavior in any major way in such brief sessions. Because of insufficient time and consumer expectation, regular health supervision visits are inappropriate times to attempt to solve complex behavioral and developmental problems. If identified during such a visit, a return level 2 or level 3 appointment should be offered or the patient referred to a mental health professional for further care.

Level 2 care is that given by *pediatricians who have areas of special interest,* either biomedical or psychosocial, e.g., allergy, gastroenterology, child development, behavior, developmental disabilities, learning problems, or adolescent health. The percentage of time spent by pediatric practitioners in level 1 or level 2 care will vary, depending on their special competencies, the needs of the patients, and the setting in which the pediatrician works. In the future, pediatric practitioners, especially those in group practice and those who have a special interest, will likely devote additional time to level 2 care.

Pediatric level 2 care for behavioral or developmental problems may be provided (1) by the interested and prepared pediatrician; (2) jointly by a pediatrician, pediatric nurse, child development associate, social worker, and/or psychologist working part- or full-time in the physician's office; or (3) through collaboration with these and others, such as the child psychiatrist or special educator in other office, agency, school, or hospital settings. Level 2 behavioral pediatric services include counseling in relation to family crises such as death, separation, divorce, or remarriage; the care of children with long-term illness or disability; developmental delay; learning disabilities; school failure; and behavioral problems and symptoms such as failure to thrive, out-of-control toddler, a persistent sleep problem, separation problems, hyperactivity, chronic headaches, recurrent abdominal pain, and chest pain.

Level 3 care, provided by the *pediatrician with fellowship or postgraduate training,* may be given in academic settings, community or regional diagnostic and treatment centers, large group practices, and occasionally in solo practice. To pursue the clinically relevant but highly complex lines of psychobiological investigation and to extend the data base in this field, a new generation of pediatric psychobiological investigators must be developed. The research level 3 pediatrician will devote most of his time to basic research but also be available to collaborate and to consult with clinical colleagues. The consultant generalist who is competent in several areas of general pediatrics such as child development, chronic disease or handicap, behavior, adolescent health, or school problems represents another type of level 3 pediatrician. Fellowship training programs to provide the clinical and research skills needed by such master generalists require at least 3 years.

6. Looking to the Future

The pediatric office of tomorrow needs to represent a parent and child resource center with some of the following roles: (1) pediatric health promotion; (2) biomedical (acute and chronic), developmental, psychological, cognitive, and social problem management; (3) help in adapting to family crises; (4) advocacy and community information; (5) research in practice; and (6) depending on the setting, as a site for pediatric resident education.

Teaching parents and children to lead healthy lives may evolve as an increasing pediatric activity. The agenda of health promotion includes the promotion of physical activity, good nutrition, and dental health; avoidance of smoking, obesity, alcohol and other substance abuse, adolescent pregnancy, and risk-taking behaviors; coping with anticipated or unanticipated stressors; training in social skills; developing a supportive social network; and education in conflict resolution. How the pediatrician can best help children acquire and maintain such good health habits remains incompletely answered. Group sessions for parents and for adolescents and collaboration with health education programs offered by schools, hospitals, churches, civic organizations, and other social agencies offer potential ways to complement and supplement the individual practitioner's efforts.

Physicians with expertise in biobehavioral pediatrics can help children and parents identify and use their strengths and potentialities through the physician–patient relationship, patient education, behavioral therapy, crisis intervention, and the fostering of personal, family, and community supports. As part of periodic health promotion visits, the pediatrician has an open opportunity to encourage family communication, especially among high-risk groups such as those who have a child with a major handicap, working parents who are absent from the home much of the time, parents who are depressed or alcoholic, and those who head a single-parent household.

Health promotion visits also provide potentially fruitful opportunities to enhance parent–child interactions. Some parents simply need to learn how to interact positively with their children, be encouraged to enjoy and play with them, helped to understand and meet their developmental needs, and coached to contribute to their self-esteem. Parents identified during health supervision visits as not doing well, e.g., the mother who is depressed or who has no social supports, should receive prompt help. Likewise, infants and children who are not thriving developmentally, e.g., those who are apathetic, highly irritable, or at risk of abuse and neglect, require urgent intervention.

In addition to health promotion, the need for preventive, early intervention, and therapeutic services will continue. Unfulfilled potential, emotional morbidity and mortality, limitations in our present understanding of the causal connections involved, and, in many cases, a lack of effective interventions will not soon disappear. The extent to which pediatricians will respond to the opportunities to address these needs seems much more promising now than just a few years ago. Both pediatric residents and practitioners are increasingly interested in learning more about this aspect of pediatrics, the number of prepared faculty has grown, pediatric psychobiological research has begun to flourish, and the relevant literature has become extensive.

Education of the resident in psychobiological pediatrics, though much improved in recent years, needs to be further enhanced. The continuing education of the practitioner must also be greatly strengthened through close collaboration between academic departments of pediatrics and the American Academy of Pediatrics.

In the face of growing consumer demand and the pediatrician's increasing psychobiological competence, the question of remuneration for these services remains incompletely answered. In many instances, services may be billed to third-party payers or to the patients themselves; however, pediatricians must energetically articulate the case for inclusion of this aspect of care in health care plans. If services are not given by pediatricians, they will be offered for a comparable or larger fee by some other discipline less prepared to integrate the biological and the psychological. The danger and the opportunity lie not so much in the oft-stated uncertainty of remuneration as in the lack of the acceptance of psychobiological care as an important daily role of the pediatric practitioner.

Suggested Reading

Green, M., 1982, Training the pediatrician in the psychosocial aspects of child health, *Zero To Three* **2:**5–7.

Green, M., 1983, Pediatric graduate medical education: Psychosocial aspects of child and family health, in: *The Study Group on Pediatric Education,* pp. 3–10, American Academy of Pediatrics, Evanston, IL.

Green, M., 1983, Coming of age in general pediatrics, *Pediatrics* **72:**275–282.

Green, M., 1985, The adaptation of children and families: The new pediatric agenda, in: *The Psychosocial Aspects of the Family: The New Pediatrics* (M. Green, ed.), pp. 1–12, Lexington Press, Lexington, MA.

Green, M., 1985, The role of the pediatrician in the delivery of behavioral services, *J. Dev. Behav. Pediatr.* **6:**190–193.

Green, M. (ed.), 1985, *Guidelines for Health Supervision,* American Academy of Pediatrics, Elk Grove Village, IL.

Green, M., 1986, Pediatric education and the care of the person, *Pediatrics* **78:**431–437.

Green, M., 1986, Behavioral and developmental components of child health promotion: How can they be accomplished? *Pediatr. Rev.* **8:**133–141.

CHAPTER 11

Long-Range Management Strategies for Adolescents and Adults with Developmental Disabilities

JONATHAN J. HALPERT

1. Introduction

After years of struggle and controversy, a constellation of factors, including court suits, research, civil rights advocacy, and congressional mandates, have conjoined to force systems throughout the United States to move away from segregated institutional settings to community-based systems of care. This redirection has led to the development of a continuum of community-based residential programs that provide the handicapped with a living arrangement within the community. This process of deinstitutionalization theorized that handicapped individuals have an inalienable right to live in an environment that is least restrictive and that will thereby maximize their normalizing experiences.

2. Intermediate Care Facility

The intermediate care facility (ICF) is one type of residential program that has evolved from this concept of deinstitutionalization. The

JONATHAN J. HALPERT • Camelot Community Residence Program, Port Jefferson Station, New York 11776.

ICF is intended to provide a cooperative group-living arrangement, as part of the larger community, rather than a small self-contained isolated community. As such, the ICF program emphasizes the development and implementation of individualized client goals that promote independence, off-site habilitation, education, recreation, and medical services.

2.1. General Goals of an ICF

Handicapped individuals living in an ICF will, depending on their level of functioning, attend an education program 5 days a week from approximately 9:00 AM to 3:00 PM. Upon their return home, the client will engage in a variety of normalizing experiences, ranging from cleaning and cooking to daily outings within the community. Many facilities provide in-house crafts, music, and movement programs in addition to recreational outings. All of these programs and activities are generated from the theoretical base that handicapped individuals should be exposed to as many normalizing experiences as possible in order that they may reach their maximum potential. Another vital factor facilitated by placement in a community residential program is the increased ability to manage and ameliorate behavioral problems. It has been well documented that living in an institution creates a repertoire of aberrant behaviors, including self-abuse, extreme passivity, violent outbursts, and eccentric tendencies. These aberrant behaviors, which evolve from institutional life and are continually reinforced by that environment, can be more effectively managed within a community residential setting. As a result of population limits of 8 to 12 clients, the ICF personnel are more capable of dealing individually with clients and implementing behavior-management programs. In addition, many undesirable behaviors observed in the institution slowly disappear because they are no longer reinforced by the community residential setting. For example, the placing of shoes under the pillow at night for fear that they will be stolen ceases once the stealing of shoes stops. Self-stimulation and hyperactive behavior such as pacing, tearing of articles, and even self-injurious behaviors also show a decline due to increased opportunities for positive attention. Within 6 months of placement in the community setting, client growth in all areas of functioning is very significant, dramatically underscoring the devastating impact that deprivation can have on human functioning. The ICF program establishes an environment in which stimulation and opportunities to interact are available. The ICF is by no means "a magical cure." Although it cannot reverse retarded cognitive functioning, it does create an environment where maximum potential can be achieved.

2.2. Impact of an ICF on Health Care Delivery

The process of deinstitutionalization and the formation of ICF programs impacts on all aspects of the community setting but is especially pronounced within the area of medical services and is therefore of special concern to the medical community. Prior to deinstitutionalization the handicapped received both routine medical and surgical care within the institutional setting. With the emergence of ICF programs, the handicapped are now being serviced in community health settings, doctors offices, and hospital wards. In addition, because of the severity of their handicaps and their prior residential history, this population comprises high-risk patients with numerous medical problems. An example of the scope and comprehensiveness of medical contracts can be found in a study conducted at the Camelot Community Residence Program that analyzed the number of medical visits by clients in 1 year. The study revealed that in a 1-year period the number of health-related visits for each client ranged from 24 to 29, with an average of 25 visits per client. These visits included trips to virtually every type of specialist in every possible medical setting and involved routine examinations, sick visits, and emergency surgery. It is obvious that a new high-risk population has entered the medical setting and is presenting a number of practical and philosophical problems to the medical community.

On a practical level physicians are now being asked to treat and diagnose patients who may be nonverbal and unable to assist in their own diagnostic process. In addition, these patients can present some rather bizarre behaviors that can only make the diagnostic and treatment process that much more difficult. Postoperative care in the hospital setting can also present some unusual problems for physicians, nursing staff, and hospital administration. The problems range from consent signatures to maintaining intravenous tubes, including requests for 24-hour staffing by the agency and the problem of who to place in the same room with a nonverbal, acting-out handicapped patient. Despite these and many more practical considerations, experience demonstrates that handicapped clients do extremely well both in the physicians's office and in the hospital. With rare exceptions even the most severe behavior problem appears to dissipate when under medical care.

Philosophical and Ethical Considerations

Deinstitutionalization has not only forced physicians to confront a host of practical concerns in their care of the handicapped, but physicians are now increasingly confronted with a range of philosophical and ethical issues including the allocation of scarce resources, the use of heroic measures, selective nontreatment, and "do not resuscitate" orders. The 1970s and 1980s have not only witnessed the deinstitutionalization of the handicapped, but also the evolution of advanced medical technology and its associated dilemmas. Each new medical advance appears to be accompanied by a new medical dilemma. By developing new techniques to extend life, science has forced society to grapple with the issue of access to this medical care and allocation of this technology. The tension between medical advances and their restrictive application impacts on many segments of society, but as the controversy intensifies it appears that the deinstitutionalized may be the population at greatest risk. At the very moment that the handicapped have finally gained access to community medical services, there is a countermovement to limit the access of the handicapped to both advanced and ordinary life-saving treatment. [It is the supreme irony that the very movement of deinstitutionalization, which was hailed as a force enhancing the civil rights of the handicapped, has unwittingly become the vehicle that threatens to strip the handicapped of their most basic civil right, *the right to life*.] The increased visibility of the handicapped, resulting from their deinstitutionalization, has not accelerated their acceptance. Paradoxically, it has confirmed the many prejudices and negative attitudes that have always existed toward the handicapped but had remained dormant. A recent study by Wolraich and Siperstein (1986) on physicians attitudes and expectations toward the retarded demonstrate that physicians, who have had extensive contact with retarded persons, have lower expectations and choose more restrictive treatment options. The negative attitudes and prejudices toward the handicapped are not a new phenomenon but are based on the belief that the handicapped are nonpersons or subhuman.

This perspective is created by developing the belief that if a person lacks certain human features, then the person is less than human. The "human feature" argument contends that conception and birth by human parents does not automatically endow one with personhood and its accompanying rights; some other characteristic or feature must also be present in the organism. Therefore, if the person lacks such human features as intelligence, self-consciousness, or human relationships, then these persons are in fact nonhumans. Another method by which the handicapped are perceived as nonhuman is the quality of life argument or the person's potential for meaningful existence. Under this approach, an arbitrary set of criteria is established to define what gives life value, meaning, and worth. If it is deemed that the person does meet this criteria, then the life is deemed to have value and the person is human. If the person fails to meet the quality of life criteria because of severe disability, then it is deemed that the life has no value and the person is judged nonhuman. It is within this context that a handicapped person may be denied enteral nutrition, ordinary life-saving measures, or placed on a plan of supportive care. A review of the legal and medical literature details how this perspective and rationalization has been applied to deny the handicapped access to the technology.

In 1973, it was reported in the *New England Journal of Medicine* that 43 infants in the special care nursery of the Yale New Haven Hospital were denied life-saving surgery that would have been performed if the babies had been normal (Duff and Campbell, 1973). The rationale for this action was that these infants faced lives that were devoid of "meaningful humanhood."

In Indiana in 1982, using the same rationale, an infant with Down's syndrome was put in a side room and starved to death over the course of 6 days (Gustafson, 1982). The infant became nationally known by the name "Baby Doe." These infants did not require life-sustaining measures, that is, measures to prolong life; rather, they merely required life-saving measures. They were also denied these services because of the belief that their lives were less than human and therefore not worth preserving. In 1979, a California Court of Appeals refused to order physicians to surgically repair the heart of Phillip Becker, a 13-year-old boy with Down's syndrome (Lusthaus, 1985). The decision ruled against the state government and favored the boy's parents who were deliberately allowing their child to die by withholding life-saving surgery. Their argument was that Phillip led a life devoid of those qualities that give it human dignity. In July 1983, a task force of the Minnesota Board of Aging found that three categories of patients should have the option to die: the terminally ill, the mentally incapacitated, and those who cannot interact in a meaningful way with their environment (Lusthaus, 1985). In January 1985, the New Jersey Supreme Court ruled that tube feeding could be withheld from terminally ill patients if the guardian was satisfied that the burdens of living outweighed the benefits (Schwartz, 1986). Bard and Fletcher (1968) wrote in their article on the newborn child's right to die that a father who placed his son with Down's syndrome in an institution with instructions that no medical care be given should feel no guilt. "Guilt" was considered only relevant when wrong is done to a person and "a Down's is not a person" (Lusthaus, 1985). Finally, Governor Lamm of Colorado in 1984 testified that "the terminally ill have a duty to die and get out of the way" (Schwartz, 1986).

This review of the literature not only demonstrates the negative attitudes held toward the handicapped, but delineates the pervasiveness of these attitudes. The literature points out that these attitudes are not limited to one segment of society, but cut across all groups, including physicians, scientists, theologians, politicians, and even parents of the handicapped.

The experiences at Camelot substantiate the literature. In one example, an anesthetist asked a surgeon who was about to perform routine surgery, "Why are you bothering?" In a second instance where a client needed a total hip replacement, a physician again asked, "Why are we using our time for this?" In a third example, a "do not resuscitate" order was automatically initiated for a client who was admitted for kidney failure. Although it is true that the review of the literature and our experience do *not* represent the attitudes of the vast majority of physicians, it is apparent that the phenomena of advanced medical technology, deinstitutionalization, and negative attitudes toward the handicapped are on a collision course. This will continue to intensify as the current deinstitutionalized population grows older and their medical problems become more acute.

2.3. Resolving Problems: Possible Strategies

Unfortunately, it is easier to identify the problem than the solution. Pontification by advocates of the handicapped serves only to convert the converted. Formation of Hospital ethics committees merely shifts the responsibility from individuals to groups without really providing any solutions. Intervention and regulation by government agencies only adds an additional source of controversy by raising the issue of the role of government in personal family decisions. The United States government's involvement in the New York "Baby Jane Doe" case is an example of how government involvement tends to deflect the issue rather than resolve the problem. In this case the Federal government attempted to force parents of a handicapped child to consent to medical intervention on behalf of the child. The resolution of this conflict can only be addressed by refocusing the debate away from the issues of quality of life and the humanity of the handicapped. The advocates of the handicapped cannot prove that the handicapped are "human" any more than the proponents of quality of life can certify that the handicapped are nonhuman. No objective criteria exist defining what is "human" and what is "quality of life" and therefore any attempt by either party to prove their point is an exercise in futility. If advocates of the handicapped are going to secure protection for the deinstitutionalized, then they must abandon this debate and develop rationales that are objective, free from religious moral preachings, and not dependent on pity.

One approach to resolving this dilemma is to stop using pejorative labels such as "handicapped," "elderly," and "terminally ill" when trying to reach decisions about equal or limited access to treatment. The handicapped as well as others represent an extremely heterogeneous group of individuals. Therefore, it is vital to emphasize that each case involves one unique individual who is not representative of the entire group. We must resist using one label to describe many people, but rather look at the many characteristics that constitute one person. The case of whether Phillip Becker should have life-saving surgery is then perceived entirely differently than ruling for or against a Down's syndrome boy. This point is best illustrated from the current tragedy that is taking place in Africa. One article on one starving child has far greater impact on our senses than numerous articles relating how thousands of Africans are starving. We do not relate well to a global label; we do identify with distinct individuals.

3. Summary

If the phenomenon of deinstitutionalization is to achieve its goal of optimal normalization, then it must guarantee that the handicapped will have equal access to advanced medical technology and the ultimate right to life. This can be accomplished if advocates of the handicapped refocus their approach and present arguments that are free from emotional and religious preachings. Such an emphasis would accelerate the needed understanding and sensitivity with the medical establishment. The twentieth century answered the challenge of space exploration, atomic energy, and unprecedented medical advancements. The challenge of the twenty-first century will be to learn how to intelligently apply these new advances. This is the challenge that awaits all concerned persons. This chapter represents one small step toward meeting this challenge.

References

Bard, B., Fletcher, J., 1968, The right to die, *Atlantic Monthly,* April, 59–64.

Duff, A., and Campbell, A., 1973, Moral and ethical dilemmas in the special-care nursery, *N. Engl. J. Med.* April, **289:**890–894.

Gustafson, J. M., 1982, Mongolism, parental desires, and the right to life, *Perspect. Biol. Med.* **16:**529–557.

Lusthaus, E., 1985, Involuntary euthanasia and current attempts to define persons with mental retardation as less than human, *Ment. Retard.* **23:**148–154.

Schwartz, William, 1986, Health care rationing explored, *Hospitals* **58** (17):15–17.
Wolraich, M., and G. Siperstein, 1986, Physicians and other professionals' expectations and prognoses for mentally retarded individuals, *American Journal of Mental Deficiency* **91**:244–249.

Suggested Reading

Engelhardt, T., 1984, Allocating scarce medical resources and the availability of organ transplantation, *N Engl. J. Med.* **311**:66–74.
Fletcher, J., 1972, Indicators of humanhood: A tentative profile of man, *Hastings Cent. Rep.* **2**:1–4.
Fletcher, J., 1974, Four indicators of humanhood—The enquiry matures, *Hastings Cent. Rep.* **4**:4–7.
Lehr, D., and Brown, F., 1985, Perspectives on severely multiply handicapped, *Am. J. Ment. Defic.* **89**:140–145.
Paris, J., and Fletcher, A., 1983, Infant Doe regulations and the absolute requirement to use nourishment and fluids for the dying infant, *Law Med. Health Care* **33**:210–213.
President's Commission for the Study of Ethical Problems in Medicine and Biomedical and Behavioral Research, 1983, *Deciding to Forgo Life-Sustaining Treatment,* Washington, DC.
Richards, G., 1984, Technology costs and rationing issues, *Hospitals* **58**:80–86.
Robertson, J., 1975, Involuntary euthanasia of defective newborns: A legal analysis, *Stanford Law Rev.* **27**:213–269.
Robertson, J., 1982, Legal aspects of withholding medical treatment from handicapped children, in: *Legal and Ethical Aspects of Treating Critically and Terminally Ill Patients* (A. E. Doudera and J. D. Peters, eds.), pp. 97–99, AUPHA Press, Ann Arbor, MI.
Rosner, R., 1983, Allocation of scarce medical resources, *NY State J. Med.* **83**:353–358.
Weir, R., 1984, *Selective Nontreatment of Handicapped Newborns,* Oxford University Press, New York.

CHAPTER 12

Right Brain, Left Brain

Practical Implications from Infancy to Adulthood

MARCEL KINSBOURNE

1. Introduction

Individuals equal in overall tested intelligence score quite diversely on mental tests that tap different domains of intellect. Some have related the resulting test profiles to variations in neuropsychological function, specifically better function in some cerebral "modules" than others. The best-known and the simplest of these formulations is the right–left brain dichotomy. It implies that there are two "packages" of intellect, each with its own hemispheric base, uncorrelated with the other (or even reciprocal).

Right–left brain theory has made a public impact because of the implication that the latent right-hemispheric abilities of many children failing in school are being ignored and left unexploited. Advocates urge that the curriculum be revised to accommodate right-hemisphere styles of thinking. These claims have outstripped knowledge, for reasons such as:

- The nature of right-hemisphere specialization is misconstrued to include value-laden attributions (holistic, empathic, creative) that lack an empirical basis
- Reciprocity between left and right hemisphere remains unproved
- Evidence for a relationship between hemispheric skills and hemispheric style is ambiguous

MARCEL KINSBOURNE • Department of Behavioral Neurology, Eunice Kennedy Shriver Center for Mental Retardation, Brandeis University, Waltham, Massachusetts 02154; and Harvard Medical School, Boston, Massachusetts 02115.

- Evidence that poor readers have an inherent right-hemisphere style (rather than a nonverbal preference secondary to their reading problem) is lacking

On these grounds, the remedial educator would do best to ignore right-brain "sales pitches" in favor of continuing empirical efforts to develop better instruction for those whose learning requirements cannot be met by traditional instruction.

Individuals differ not only in what they know, but in how readily they learn it. Whereas exposure to information and availability of instruction are necessary conditions for learning, they are not sufficient. A minimal brain-based aptitude is also required, and aptitude is to a considerable extent domain specific. Individuals with comparable overall intelligence (as reflected, for instance, in IQ) differ widely in their ability to grasp and retain information and master operations in different academic or conceptual fields. Such aptitude differential is presumably based on differences in the extent to which various parts of the brain are efficient in executing their specialized functions.

Ultimately, then, a neuropsychological account must become available for a wide range of individual differences in learning. This will reflect variation in some performance-limiting attribute of the neural substrate: number of neurons, synaptic density, pattern of interconnection between neurons, differential distribution of excitatory and inhibitory cells, degree of ascending activation (or more likely, attributes of the existence of which no one is as yet aware). At any rate, such obvious variables such as overall brain bulk or relative size of different cerebral regions have clarified neither brain power nor brain organization. Certainly, the more intelligent individuals do not possess the bigger brains. Even when brain organization differs radically between groups, as between right-handers and left-handers (Hicks and Kinsbourne, 1976), no reliable differences in cerebral configuration is known to distinguish one pattern of cerebral representation of function from another. Thus far, efforts to refer individual differences in attitude and preference (cognitive style) to the brain have concentrated on identifying behavioral distinctions that plausibly index the extent to which a person tends to use one part or another of his brain. Such efforts rely first on the known facts of cerebral specialization and subsequently on extrapolations from them. They have been organized usually around the actual or presumed differences in the specializations of the two cerebral hemispheres.

The principle of differential hemisphere specialization has been well established (Kinsbourne, 1978). Whether a single dichotomized formulation is capable of capturing the essence of hemispheric complementarity is more contentious (Bradshaw and Nettleton, 1982). Still in greater doubt is the implication for functions, if any, of hemispheric specialization. Nonright-handers are well known to have far less-circumscribed specialized ("dedicated") cerebral territories than right-handers. Yet their cognitive abilities are not thought to be inferior (Hardyck *et al.*, 1976). What are we to make of the fact that the cerebrum comes in two anatomically distinct (albeit highly interconnected) packages? Does this mean that people are constrained to use each hemisphere as a whole or even to choose between hemispheres when deploying their processing capabilities in everyday life? An immediate reaction must be that human behavioral control cannot be thought of as so crudely constrained. There are obviously many, not just two, patterns of cognitive skill. Intact people are obviously not confined to a single processing style applied routinely in all situations. Nevertheless, a scientifically approachable issue remains: Are there observable biases in behavior that represent a *tendency* to draw upon functions within a hemisphere rather than between, when either is appropriate for the task at hand, and to favor the processing mode of one hemisphere rather than the other in situations admitting of either approach? If such were the case, two opportunities might open up to enhance human behavioral potential: (1) to adapt learning environments to the individual's hemisphere of preference, thus maximizing the amount learned; and (2) to teach the individual to increase the use of his nonpreferred style where that happens to be the superior route to problem-solving.

The notion that there are vast resources of untapped intellect in the human brain is pervasive and persistent. Frequently this concept is embodied in such statements as "Use your head: Start to develop the other 80% of your brain" (in blunt advertising, "a thought-provoking guide" to how to do this). Who first said that we only use a small part of our brain, and how he (she) knew, I cannot tell (and even why *number* of brain cells is usually nominated as critical is unclear). However, the appeal of the popular right-brain/left-brain theorizing surely resides not only in the need to understand how people might approach the same issue differently. The theory also more subtly suggests that we could double our brain power if we used both hemispheres rather than only one (Galin, 1976), a prospect with an obvious, if superficial, attraction.

Educators have not been slow to capitalize on this concept. For example, a Bulgarian psychiatrist turned educator has devised a system called "Suggestopedia" (Lozanov, 1978) in which the whole brain is allegedly activated at once and locked up human resources are liberated. As for the unconscious mind, relaxation induced by Baroque music leaves it alert. Business men have not been far behind (Mintzberg, 1976).

This type of claim pervades popular science magazines (*Brain–Mind Bulletin, Science Digest*) and popular self-help books (Edwards, 1979; Blakeslee, 1980; Ferguson, 1980) to the point of reflecting a rampant dichotomania (Harris, 1988).

A major purpose of this chapter is to provide a framework for appraising hemisphere-dichotomizing claims. Such appraisals cannot be done empirically, as reliable outcome statistics never appear to be available. Therefore, the plausibility of claims has to be judged on the basis of what is known about how the brain works.

2. Two Intelligences

The current interests in right- and left-brain intelligences arise from the convergence of two long-evolving concepts that (1) there are (at least) two patterns of intellect, rather than a single dimension, along which all humans could potentially be arranged in order of mental brightness; and (2) the brain is a functionally differentiated, even "modular," device, with different areas, or at least its two cerebral hemispheres, functioning largely independently, if not reciprocally. Correspondingly, the "hemisphericity theory" (Bogen *et al.,* 1972) makes parallel claims at the level of behavior and the level of brain; claims that can be formulated either in terms of a weak theory or of a strong theory. The weak theory proposes that there are two types of intellect, essentially verbal versus visuospatial, corresponding to the better development of (or greater control of) behavior by one or the other hemisphere (Bakan, 1971). These differences dictate occupational choices (Galin and Ornstein, 1974). On the other hand, the strong version alleges that the balance between these hemispheric packages, beyond mental power, determines strategic preference, i.e., the deployment of a verbal left-hemispheric or visuospatial right-hemispheric style when a problem is open to either approach or even when the alternate approach would have been more appropriate and more likely to succeed.

In its challenge to the traditional unitary views of intellect and the brain, the hemisphericity theory makes a rather conservative appeal to multiplicity of intellects. If there is more than one pattern of intellect, there are no more than two. If one or the other hemisphere may be in the ascendant, no such rivalry is made available to patterns of problem solving that might be represented separately within one half of the brain. As for strategies of problem solving, there are as many as but not more than two. If it is right to accommodate more than one way of going about solving problems, it is also sufficient if two contrasting strategies have been accommodated.

A commonsense approach to "multiple intelligences" (Gardner, 1983), if accepted in preference to the appealing notion that there is such a thing as general intelligence ("g") or reasoning power that cuts across modalities of thinking and domains of the intellect (Jensen, 1984), is not apt to stop at postulating just two such domains packaged within alternative hemispheres. Individual variation in human aptitude surely calls for as many as seven (Gardner, 1983), nine (U.S. Dept. of Labor, 1982), or 120 (Guilford, 1959) intellects. Yet the hemisphericity theory need not contest that there can be variants within each of the two major domains. It need merely to assert, and demonstrate, that the two major domains are overriding. It would be sufficient to document the selective activation and use of one hemisphere (as a whole) at a time in problem-solving situations without denying that much if not most of the time humans use both sides and many parts of their brains. It would be damaging to this approach if within-subject correlations are as great or greater for faculties represented contralateral to each other as for faculties represented within a hemisphere.

This chapter will first briefly consider current understanding of the factorial structure of the intellect, then of the localization of function in the cerebral hemispheres. The data will then be applied to the question of coherence in power and coherence in style of mental operations, reasonably characterized in terms of the known specializations of the two sides of the brain.

3. The Structure of the Intellect

One cannot deny that some individuals have better reasoning ability than others and that some people have different intellectual strengths and aptitudes. One approach to these differences might make an overarching functional principle of general intelligence. Variations in efficiency in applying general intelligence to issues in different modalities or modes may be a matter of detail to which differences in environmental opportunity and motivation substantially contribute. A contrasting approach would deny the existence of such a factor as generalized reasoning ability, postulating that each type of intellect (be there 2 or 100 types) has its own reasoning power and the excellence of which can vary independently of that of other intellects represented within that individual. A third point of view would combine these positions. Specific domains, notably language, have their own problem-solving facilities. Independent of that and not localized in the same way, but diffusely represented, is a general problem-solving ability that is supramodal in its approach to anything that is novel and not immediately understood.

For present purposes, the differential merits of these three positions need not be explored, so as to avoid a controversy that is thoroughly unresolved. Hemisphericity is a variant of the second approach. It does not accommodate reasoning power as a general principle, but must explain the existence of differential levels of understanding that cut across domains by appealing to separate mental facilities that, for whatever biological reason, have differentiated more finely in one individual than another. However, when the other two perspectives are considered, a major limitation of the hemisphericity theory is noted. By insisting on lateral differentiation, it implicitly ignores differentiation in the anterior–posterior dimension.

The various modules, or categorically limited forms of intelligence, are most reminiscent of the type of specializations that have been demonstrated for the posterior, parietooccipital, and superior temporal parts of the cerebrum. Ability to reason, to accommodate to novelty, flexibly shift mental set, and weigh simultaneously multiple perspectives on an issue conform much better to what little is so far understood of the functions of the prefrontal and anterior temporal lobes. In response, the hemisphericity theory would argue that the front temporal systems themselves are laterally differentiated, each bestowing reasoning power on the specializations of its own side. To some extent, this appears to be so (Petrides and Milner, 1982), but the communalities between the right and left prefrontal area have so far more impressed the investigator than the differences between them (Luria, 1973).

4. Specializations of the Hemispheres

Once, in the 1940s, it was appreciated that the right hemisphere had its specializations complementary to the well-known verbal specialization of the left hemisphere (Paterson and Zangwill, 1944), it became open season on overarching formulations of the contributions of the two hemispheres to mental life. Although there is no biologically founded reason to assume that the specializations of one cerebral hemisphere will share a single underlying principle, this assumption has only rarely been mentioned (DeRenzi, 1982), let alone been questioned. It is usually taken for granted in the context of numerous dichotomies offered to characterize the presumed differences between the guiding principles of function of each hemisphere. Beyond the early verbal–nonverbal formulations, left-hemisphere function has been described as successive, analytic, and serial. On the other hand, the right-hemisphere's guiding principle has been termed simultaneous, synthetic or holistic, or parallel. Other formulations include digital versus analog and a propensity for left-sided automatization versus right-sided orientation to novelty. Taking a more biological view, I have stressed the approach tendencies of the left and withdrawal tendencies of the right hemisphere (Kinsbourne, 1978), and more recently the control by the left hemisphere of ongoing behavior versus the arrest of ongoing behavior by the right (Kinsbourne, 1988).

Each of these formulations probably captures some aspect of the truth. Each formulation, however, also overemphasizes the degree to which the functional specialization of the hemispheres can truly be taken to be disparate. Differentiation is most pronounced in the verbal domain and even there it is really in the speech output function that lateralization is thought to be absolute. The right hemisphere is not only thought to have a significant role in the comprehension of relational concepts verbally expressed, as well as verbal humor (Gardner *et al.*, 1975), but it is known to have major compensatory potential relative to left-hemisphere damage particularly with respect to input aspects of language function (Code, 1987). It appears that if the pattern of functioning of the right hemisphere is in some fundamental way different than that of the left, as it has been alleged (Semmes, 1968), this does not preclude the right hemisphere in certain pathological circumstances from programming language behavior (and language development) of a type that is indistinguishable from the normal left-hemisphere-based activity in its general characteristics (although it has been asserted that there are certain syntactic formulations of which the right hemisphere does not become capable) (Dennis and Kohn, 1975).

Fortunately, for present purposes a decision between rival formulations of hemisphere specialization need not be made, because when hemispheric styles are considered, they come in two types of formulation only. One is simply a verbal versus nonverbal (e.g., visuospatial) strategy. The other is a set of distinctions between hemispheric styles that are generally not based on empirical findings. Rather, the distinctions are based on the surplus meaning of terms that have been used legitimately in more mundane connotations; distinctions between an allegedly *left-hemisphere style* that is concrete, detail-oriented, and materialistic and a *right-hemisphere style* that is more abstract, intuitive, and spiritual. No evidence for any such distinctions exists. For instance, when patients sustain major damage to one hemisphere, they do not experience the expected personality change in the direction attributed to the other. By and large these attributions evolved from the old and primitive verbal–nonverbal distinction on the assumption that what is not verbal is likely to be ineffable. In fact, those cognitive specializations that have been demonstrated for the right hemisphere (face recognition, judgment of the orientation of lines, map reading) are no more spiritual or amenable to expansion than are the classical verbal functions. Nevertheless, some support for the notion of "hemisphericity" has been mustered by use of the paradigms that appear to index the selective activation of a particular hemisphere in the act of problem solving. Such paradigms are usually behavioral, though some psychophysiological studies have also been performed.

5. Is a Hemisphere Used as a Whole?

Implicit throughout the hemisphericity debate is an assumption that is rarely specifically addressed; that is, when one part of a hemisphere is used, for some specialized purpose, essentially the whole of that hemisphere is deployed for action. As an extension of this concept, it is sometimes suggested and taken for granted that the opposite hemisphere is actually suppressed. What evidence can be mustered to support these concepts?

Classical connectionistic neuropsychological theory (Geschwind, 1965) makes no provision for this phenomenon. It essentially relies on private lines of communication between specialized cerebral loci ("centers"). Any neural area not included in the relevant "channel" is irrelevant, whether it is anatomically close or distant, ipsilateral or contralateral. This static model is too limited to serve as a basis for investigating cognitive preference (cognitive style). However, the private unidirectional communication channels of the connectionists are not apparent in the cortical neuronal network and continuity rather than disparity characterizes the cortical mantle (Pribram, 1971). Recently developed methodologies for imaging event-related cerebral activity suggest a wide ranging of cortical involvement, even in specific tasks for which discrete cerebral specialization is usually assumed.

How can one reconcile the massive evidence for selective cognitive deficits arising from discrete limited cerebral lesions with documented widespread cerebral activation while such activities are carried out? It appears that focally represented cerebral "generators" initiate the appropriate pattern of neuronal firing but engage wide areas of "neuronal computational space" in the activity in question. There is certainly ample evidence that if one part of a hemisphere is engaged in processing, other ipsilateral areas manifest their concurrent activation in an observable fashion. Laterality phenomena can therefore be interpreted in terms of relative hemisphere balance (Kinsbourne, 1970), a concept of direct relevance to the issues of hemisphericity.

6. Hemisphere Styles

Differential hemisphere styles can be demonstrated either by a between- or a within-subject experimental design. Between subjects, one could attempt to demonstrate subgroups that tend to rely on one or the other hemisphere when performing a particular task. Within subjects, one may demonstrate differences in the way the person undertakes a task, depending on the use of manipulations that favor selective activation of one or the other hemisphere.

Various methods attempt to determine whether subjects use one or the other hemisphere more for a given task. Thus they look for interindividual differences in hemisphere usage, making inferences from evidence of greater activation or alerting of one rather than the other hemisphere based on a laterality paradigm (Kinsbourne, 1970). The behavioral methods are divided into the widely used (1) dichotic and hemifield viewing paradigms (looking for differences in a degree or direction of any ear or field advantage), and (2) lateral-orienting paradigms (looking for relationships between style of performance and differential hemisphere activation as inferred from lateral shifts of attention). Arndt and Berger (1978), in a visual laterality study, suggested that lawyers and potters tend to activate the left and the right hemisphere, respectively, more of the time.

In the case of dichotic listening paradigms, the right-ear and right-field advantage with verbal input is relatively robust. There has been little success in demonstrating deviations from this pattern, except in pathological populations such as the language disordered, who usually fail to show the expected asymmetries. Some research has attempted to demonstrate that there are differences in results depending on the language used by the subjects. Studies have been conducted of laterality performance by the Navajo Indians, both in their own language and in English. One study reported that Navajo speakers obtain a left-ear advantage for verbal input in their language (Scott *et al.*, 1979). This finding was predicted from (1) a consideration of the Navajo language and (2) mentality as being concrete and holistic (as allegedly is the Navajo cast of mind). However, McKeever (1981) failed to confirm this. The study is open to the criticism that the Navajo speakers in McKeever's study were somewhat assimilated to the more common English/American way of proceeding. Studies of English speakers of various types have failed to reveal any reversal of the right-ear advantage for verbal material. Arguments with respect to the degree of a rightward laterality bias are complicated by the fact that (1) this measure is quite variable in general populations; (2) irregularly subject to age and gender effects; and (3) seriously confounded by such variables as aptitude and task difficulty. A more promising approach would seem to derive from use of the alternate type of paradigm in which hemispheric orienting is inferred from lateral attentional shifts.

When subjects engage in a task for which one hemisphere is specialized, it has been possible to show that they tend to shift head and eyes in a direction away from the side of the hemisphere in use. Thus right-handers, when considering the answer to verbal questions, tend to turn their head and eyes to the right (Kinsbourne, 1972; Gur *et al.*, 1975a). When engaged in visuospatial thought, the lateral shift is more in the leftward direction. Conversely, when subjects turn their head and eyes to the right, there is evidence that their ability to perform verbal task such as verbal memory is enhanced relative to head turn in the opposite direction (Lempert and Kinsbourne, 1982).

Day (1964) was the first to observe that people tend to have a characteristic direction of lateral gaze while considering the answer to questions susceptible of either visual or spatial resolution. He subtyped individuals into "right-movers" and "left-movers" and attributed divergent styles on a variety of dimensions to them. A considerable literature base has subsequently resulted. In general this concept attributes to right-movers a more detailed, analytic, and material approach to problems, an obsessive and externalizing style, the choice of occupations in verbal, intellectual fields, and subjects for study including the physical sciences and mathematics. In contrast, left-movers are thought to be more holistic in their approaches, have a more hysterical and internalizing style, be more likely to engage in the arts and literature, and to gravitate toward the humanities in college (Parrott, 1984). Students may tend to sit at the left side of the classroom when analytic topics are being discussed and at the right side when the issues are more artistic and integrated (Gur *et al.*, 1975b). There is some empirical support for the prediction that left-movers are superior on visuospatial tasks (Otteson, 1980; Swinnen, 1984; Hiscock and MacKay, 1985).

A striking example of disinhibited theorizing is neurolinguistic programming. This doctrine proposes that direction of gaze reveals the modality of information intake: visual, upward; auditory, horizontal; tactile, downward (Bandler and Grinder, 1975, 1979). Experimental tests fail to confirm these claims (Peffel and Gross, 1985; Farmer *et al.*, 1985). Like much of right-brain/left-brain theory, this extrapolation from scientific fact loses contact with empirical evidence.

Drake (1984) has applied the approach of using "induced lateral orientation" to demonstrate within-subject differences in personality characteristics. He has reported that undergraduates, when questioned while their heads and eyes are turned rightward, will tend to be more optimistic about themselves, derogatory of others, and firm in their existing belief than when they look and turn toward the left. In the latter posture, they appear to be more open to new concepts and disconfirmatory ("counterattitudinal") arguments. Several studies have also suggested that emotional information when presented from the left side of space is more appreciated, has a greater effect on the subjects' arousal systems, and is more likely to be internalized than the same input coming from the right side of space (Kinsbourne and Bemporad, 1984). If confirmed, these findings suggest that each hemisphere has its own set of priorities with respect to the interpretation of the same type of information. Certain findings from study of callosally sectioned ("split-brain") patients can be similarly interpreted (Gazzaniga, 1986). It remains an open question whether the differences elicited from each of the two disconnected hemispheres in reaction represent different evaluation of the same information or differential hemispheric sensitivity to particular aspects of incoming stimuli.

In the realm of psychophysiology, several studies have been performed that scrutinize electrophysiological indices of hemisphere arousal as they might differentiate, for instance, different occupational groups. The results have been inconclusive (Dumas and Morgan, 1975; Ornstein and Galin, 1976).

Finally, questionnaires have been used to determine profiles of subjects' preference using questions intended to tap preferences indicative of right versus left hemisphericity. The validity of these instruments remains to be established. This is a difficult task, as other measures of hemisphericity that might be used as standards are themselves short on validity. A further reason for caution derives from the low correlations between different questionnaire measures of the same construct (Payne and Evans, 1987).

7. Hemispheric Profiles of Mental Abilities

A more direct way of ascertaining the predominance of right- and left-hemisphere function would seem to be to administer neuropsychological tests thought to be differentially sensitive to the participation of each hemisphere. Certainly, within the general population, people vary widely in the relative balance of their left- and right-hemispheric skills, and this appears to have impact on occupational choices (Gordon *et al.*, 1982; Harpaz, 1983, Gordon and Krontz, 1984). At its extremes, between-hemisphere discrepancy in mental skills is thought to relate to, and possibly explain, such contrasting selective problems as dyslexia (Gordon, 1980) and "nonverbal learning disability" (Badian, 1985). The fact that the profile of intellectual abilities varies widely across people within a comparable level of general intelligence is hardly new and there is no reason to assume that the divergent patterns fall neatly into two (hemispheric) domains. An important question is whether differences in intellectual profile have anything to do with preferential utilization of one or the other hemisphere, or whether they simply reflect the extent to which each hemisphere has developed sophistication in its own specialization independent of each development of the opposite side. Various questionnaires have been designed, attempting to probe for subject's preference in terms of what is taken to be hemispheric style (Torrance *et al.*, 1977; Torrance and Mourad, 1979). The data have not shown a significant correlation with neuropsychometric profiles intended to delineate the relative efficiency of right- and left-hemisphere functioning (Knolle *et al.*, 1987), but this is not a universal finding (Zenhausern *et al.*, 1981). In essence, there is no evidence that subjects fail in tasks proper to a particular hemisphere because of maladaptive propensity to overutilize the other; that is, to extend its use beyond its proper domain. Were it the case, this latter possibility would have a major implication for educational remediation.

Instead, in so far as a pathological group exhibits hemisphericity, this is probably secondary to weakness in the functioning of the nonpreferred hemisphere. Caplan and Kinsbourne (1981) assessed verbal versus spatial preference in normal and reading-disabled children. Briefly, the preponderance of verbal over nonverbal preference increased with increasing age, was greater in females at a given age, and was lower in backward than normal readers (Caplan and Kinsbourne, 1982). It appears that those children who had the greater verbal facility (as a correlate of age, gender, or learning ability states) were more apt to resort to a verbal means for problem solving.

Further cause to doubt the relevance of hemisphericity indices for programming education has been provided (Brog, 1985; Bender, 1987). The history and current status of "right-brain training" has been reviewed comprehensively by Harris (1988).

Nevertheless, some suggestions have been made that "dominance training" could help in achieving educational objectives. Whereas early attempts (Delacato, 1959) were theoretically primitive and ill-documented in their outcome (Cohen *et al.*, 1970), recent work by Bakker and his colleagues (1985) has reviewed interest in this practical possibility. They attempt to identify children whose reading disorder is due to the too-exclusive use of one hemisphere. They then present the child with visual–verbal material projected to the other hemisphere in an attempt to redress the hypothesized imbalance. Some preliminary findings suggest encouraging results of such training (Bakker and Vinke, 1985).

8. Summary

In conclusion, the view that a trait preference for use of one hemisphere for tasks that could be processed by either (or both) accounts for major individual differences in learning ability has generated a rich experimental literature but few consensual conclusions. Faced with what appears to be relentless neuroanatomy, the student of learning cannot help but be captivated by the possibility that simple and noninvasive behavioral maneuvers could enhance abilities thought "genetic" and presumably limited by considerations of neuronal circuitry. A dynamic view of brain function must and should encourage attempts to modify brain function. With the advent of dynamic neuroimaging techniques, we can expect such efforts to be based on a much more powerful diagnostic base in the future, so that the currently unsettled question of their validity can be answered once and for all.

References

Arndt, S., and Berger, D., 1978, Cognitive mode and asymmetry in cerebral functioning, *Cortex* **14:**78–86.

Badian, N. A., 1985, Dyscalculia and nonverbal disorders of learning, in: *Progress in Learning Disabilities* (H. Mykelbust, ed.), pp. 235–264, Grune & Stratton, New York.

Bakan, P., 1971, The eyes have it, *Psychol. Today* **96:**64–67.

Bakker, D. J., and Vinke, J., 1985, Effects of hemisphere-specific stimulation on brain activity and reading in dyslexics, *J. Clin. Exp. Neuropsychol.* **7:**505–525.

Bandler, R., and Grinder, J., 1975, *The Structure of Magic,* Science and Behavior Books, New York.

Bandler, R., and Grinder, J., 1979, *Frogs into Princes; Neurolinguistic Programming,* Real People Press, Motab, UT.

Bender, W. N., 1987, Inferred brain hemispheric preference and behavior of learning disabled students, *Percept. Mot. Skills* **64:**521–522.

Blakeslee, T. R., 1980, *The Right Brain: A New Understanding of the Unconscious Mind and Its Creative Powers,* Anchor Press/Doubleday, Garden City, NY.

Bogen, J. E., Dezure, R., Tenhouten, W. D., *et al.,* 1972, The other side of the brain: IV. The A/P ratio. *Bull. Los Angeles Neurol. Soc.* **37:**49–61.

Bradshaw, J. L., and Nettleton, N. C., 1982, The nature of hemispheric specialization in man, *Behav. Brain Sci.* **4:**51–63.

Brog, M. J., 1985, Hemisphericity, locus of control, and grade point average among middle and high school boys and girls, *Percept. Mot. Skills* **60:**39–45.

Caplan, B., and Kinsbourne, M., 1981, Cerebral lateralization preferred cognitive mode, and reading ability in normal children, *Brain Lang.* **14:**349–370.

Caplan, B., and Kinsbourne, M., 1982, Cognitive style and dichotic asymmetries of disabled readers, *Cortex* **32:**177–228.

Code, C., 1987, *Language, Aphasia and the Right Hemisphere,* Wiley, New York.

Cohen, H. J., Birch, H. G., and Taft, L. T., 1970, Some considerations for evaluating the Doman–Delacato "patterning" method, *Pediatrics* **45:**302–314.

Day, M. E., 1964, An eye movement phenomenon relating to attention, thought and anxiety, *Percept. Mot. Skills* **19:**443–446.

Delacato, C. H., 1959, *Neurological Organization and Reading,* Charles C. Thomas, Springfield, IL.

Dennis, M., and Kohn, B., 1975, Comprehension of syntax in infantile hemiplegics after cerebral hemidecortication: Left hemisphere superiority, *Brain Lang.* **2:**472–482.

DeRenzi, E., 1982, *Disorders of Space Exploration and Cognition,* Wiley, New York.

Drake, R., 1984, Lateral asymmetry of personal optimism, *J. Res. Pers.* **18:**497–507.

Dumas, K., and Morgan, A., 1975, EEG asymmetry as a function of occupation, task and task difficulty, *Neuropsychologia* **13:**279–288.

Edwards, B., 1979, *Drawing on the Right Side of the Brain. A Course in Enhancing Creativity and Artistic Confidence,* Tarcher, Los Angeles.

Farmer, A., Rooney, R., and Cunningham, J. R., 1985, Hypothesized eye movements of neurolinguistic programming: A statistical artifact, *Percept. Mot. Skills* **61:**717–718.

Ferguson, M., 1980, *The Aquarian Conspiracy: Personal and Social Transformation in the 1980s,* Tarcher, Los Angeles.

Galin, D., 1976, Educating both halves of the brain, *Child. Educ.* **53:**17–20.

Galin, D., and Ornstein, R., 1974, Individual differences in cognitive style. I. Reflective eye movements, *Neuropsychologia* **12:**367–376.

Gardner, H., 1983, *Frames of Mind: The Theory of Multiple Intelligences,* Basic Books, New York.

Gardner, H., Lang, P. K., Flamm, L., *et al.,* 1975, Comprehension and appreciation of humor in brain-damaged patients, *Brain* **98:**399–412.

Gazzaniga, M., 1986, *The Social Brain: Discovering the Networks of the Mind,* Basic Books, New York.

Geschwind, N., 1965, Disconnection syndromes in animals and man, *Brain* **88:**237–294, 585–644.

Gordon, H. W., 1980, Cognitive asymmetry in dyslexic families, *Neuropsychologia* **18:**645–656.

Gordon, H. W., and Krontz, K., 1984, *Cognitive Asymmetry and Occupations: Computer Programmers, Students and Bank Personnel,* Office of Naval Research Technical Report 09-84-03, Chesapeake, Maryland.

Gordon, H. W., Silverberg-Shalev, R., and Czernilas, J., 1982, Hemispheric asymmetry in fighter and helicopter pilots, *Acta Psychol.* **52:**33–40.

Guilford, J. P., 1959, *Personality,* McGraw-Hill, New York.

Gur, R. E., Gur, R. C., and Harris, L. J., 1975a, Cerebral activation, as measured by subjects' lateral eye movements, is influenced by experimenter location, *Neuropsychologia* **13:**35–44.

Gur, R. E., Gur, R. C., and Marshalek, B., 1975b, Classroom seating and functional brain asymmetry, *J. Educ. Psychol.* **67:**151–153.

Hardyck, C., Petrinovitch, L., and Goldman, R., 1976, Left-handedness and cognitive deficit, *Cortex* **12:**266–279.

Harpaz, I., 1983, Asymmetry of cognitive functioning as a possible predictor for vocational counseling and personnel classification, *J. Vocat. Behav.* **23:**305–317.

Harris, L. J., 1988, Right-brain training: Some reflections on the application of research on cerebral hemisphere specialization, in: *The Developmental Implications of Cerebral Lateralization* (D. Molfese and S. Segalowitz, eds.), pp. 202–235, Gulford Press, New York.

Hicks, R. E., and Kinsbourne, M., 1976, On the genesis of human handedness: A review, *J. Mol. Behav.* **8:**257–266.

Hiscock, M., and MacKay, D., 1985, Neuropsychological approaches to the study of individual differences, in: *Methodological and Statistical Advances in the Study of Individual Differences* (C. Reynolds and V. Willson, eds.), pp. 117–176, Plenum Press, New York.

Jensen, A. R., 1984, Test validity: g versus the specificity doctrine, *J. Soc. Biol. Struct.* **7:**93–118.

Kinsbourne, M., 1970, The cerebral basis of lateral asymmetries in attention, *Acta Psychol.* **33:**193–201.

Kinsbourne, M., 1972, Eye and head turning indicates cerebral lateralization, *Science* **176:**539–541.

Kinsbourne, M., 1978, Biological determinants of functional bisymmetry and asymmetry, in: *Asymmetrical Function of the Brain* (M. Kinsbourne, ed.), pp. 3–13, Cambridge University Press, Cambridge, UK.

Kinsbourne, M., 1988, Hemisphere interactions in depression: Methods and theory, in: *Cerebral Hemisphere Function in Depression* (M. Kinsbourne, ed.), pp. 133–162, American Psychiatric Association, Washington, D.C.

Kinsbourne, M., and Bemporad, B., 1984, Lateralization of emotion: A model and the evidence, in: *The Psychobiology of Affective Development* (N. Fox and R. J. Davidson, eds.), pp. 259–292, Erlbaum, Hillsdale, NJ.

Knolle, L., Gordon, H. W., and Gwany, D., 1987, Relationships between performance and preference measures of cognitive laterality, *Psychol. Rep.* **61:**215–223.

Lempert, H., and Kinsbourne, M., 1982, Effect of laterality of orientation on verbal memory, *Neuropsychologia* **20:**211–214.

Lozanov, G., 1978, *Suggestology and Outlines of Suggestopedy,* Gordon and Breach, New York.

Luria, A. R., 1973, *The Working Brain,* Penguin Books, New York.

McKeever, W. F., 1981, Evidence against the hypothesis of right hemisphere language dominance in the Native American Navajo, *Neuropsychologia* **19:**595–598.

Mintzberg, H., 1976, Planning on the left side and managing on the right, *Harvard Bus. Rev.* **54:**49–58.

Ornstein, R., and Galin, D., 1976, Physiological studies of consciousness, in: *Symposium on Consciousness* (P. Lee, R. Ornstein, D. Galin, A. Deikman and C. Tart, eds.), Viking Press, New York.

Otteson, J. P., 1980, Stylistic and personality correlates of lateral eye movements: A factor-analytic study, *Percept. Mot. Skills* **50:**995–1010.

Parrot, C. A., 1984, Personality characteristics associated with lateral eye-movement patterns, *Percept. Mot. Skills* **58:**867–874.

Paterson, A., and Zangwill, O. L., 1944, Disorders of visual space perception associated with lesions of the right cerebral hemisphere, *Brain* **67:**331–358.

Payne, D. A., and Evans, K. A., 1987, Interrelationships among three measures of preference for cognitive style based on hemisphere specialization theory, *Percept. Mot. Skills* **63:**19–25.

Petrides, M., and Milner, B., 1982, Deficits on subject-ordered tasks after frontal and temporal-lobe lesions in man, *Neuropsychologia* **20:**249–262.

Peffel, S. A., and Gross, H. J., 1985, Neurolinguistic programming: A test of the eye-movement hypothesis, *Percept. Mot. Skills* **61:**1262.

Pribram, K. H., 1971, *Languages of the Brain,* Prentice-Hall, Englewood Cliffs, NJ.

Scott, S., Hynd, G., and Hunt, L., *et al.,* 1979, Cerebral speech lateralization in the native American Navajo, *Neuropsychologia* **17:**89–92.

Semmes, J., 1968, Hemispheric specialization: A possible clue to mechanism, *Neuropsychologia* **6:**11–62.

Swinnen, S., 1984, Some evidence for the hemisphere asymmetry model of lateral eye movements, *Percept. Mot. Skills* **58:**79–88.

Torrance, E. P., and Mourad, S., 1979, Role of hemisphericity in performance on selected measures of creativity, *Gifted Child Q.* **23:**44–45.

Torrance, E. P., Reynolds, C. R., Riegel, T., *et al.,* 1977, Your style of learning and thinking, Forms A and B: Preliminary norms, abbreviated notes, scoring keys and selected references, *Gifted Child Q.* **21:**563–573.

United States Department of Labor, 1982, *Manual for the USES General Aptitude Test Battery,* U.S. Employment Service, Washington, D.C.

Zenhausern, R., Nataro, J., and Schiano, P., 1981, The interaction of hemispheric preference, laterality and sex in the perception of emotional tone and verbal context, *Int. J. Neurosci.* **13:**121–126.

CHAPTER 13

Enhancing Pediatric Compliance in Primary Care

JUDITH R. MATHEWS
AND EDWARD R. CHRISTOPHERSEN

1. Introduction

As pediatric health care has expanded to include not only the treatment of disease but also the prevention of disease and disability, the effectiveness of health care depends on medical compliance by parents and their children. Numerous studies have documented the problem of noncompliance with regimens for the treatment of acute illnesses (Bergman and Werner, 1963; Charney *et al.*, 1967), for chronic diseases (Gordis *et al.*, 1969; Lund *et al.*, 1964), and for preventive strategies to protect and promote child health (Reisinger *et al.*, 1981). Medical compliance (Dunbar and Stunkard, 1979; Haynes *et al.*, 1979; Rapoff and Christophersen, 1982a) and *parental* compliance (Mathews and Christophersen, 1988; Rapoff and Christophersen, 1982a,b) have been reviewed in the literature. This chapter will be devoted to a brief review of the literature on *children's* compliance with medical procedures and regimens. The goal is to provide the busy pediatrician with a summary of strategies that have been shown to produce the most beneficial effects on compliance.

JUDITH R. MATHEWS • Department of Behavioral Pediatrics, University of Kansas Medical Center, Kansas City, Kansas 66103. **EDWARD R. CHRISTOPHERSEN** • Department of Behavioral Pediatrics, The Children's Mercy Hospital, Kansas City, Missouri 64108.

2. Child and Adolescent Compliance

2.1. Compliance with Medical Procedures

Compliance with medical procedures is directly related to the child's age. Children younger than 6 or 7 years tend to exhibit more physical resistance, particularly if the procedure is painful (Jay and Elliott, 1983; Katz *et al.*, 1980). At very young ages, children are more likely to generalize their fears across settings and people, sometimes resulting in overall resistance to all procedures and personnel (Traughber and Cataldo, 1983). As children get older, they are better able to discriminate between invasive and noninvasive occurrences. In addition, older children are more likely to be under better instructional control, to be influenced by peer and adult expectations of compliance, and to have developed some sort of coping strategies (Baron and Galizio, 1983; Ross and Ross, 1984). The manner in which instructions are delivered may influence a child's compliance. Baron and Galizio (1983) suggest that instructions can control behavior, particularly if the child has been reinforced for compliance to instructions in the past. Instructions are most effective if detail is kept to a minimum.

Parents have a direct effect on their child's compliance with medical procedures. They act as a model of appropriate or inappropriate behavior (Jay and Elliott, 1983). In 4- to 10-year-olds undergoing venipuncture, Gross *et al.* (1983) found that while there was no difference in resistance or aggression, there was significantly more crying in children whose mothers were present. Shaw and Routh (1982) also reported more negative behavior in children whose mothers were present during immunizations. Gross *et al.* (1983) suggested that increased negative behavior in children whose parents are present may not be a function of modeling inappropriate behavior. They speculated that most children have learned to identify their parents as a potential means of escape from aversive events. When parents do not protect their children from unpleasant procedures, it may be that the children react to this change in their parents' pattern of behavior by resisting the procedure. Thus, if parents are present when their child is undergoing an unpleasant or aversive procedure, it must be with the understanding that the parents will not interfere with the procedure and will not be supportive of disruptive or inappropriate behavior from their child.

Similarly, professionals can influence a child's compliance. Hyson *et al.* (1982) looked at the doctor–patient relationship in preschoolers undergoing routine check-ups and concluded that children responded most positively to a physician's "warmth" (defined as close physical proximity, verbal expressions of empathy, and hugs or gifts at the end of the appointment). In another study, Weinstein (1982a) reported that children engaged in fewer "fear behaviors" (i.e., crying, physical resistance, screaming, whimpering, protest, and expressions of hurt or discomfort) if the physician used precise and immediate directions, positive reinforcement of specific behaviors, physical touch, and frequent queries to determine if the child was experiencing pain. In contrast, coercion, coaxing, put-downs, and stopping treatment to manage behavior resulted in increased fear behaviors. In a subsequent study, the authors noted a circular response pattern, where doctors responded to child fear behaviors with the very responses that evoked increased fear behaviors (Weinstein *et al.,* 1982b). They concluded that providers must be aware of their own behavior and how it affects the behavior of their patients.

2.2. Noncompliance with Medical Regimens

Parents are usually responsible for implementing regimens with younger children. It is not surprising that children with general behavior problems at home are less likely to receive medical regimens as prescribed (Firestone, 1982). Parents of diabetics have attributed their children's noncompliance to various social pressures, personality characteristics, and temporary physical conditions (Allen *et al.,* 1983). Children with increased responsibility for their regimens appeared to cope better. However, those who gave their own injections tended to have poorer control, presumably because of (1) inadequate knowledge of the regimen or (2) other activities were more enjoyable. Additional factors making noncompliance more likely are regimens that result in physical discomfort (Rapoff *et al.,* 1985) and that are long-term and initiated at an older age (Litt and Cuskey, 1981). In another study with diabetic children at a summer camp, 33% reported falsifying their urine tests in order to gain access to increased activity or sweets or to avoid being punished (Simonds, 1979). Rapoff *et al.* (1984) surveyed parents of children with juvenile rheumatoid arthritis to ascertain the frequency and types of compliance problems they encountered. They reported that children had the most negative reaction (i.e., crying, complaining, and noncompliance) to range-of-motion exercises, splint-wearing, and medication (in that order). They suggest that higher noncompliance to exercises is related to the pain or discomfort resulting from following the regimen.

Adolescents tend to have higher rates of noncompliance with regimens than younger children (Litt and Cuskey, 1980). This may well be due to a changing role in assuming responsibility for their own regimen

(Sallis, 1985). In addition, Litt *et al.* (1982) found that diabetic adolescents who had difficulty resisting peer pressure and who had been diabetic for a longer time were more noncompliant. Barnard *et al.* (1987) suggest that a major factor contributing to adolescent noncompliance may be inaccurate knowledge of their illness or regimen. They noted that 92% had inadequate knowledge of their illness, 90% tested their blood and/or urine inaccurately, 85% timed their insulin injections incorrectly, and 79% had inadequate nutritional information. Studies of compliant adolescents revealed that their families had had more experience with illness and were more supportive than families of noncompliant adolescents (Litt and Cuskey, 1980). In addition, compliant adolescents had more responsibility for their regimen (Litt *et al.*, 1982), but did better if supervised by a professional (Litt and Cuskey, 1980).

3. Strategies for Enhancing Child and Adolescent Compliance

Physicians can serve a crucial role in enhancing compliance. In attempting to improve compliance, it is important to examine how environmental factors affect the childrens' and adolescents' compliance and then to manipulate those factors that may interfere with following medical directions.

3.1. Improving Compliance with Medical Procedures

Young age is a strong predictor of noncompliance (Gross *et al.*, 1983). It is therefore important for physicians to adapt their explanations and directions accordingly. The inability of younger children to think in abstractions (Christophersen, 1986) necessitates short and concrete explanations about the child's illness or impending procedures (Steward and Steward, 1981). For example, peer modeling and rehearsal have been shown to improve compliance (Stokes and Kennedy, 1980). The use of filmed (Melamed and Siegel, 1975) and live peer models (Stokes and Kennedy, 1980) has successfully decreased uncooperative behavior during dental procedures and hospitalization. Melamed *et al.* (1982) suggested that increased compliance may be a function of exposure to the specific modeling. Based on extensive research examining such factors as specific peer model characteristics, age of the child, and length of time between exposure to the model and the actual procedure, Melamed *et al.* (1982) concluded that the same film cannot be used with children of different ages and different medical experiences. Research also demonstrates that even though peer modeling helps the first time that a child undergoes a procedure, the use of modeling for subsequent procedures can actually contribute to undesirable behavior on the child's part.

With very young children, two apparently contradictory approaches may be needed, depending on the circumstance. During medical procedures, it may be desirable to teach the child to generalize from one setting to another and from one person to another (e.g., from inpatient to outpatient clinics). This can be accomplished by teaching the child in several locations with several different personnel or by intentionally being inconsistent with instructions and rewards (Stokes and Baer, 1977). For very young children, however, such inconsistencies may lead to learned helplessness or suppression of all behavior (Maier and Seligman, 1976); consequently it may be more appropriate to provide an extremely consistent environment so that the child can discriminate between invasive and noninvasive interactions. Once children have adapted to the procedure, they then can be taught systematically to comply in new situations and with new people. Positive interaction with medical personnel, at times when procedures are not performed, is essential to prevent the child from always associating personnel with aversive procedures (Traughber and Cataldo, 1983). Although older children are not as likely to overgeneralize, it is important to make sure that information about procedures be kept simple and at a level consistent with their cognitive development.

In an interesting case study, a 17-month-old burned child's crying had generalized to approach by any hospital staff (Shorkey and Taylor, 1973). A different color gown was worn by the staff and the room lighting was changed for social interactions and invasive procedures. As a result, there was a decrease in crying during social times, while there was understandably no change in crying during medical treatments. This study implies that careful arrangement of the environment can help to prevent the generalization of the aversiveness of some procedures to the entire hospital experience. Adaptation of this approach could include undergoing invasive medical procedures only in the treatment room when the nurse is wearing a gown of a particular color. Once the child has adapted to a procedure, he/she can be systematically taught to comply in new situations and with new people.

Surprisingly, few children report using any kind of coping strategy when dealing with pain (Ross and Ross, 1984). Distraction was among the most frequently mentioned approaches. While distraction has an intuitive appeal, its effectiveness has not been systematically investigated with children. Distraction had been shown to be effective in reducing crying during painful burn procedures, when combined with positive reinforcement and planned ignoring (Kelley *et al.*, 1984). Another study revealed more compliance during hospitalization in children who (1) learned to use distraction in combination with relaxation and comforting self-talk and (2) viewed a filmed model, in contrast to children who learned a single coping strategy or who were given simple information about their upcoming surgery (Peterson and Shigetomi, 1981).

In laboratory pain tests with adults, McCaul and Malott (1984) reported that distraction appeared to be most effective if the procedure was not severe or did not last a long time. In another study, it was found that some adults prefer to monitor every aspect of a medical procedure and do *not* want to be distracted (Miller, 1980). Further study is needed to explore how children cope with painful procedures and how distraction can be used effectively.

Children who are hospitalized may feel that they have no control in this unfamiliar environment (Cataldo *et al.*, 1982). In addition, they have moved from a fairly predictable home environment to one filled with new (and often unpleasant) experiences, occurring in what may appear to the child to be an organized manner. Children who lose a sense of control and predictability may react by withdrawing into a depressed state or may become aggressive (Cataldo *et al.*, 1982). It is important, therefore, to provide as much structure and order for the child as possible. Informing children immediately prior to procedures and offering explanations and expectations consistent with their developmental level can help to provide a more predictable environment. In addition, while many medical decisions cannot be made by children, they can participate in small ways that provide a sense of some control. For example, children can choose where they take their medication or whether they use a straw or drink directly from a cup. Some children prefer to lie down when an intravenous line is being started, while others prefer to sit up. In addition, in the authors' experience, giving a child one chance to comply with a procedure before being physically restrained (even if the child has a past history of noncompliance) gives the child an opportunity to learn self-control. However, physicians should place a short, clearly defined time limit before restraining a child and proceeding with a minimum of reprimanding or negative attention. Repeated delays of procedures in response to noncompliance may result in an increased likelihood of noncompliance in the future.

Physicians should explore routinely the child's behavior at home, as well as management strategies utilized by the parents. For example, if parents report that they have difficulties with bedtime, eating, aggression, general noncompliance, or high activity level, the provider may recommend they read about child management strategies (e.g., Christophersen, 1988). In more severe cases parents may be referred for professional counseling. It is not surprising that children with general behavior problems at home are less likely to receive the prescribed regimens (Firestone, 1982; Kaplan *et al.,* 1985). Early identification and treatment of problems of this nature may well prevent excessive noncompliance, if hospitalization or medical treatment becomes necessary. If the child presents with behavior problems (independent of any medical procedures), then the professional may want to treat behavioral noncompliance before treating the medical noncompliance. This strategy may remove the potential confound of behavioral and medical noncompliance.

Child compliance can be greatly improved by teaching the child to comply consistently with adult instruction (Baron and Galizio, 1983). One interesting report (Hedberg and Schlong, 1973) noted that when school-aged children were simply given the instruction not to faint, both fainting and disruptive behavior decreased while they were being inoculated. Parent-training research has demonstrated that clear, concise instructions can be effective in increasing compliance in the home (Roberts *et al.,* 1978), particularly if eye contact precedes an instruction (Hamlet *et al.,* 1984). Table 1 provides an example of a protocol used in our clinic for teaching parents to give clear instructions in order to improve compliance.

Gearing instructions to the developmental level of the child must also be considered; that is, complicated instructions are ineffective in changing young children's behavior (Roberts, 1984). In order to achieve instructional control in the classroom, Etzel and LeBlanc (1979) suggest that four environmental components be examined: "(1) the motivational system; (2) the possible presence of child responses that are incompatible with learning; (3) the presence of prerequisite skills; and (4) the effectiveness of teacher instructions, feedback, and other environmental stimuli in the learning environment" (pp. 363–364). Furthermore, they suggest that instructions are most effective if detail is kept to a minimum. While intended for an educational setting, these suggestions might be useful in a medical environment.

Once the provider has obtained consistent compliant behavior from a family, then simple behavioral strategies, such as those detailed in Table 2 may be all that is needed in order to obtain medical compliance.

Table 3 describes the steps that Blount *et al.* (1984) used in teaching children to accept pills. They taught the children to swallow tiny cake sprinkles and then slowly increased the candy size until the candy ap-

Table 1. Teaching Your Child to Follow Instructions: Guidelines for Parents[a]

Parents frequently have problems getting their children to follow instructions. Your child's compliance can improve if you follow the suggestions given below.

A. Giving instructions or commands
   1. Get your child's attention when giving a direction. Say the child's name and request that he/she look at you (for example, "Bob, look at me")
   2. Thank the child when he/she has complied by looking at you
   3. Give the child a simple command ("Please shut the door")

   Things to remember
   - Be realistic. Give your child instructions that you know he/she is *physically* and *developmentally* capable of following
   - Be direct. ("Joey, please put your shoes in the closet" "Open the door") Avoid questions that imply choice when there really is no choice ("Won't you go to your room?" or "Don't you want to go downstairs?")
   - Be specific. "Put your bear in the toy box." Take off your shoes." Avoid abstractions: "*Be careful*" or "Get *ready* to go"
   - Give one instruction at a time and allow your child 5 seconds to begin to obey. Do not repeat the same instruction a second time
   - Avoid interrupting your child's attempt to comply by giving a second command while he/she is working on the first command
   - *Avoid giving your child a command unless you are prepared to use time-out for not minding*

B. When your child obeys
   1. When your child *begins* to comply, praise and encourage him/her so he/she will continue the desired behavior
   2. Thank the child immediately for following the direction ("Thank you for putting your bear in the toy box, Joey")
   3. Kids love hugs and pats, so be sure to touch your child as well as praise his/her behavior

C. If your child does not begin to obey within 5 seconds
   1. Put him/her in time-out immediately (see time-out handout)
   2. Be careful not to unintentionally give your child attention for not obeying or for behaving unacceptably
   3. After time-out, require that your child complete the requested task. This will give him/her a chance to receive attention when he/she obeys, and will teach him/her that you are serious when you give a command

[a]Linda V. Ross, Stephen G. Glasscock, and Edward R. Christophersen, 1985, University of Kansas Medical Center.

proximated the capsule size. Subsequently, placebo capsules were introduced. An important component of the training program is to frequently reinforce the child for each step in the program.

Mathews and Grantmyre (1985) also improved a 2-year-old child's compliance with radiation therapy by teaching her the necessary components slowly and in small, graded steps. They determined that the three most difficult components of the procedure were (1) lying still for up to

Table 2. Some Tips for Giving Medication[a]

A. Getting ready
Give medication at the same time every day; work the times into your routine and post reminders (e.g., if giving them at mealtimes, post a reminder or recording sheet on the refrigerator)

B. Giving medication
1. Ask your child to come get the medication.
2. Give him/her small amounts of medication at a time, followed with sips of a chaser of the child's choice (water, milk, pop—check with your doctor to make sure the particular liquid can be given with the specific meds)
3. *Praise* taking medication without a fuss
4. *Use time-out immediately* (see separate handout) for
   - Refusals or stalling; avoid coaxing
   - Spitting out medication
   - Vomiting

   (discuss with your doctor whether or not to give medication again if he/she vomits or spits out the medication)
5. *Ignore* gagging.

C. Afterwards
1. *If he/she has taken medication without any problem*
   - Praise and give a hug
   - Give 15 minutes specialtime to do an activity of his/her choice with the parents
2. *If he/she has had to go to time-out*
   - Praise taking the medication
   - Do not comment on time-out or noncompliance
3. *If you have repeated problems with refusals or vomiting, consult your physician*

[a]Judith R. Mathews, Linda V. Ross, and Edward R. Christophersen, 1987, University of Kansas Medical Center.

2 minutes, (2) being separated from her mother, and (3) having the equipment positioned above her. Consequently, they first taught the child to lie still on a platform outside of the treatment room for progressively longer periods of time. The authors then faded the mother's presence while maintaining the mother's verbal contact with a microphone. Finally, they practiced in the treatment room with the machinery. One interesting observation was that tears in the eyes always preceded noncompliant behavior. Consequently, they were able to avoid noncompliance by using a verbal reprimand for tears in the child's eyes.

The physical arrangement of the environment may be important in determining a child's compliance. For example, Swallow *et al.* (1975) reported that children undergoing a dental procedure show less "anxiety" if they were first interviewed in a neutral room and then treated in a "modified surgery" room (i.e., one in which all apparatus and instruments were kept out of sight). Anecdotally, Beales (1983) reported that exposure to instruments with younger children on a burn unit and the

Table 3. Teaching Pill-Swallowing[a,b]

A. Model for your child the steps in swallowing a pill
   1. Place pill on the back of the tongue
   2. Keep the tongue flat
   3. Take liquid into the mouth
   4. Tilt the head backwards slightly
   5. Swallow

B. Gradually increase the size of the pill in the following order
   1. Oblong, multicolored "sprinkle" used for cake decoration
   2. Spherical, silver cake decoration
   3. Round, multicolored candy (0.3 cm × 0.7 cm diameter)
   4. Red licorice "whip" cut to 1-cm length
   5. Capsule-shaped candy, multicolored, sold as "Tic Tacs" or "Dynamints"
   6. Vitamin (red, enteric coated): consult with physician and do not exceed recommended daily dose
   7. Normal-sized capsule: child's actual pills

[a]Adapted from Blount (1984).
[b]Judith R. Mathews, Linda V. Ross, & Edward R. Christophersen, 1987, University of Kansas Medical Center.

sight of the wound with all ages increased children's report of pain. It was not reported if pain behavior was also correlated with increased noncompliance, although an association between pain complaints and noncompliance has been documented elsewhere (Varni *et al.,* 1980).

As discussed previously parental presence may result in increased crying (Gross *et al.,* 1983). However, whether parents should be present during procedures has yet to be established. Parental participation may serve an important function for parents, who themselves may feel helpless in a hospital setting. For parents who wish to participate in their child's medical care, specific instruction and feedback should be provided regarding their appropriate behavior during the course of various procedures. If parents prefer not to be present, their wishes should be accommodated. If parents will be required to continue the treatment at home, however, slow and systematic exposure of the parent to the treatment protocol will be necessary. Parental expressions of anxiety regarding medical procedures are an indicator that professionals should provide information about the illness, procedure, and the parent's specific role. Table 4 outlines examples of suggestions useful for parents in helping their children during medical procedures. Reading material regarding preparation of children for doctor's appointments or hospitalization (e.g., Kellerman, 1981) may also be appropriate.

In summary, instructions to the child should be brief and clear, geared to his/her developmental level, and home behavior problems

Table 4. Coping with Fears about Medical Procedures and Doctor Visits: Guidelines for Parents[a]

General guidelines

1. Parents can model appropriate coping behaviors. Show your child how you cope with fears (not just tell them)
2. *Do not* use medical procedures as a threat of punishment (e.g., "If you don't behave, the doctor will give you a shot")
3. Give accurate explanations about medical procedures. Give as much information as your child requests and that you can supply. Ask the doctor or nurse to explain things to you and your child if you have questions
4. Answer questions about "hurts" honestly. It does hurt, but it doesn't last long, etc.
5. Prepare your child for what will happen and how to cope. Use some or all of the specific strategies listed below
6. Give your child positive feedback for cooperation (such as praise), and ignore minor disruptive behavior. In cases of more serious disruptive behavior, a brief "time-out" period may be necessary. It's important that the child not be allowed to avoid the test or procedure completely

Specific guidelines

The following are three specific methods to reduce anxiety and pain associated with medical procedures. These have been used to prepare children for surgery, bone marrow aspirations, and blood sticks. There are spaces for you and your child to list things he/she may find helpful.

A. Relaxation

One of the simplest ways of minimizing fear and anxiety is to relax the muscles in the body. It is difficult to feel very scared inside if the muscles outside are completely relaxed.

A quick and easy way of helping a child's muscles to relax is to have him/her stretch the muscles in the arms and legs until they are relaxed. This is done by tensing the muscles (for 5 seconds) and then allowing them to go completely limp.

It is best to practice this with the child lying down. You can practice this with your child by following these steps:

1. Eyes lightly closed (not too tight, this creates tension)
2. Take three *slow* deep breaths (not too fast or the child will hyperventilate). Remind your child to think the word "calm" or "relax" to himself/herself as he/she breathes.
3. Tense the arms and legs (make a fist with both hands, tightened legs and point toes up), hold for 5 seconds and then relax all muscles at once (letting them go completely limp)
4. Repeat this tense/relax cycle 3 to 5 times minimum
5. Practice this with your child at least once a day. In some cases tensing is not appropriate. When in doubt ask your doctor.

B. Imagination

This method uses the child's ability to "make believe" to control fear or pain temporarily. It is a well-known fact that fear or pain is experienced differently in dissimilar situations. For example, most people have experienced going to a movie or a restaurant with a headache and forgetting all about the headache until the movie or dinner is over. Or take the case of a small cut on the finger. If you cut yourself while

(continued)

Table 4. *(Continued)*

rushing through the grocery store to make some last minute purchases, would you notice it as much as if you cut your finger in the middle of a long, boring meeting? We tend to forget pain or anxiety if something more interesting or absorbing is going on. This principle of distraction can be very useful to children when they are afraid.

The first step of this technique is for you and your child to select something to imagine. It is best to select a scene or activity that is happy, clear in your child's mind, and interesting and/or peaceful. It is better, for example to use the scene of lying on the beach rather than riding on a bucking bronco. You want the scene to bring out feelings that are the opposite of fear—peaceful, quiet feelings or fun activities. Try to describe the scene in a clear and soothing voice.

Once you and your child have selected an appropriate scene to imagine, work on all aspects of the picture. If the imagining is to distract the child, it must be real to him/her. Help your child describe and imagine how the scene looks, what colors and textures are present. Help him/her imagine how it feels to be there, how warm or cool it is, whether a breeze is blowing, and so on. Even imagining smells and sounds helps to complete the picture. The steps to practice are as follows

1. Lie down, eyes shut lightly
2. Body relaxed. Follow relaxation instructions
3. Imagine a clear picture of the favorite place or event
   Describe the sights, feelings, sounds, smells, or anything else to help the picture be more clear and real
4. Practice this with your child until he/she can easily imagine the scene. Then practice once a day

C. Self-talk

There are many comforting things you may wish to say to your child when he/she is anxious or upset. It is often helpful if the child can think (or "say to himself/herself") comforting thoughts. The following are simple messages which your child can tell himself/herself whenever he/she feels afraid or hurt. You can help your child practice them by saying each of them aloud with him/her twice, then requesting him/her to think them one by one himself/herself as you say them aloud. Finally, have him/her say them to himself/herself while you say nothing. You can repeat and have your child think the following things after you say them:

"I will feel better in a little while."
"Everything is going to be all right."

Adding your own examples

Pleasant and/or fun images: ______________________

____

Self-talk: ______________________

____

[a]Adapted from materials by Lizette Peterson, Ph.D., and Jonathan Kellerman, Ph.D.

should be addressed. The child's preexisting coping strategies should be incorporated wherever possible. Parental involvement in procedures should be determined by previous experience with the parent, their expressions of anxiety regarding the procedure, and the future necessity and practicality of their involvement. Finally, identifying and arranging consistent indicators in the physical environment of upcoming procedures can prevent very young children from overgeneralizing across all settings and people.

3.2. Improving Compliance with Medical Regimens

With the exception of those adolescent intervention studies on child compliance with medical regimens, most instruction teaches the parent to implement a particular strategy. For example, Lowe and Lutzker (1979) improved compliance in a diabetic 9-year-old by teaching the parents to implement a point system. Although ineffective for urine testing and foot care, when parents simply put a reminder in a prominent place in the house, it improved the child's dietary compliance. Rapoff *et al.* (1984) reported improved regimen compliance in a 7-year-old girl with juvenile rheumatoid arthritis by teaching the parents to use a token reinforcement program.

Parental instruction in the simple behavioral procedures that may reduce noncompliance is appropriate. For example, Table 2 outlines some suggestions for parents who will be administering medications to their child. For children with a history of noncompliance, a "star chart" can be used for short- or long-term regimens. Initially, stars can be followed with a more concrete reward, which are gradually decreased until the rewards occur infrequently. Eventually, the entire chart can be discontinued or adapted into a simple recording sheet. Other reward systems that have been used are grab-bags, dot-to-dot pictures, and advent calendars. Instructions in appropriate use of "time-out" as a disciplinary procedure may also be necessary (Rapoff and Christophersen, 1982a).

Adolescents exhibit better regimen compliance if they are provided increased regimen responsibility with professional supervision (Litt and Cuskey, 1980). Sallis (1985) suggests that responsibility should be designed according to the child's developmental level. Specifically, it has been suggested that parent and child involvement be adapted on a scale from "high" to "low" in any of the following regimen components: (1) "scheduling/cueing; (2) medication administration; (3) monitoring adherence; and (4) rewards" (p. 120). A clear delineation of responsibility is necessary from the outset of prescribing a regimen, with a gradual shift toward the child assuming increasing responsibility. Monitoring is necessary, however, to ensure that the child is carrying out the regimen appropriately.

Consistent with findings on compliance with adults, Kaplan *et al.* (1985) noted that improved knowledge about diabetes had no effect on metabolic control in adolescents. They found, however, that teaching social skills to diabetic adolescents and how to resist peer pressure had more impact on improving their metabolic control than education about diabetes per se.

Finding effective intervention strategies may be very complex and requires individual components geared to the adolescent's family relationships, style of learning, and unique motivators (e.g., Schafer *et al.*, 1982). It is likely (although not documented by research studies) that, as with adults, adolescent compliance may improve by tailoring the regimen to their routine (e.g., Rapoff and Christophersen, 1982b). For instance, exercises may be scheduled immediately after school or while watching a regular television program. Self-recording on a calendar has improved medication giving in parents (Finney *et al.*, 1985) and can be adapted by adolescents who should assume responsibility for their own regimens.

In essence, child compliance with medical regimens has been improved by teaching parents to use behavior management strategies such as token systems. Adolescents, who tend to assume greater responsibility for their regimens, present a complex problem. While increasing responsibility is associated with better compliance, adolescents require adult supervision (preferably not from a family member). Instruction in ways to resist peer pressure is particularly appropriate for this age group. Intervention strategies must be adapted to the individual needs of the adolescent. Approaches such as tailoring to the adolescent's routine, self-monitoring calendars, and posted reminders can improve compliance.

4. Suggestions for the Medical Community

4.1. Medical Personnel

Warm and positive pediatricians are much more effective in obtaining compliance from children and their parents. Table 5 is a list of specific recommendations for physicians based on various studies of child compliance with medical procedures and regimens.

Table 5. Suggestions for Medical Personnel[a]

Medical procedures
1. Explore the child's behavior at home and suggest behavior management strategies to the parent if appropriate
2. Examine the physical set-up of the office or treatment room and minimize the number of visible instruments that might be frightening
3. Make the environment as predictable as possible
4. Introduce potentially aversive procedures gradually when possible
5. Use clear, concise instructions
6. Adapt information and instructions to the child's developmental level
7. Give the child choices whenever possible
8. Discuss parental presence during procedures beforehand and give clear guidelines for appropriate parental behavior

Medical regimens with adolescents
1. Determine the responsibility of the parent and adolescent in implementing the regimen
2. Provide written information on the regimen components and clear instructions regarding their implementation
3. Discuss the adolescent's routine and tailor the regimen to his/her schedule
4. Provide self-monitoring sheets and discuss posting them in a prominent place in the adolescent's home
5. Arrange for supervision from an adult other than the parents (e.g., a nurse practitioner or school nurse)

[a]Judith R. Mathews and Edward R. Christophersen, 1987, University of Kansas Medical Center.

4.2. Organizational Changes

The need for intervention strategies designed to decrease aversiveness to hospitalization has been recognized (Cataldo *et al.*, 1979). However, not all decisions aimed at improving hospital conditions for children have been empirically evaluated. One well-documented approach that has been adopted by many hospitals is the use of preparatory films prior to hospitalization. Other hospital programs, such as parent rooming-in and/or presence during procedures, require further evaluation to determine if they are actually beneficial. Another important area for future research is the physical arrangement of patient rooms, waiting rooms, and treatment rooms. Finally, the training of medical personnel in appropriate interactions with the child and parent is of vital significance in preventing compliance problems.

5. Conclusion

Child noncompliance with medical regimens and procedures may have serious repercussions, both medically and financially. In many instances medical professionals can prevent problems by anticipating them, when implementing a prescribed procedure or regimen.

In order for health care professionals to utilize this literature, they must be cognizant of factors that are known to improve or reduce compliance. Some of these factors, such as the use of written handouts and monitoring sheets, can be addressed by keeping a ready supply of handouts available in the treatment area. Other factors, such as tailoring regimens to the adolescent's life-style or adapting instructions to the child's developmental level, must be addressed during the office visit.

Younger children with behavior problems at home are more likely to be noncompliant with medical procedures. Professionals should therefore routinely address home discipline problems with their new patients. Physicians must consider the manner in which children are prepared for procedures, the environmental factors that may make the child more fearful, and whether parent presence is appropriate. Expectations should be adapted to the child's developmental level and children should be provided with as predictable and controllable an environment as possible.

Compliance with medical regimens is complicated by the necessity of using the parent as the implementor. This necessitates ensuring that parents understand and are able to follow through on recommendations and that they can implement behavior management strategies when their children are noncompliant. Adolescents provide a particular challenge and physicians should deal directly with adolescents rather than communicating primarily through their parents. Nonetheless, supervision is required—a role that perhaps can be accomplished through nurse specialists. Regimen compliance is further complicated by the long-term nature of many illnesses. Maintenance over many months or years is difficult for even the most conscientious parent or child. Routine contact and nonjudgmental problem solving, when compliance deteriorates, are important for the physician to maintain.

In many instances, noncompliance is not the result of willful resistance to a physician's recommendations. Instead, regimen noncompliance may result from incomplete understanding of the recommendations, inability to find ways to eliminate barriers in the home, or inability to deal with social pressures. Procedure noncompliance may result from a child's developmental inability to anticipate and cope with stressful and often painful circumstances. The medical professional's role, then, should be one of teacher for both the parent and child. Careful observation, anticipation of potential problems, and prophylactic intervention are extremely valuable in providing optimum care for children with health problems.

ACKNOWLEDGMENTS. Preparation of this manuscript was partially supported by grants from NICHD (Grants HD 03144, HD 18435, and HD 02528) to the University of Kansas Medical Center.

JRM submitted this chapter as partial fulfillment for the Ph.D. requirements in the Developmental and Child Psychology program at the University of Kansas.

References

Allen, D. A., Tennen, H., McGrade, B. J., *et al.*, 1983, Parent and child perceptions of the management of juvenile diabetes, *J. Pediatr. Psychol.* **8:**129–141.

Barnard, M. U., Moore, W. V., Russo, L. L., *et al.*, 1987, *Noncompliance or Pseudo-noncompliance,* unpublished manuscript.

Baron, A., and Galizio, M., 1983, Instructional control of human operant behavior, *Psychol. Rec.* **33:**495–520.

Beales, J. G., 1983, Factors influencing the expectation of pain among patients in a children's burn unit, *Burns Therm. Injury* **9:**187–192.

Bergman, A. R., and Werner, R. J., 1963, Failure of children to receive penicillin by mouth, *N. Engl. J. Med.* **268:**1334–1338.

Blount, R. L., Dahlquist, L. M., Baer, R. A., *et al.*, 1984, A brief effective method for teaching children to swallow pills, *Behav. Ther.* **15:**381–387.

Cataldo, M. F., Bessman, D. A., Parker, L. H., *et al.*, 1979, Behavioral assessment for pediatric intensive care units, *J. Appl. Anal.* **12:**83–97.

Cataldo, M. F., Jacobs, H. E., and Rogers, M. C., 1982, Behavioral/environmental considerations in pediatric inpatient care, in: *Behavioral Pediatrics: Research and Practice* (D. C. Russo and J. W. Varni, eds.), pp. 271–298, Plenum Press, New York.

Charney, E., Bynum, R., Eldredge, D., *et al.*, 1967, How well do patients take oral penicillin? A collaborative study in private practice, *Pediatrics* **40:**188–195.

Christophersen, E. R., 1988, *Little People: Guidelines for Commonsense Child Reading,* Westport Publishers, Kansas City, MO.

Christophersen, E. R., 1986, Anticipatory guidance on discipline, *Pediatr. Clin. North Am.* **33:**789–798.

Dunbar, J. M., and Stunkard, A. J., 1979, Adherence to diet and drug regimens, in: *Nutrition Lipids, and Coronary Heart Disease* (R. Levy, B. Rifkind, S. Dennis, *et al.*, eds.), Raven Press, New York.

Etzel, B. C., and LeBlanc, J. M., 1979, The simplest treatment alternative: The law of parsimony applied to choosing appropriate instructional control and errorless-learning procedures for the difficult-to-teach child, *J. Autism Dev. Disord.* **9:**361–382.

Finney, J. W., Friman, P. C., Rapoff, M. A., *et al.*, 1985, Improving compliance with antibiotic regimens for otitis media, *Am. J. Dis. Child.* **139:**89–95.

Firestone, P., 1982, Factors associated with children's adherence to stimulant medication, *Am. J. Orthopsychiatry* **52:**447–457.

Gordis, L., Markowitz, M., and Lilienfeld, A. M., 1969, Why patients don't follow medical advice: A study of children on long-term antistreptococcal prophylaxis, *J. Pediatr.* **75:** 959–968.

Gross, A. M., Stern, R. M., Levin, R. B., *et al.*, 1983, The effect of mother–child separation on the behavior of children experiencing a diagnostic medical procedure, *J. Consult. Clin. Psychol.* **51:**783–785.

Hamlet, C. C., Axelrod, S., and Kuerschner, S., 1984, Eye contact as an antecedent to compliant behavior, *J. Appl. Behav. Anal.* **17:**553–557.

Haynes, R. B., Taylor, D. W., and Sackett, D. L. (eds.), 1979, *Compliance in Health Care,* John Hopkins University, Baltimore.

Hedberg, G., and Schlong A., 1973, Eliminating fainting by school children during mass inoculation clinics, *Nurs. Res.* **22:**352–353.

Hyson, M. C., Snyder, S. S., and Andujar, E. M., 1982, Helping children cope with checkups: How good is the "good" patient? *Child. Health Care* **10:**139–144.

Jay, S. M., and Elliot, C. H., 1983, Behavioral observation scales measuring children's distress. The effects of increased methodological rigor, *J. Consult. Clin. Psychol.* **52:** 1106–1107.

Kaplan, R. M., Chadwick, M. W., and Schimmel, L. E., 1985, Social learning intervention to promote metabolic control in type 1 diabetes mellitus: Pilot experiment results, *Diabetes Care* **8:**152–155.

Katz, E. R., Kellerman, J., and Siegel, S. E., 1980, Behavioral distress in children with cancer undergoing medical procedures: Developmental considerations, *J. Consult. Clin. Psychol.* **48:**356–365.

Kellerman, J., 1981, *Helping the Fearful Child,* Contemporary Books, Chicago.

Kelley, M. L., Jarvie, G. J., Middlebrook, J. L., *et al.*, 1984, Decreasing burned children's pain behavior: Impacting the trauma of hydrotherapy, *J. Appl. Behav. Anal.* **17:**147–158.

Litt, I. F., and Cuskey, W. R., 1980, Compliance with medical regimens during adolescence, *Pediatr. Clin. North Am.* **27:**3–15.

Litt, I. F., and Cuskey, W. R., 1981, Compliance with salicylate therapy in adolescents with juvenile rheumatoid arthritis, *Am. J. Disabled Child* **135:**434–436.

Litt, I. F., Cuskey, W. R., and Rosenberg, A., 1982, Role of self-esteem and autonomy in determining medication compliance among adolescents with juvenile rheumatoid arthritis, *Pediatrics* **69:**15–17.

Loew, K., and Lutzker, J. R., 1979, Increasing compliance to a medical regimen with a juvenile diabetic, *Assoc. Advance. Behav. Ther.* **19:**57–64.

Lund, M., Jorgensen, R. S., and Kuhl, V., 1964. Serum diphenylhydantoin (Phenytoin) in ambulant patients with epilepsy, *Epilepsia* **5:**51–58.

Maier, S. F., and Seligman, M. E. P., 1976, Learned helplessness: Theory and evidence, *J. Exp. Psychol.* **105:**3–46.

Mathews, J. R., and Christophersen, E. R., 1988, Measuring and preventing noncompliance in pediatric health care, in: *Handbook of child health assessment* (P. Karoly ed.), Wiley, New York

Mathews, J. R., and Grantmyre, J. D., 1985, *Increasing Compliance to Radiation Therapy in a Two-Year-Old Child,* paper presented at the meeting of the Association for the Advancement of Behavior Therapy, Houston, Texas.

McCaul, K. D., and Malott, J. M., 1984, Distraction and coping with pain, *Psychol. Bull.* **95:** 516–533.

Melamed, B. G., and Siegel, L. J., 1975, Reduction of anxiety in children facing hospitalization and surgery by use of filmed modeling, *J. Consult. Psychol.* **43:**511–521.

Melamed, B. G., Robbins, R. L., and Graves, S., 1982, Preparation for surgery and medical procedures, in: *Behavioral Pediatrics: Research and Practice* (D. C. Russo and J. W. Varni, eds.), pp. 225–267, Plenum Press, New York.

Miller, S. M., 1980, When is a little information a dangerous thing? Coping with stressful events by monitoring vs. blunting, in: *Coping and Health* (S. Levine and H. Ursin, eds.), pp. 145–169, Plenum Press, New York.

Peterson, L., and Shigetomi, C., 1981, One-year follow-up of elective surgery child patients receiving preoperative preparation, *J. Pediatr. Psychol.* **7**:43–48.

Rapoff, M. A., and Christophersen, E. R., 1982a, Improving compliance in pediatric practice, *Pediatr. Clin. North Am.* **29**:339–357.

Rapoff, M. A., and Christophersen, E. R., 1982b, Compliance of pediatric patients with medical regimens: A review and evaluation, in: *Adherence, Compliance, and Generalization in Behavioral Medicine* (R. B. Stuart, ed.), pp. 79–124, Brunner/Mazel, New York.

Rapoff, M. A., Lindsley, C. B., and Christophersen, E. R., 1984, Improving compliance with medical regimens: Case study with juvenile rheumatoid arthritis, *Arch. Phys. Med. Rehab.* **65**:267–269.

Rapoff, M. A., Lindsley, C. B., and Christophersen, E. R., 1985, Parent perceptions of problems experienced by their children in complying with treatments for juvenile rheumatoid arthritis, *Arch. Phys. Med. Rehab.* **66**:427–429.

Reisinger, K. S., Williams, A. F., John, C. F., *et al.*, 1981, Effects of pediatricians' counseling on infant restraint use, *Pediatrics* **67**:201–206.

Roberts, M. W., 1984, An attempt to reduce time-out resistance in young children, *Behav. Ther.* **15**:210–216.

Roberts, M. W., McMahon, R. J., Forehand, R., *et al.*, 1978, The effect of parental instruction-giving on child compliance, *Behav. Ther.* **9**:793–798.

Ross, D. N., and Ross, S. A., 1984, Childhood pain: The school-aged child's viewpoint, *Pain* **20**:179–191.

Sallis, J. F., 1985, Improving adherence to pediatric therapeutic regimens, *Pediatr. Nurs.* **11**:118–120, 148.

Schafer, L. C., Glasgow, R. E., and McCaul, K. D., 1982, Increasing the adherence of diabetic adolescents, *J. Behav. Med.* **5**:353–362.

Shaw, E. G., and Routh, D. K., 1982, Effect of mother presence on children's reaction to aversive procedures, *J. Pediatr. Psychol.* **7**:33–42.

Shorkey, C. T., and Taylor, J. E., 1973, Management of maladaptive behavior of a severely burned child, *Child Welfare* **52**:543–547.

Simonds, J. F., 1979, Emotions and compliance in diabetic children, *Psychosomatics* **20**:544–551.

Steward, M. S., and Steward, D. S., 1981, Children's conceptions of medical procedures, in: *Children's Conceptions of Health, Illness, and Bodily Functions* (R. Bibace and M. E. Walsh, eds.), pp. 67–84, Jossey-Bass, San Francisco.

Stokes, T. F., and Baer, D. M., 1977, An implicit technology of generalization, *J. Appl. Behav. Anal.* **10**:349–367.

Stokes, T. F., and Kennedy, S. H., 1980, Reducing child uncooperative behavior during dental treatment through modeling and reinforcement, *J. Appl. Behav. Anal.* **13**:41–49.

Swallow, J. N., Jones, J. M., and Morgan, M. F., 1975, The effect of environment on a child's reaction to dentistry, *J. Dent. Child.* **42**:42–44.

Traughber, B., and Cataldo, M. F., 1983, Biobehavioral effects of pediatric hospitalization, in: *Pediatric and Adolescent Medicine: Issues in Treatment* (P. J. McGrath and P. Firestone, eds.), pp. 107–131, Springer, New York.

Varni, J. W., Bessman, C. A., Russo, D. C., *et al.*, 1980, Behavioral management of chronic pain in children: Case study, *Arch. Phys. Med. Rehab.* **61**:375–379.

Weinstein, P., Getz, T., Ratener, P., *et al.*, 1982a, The effect of dentists' behavior on fear-related behaviors in children, *J. Am. Dent. Assoc.* **104:**32–38.
Weinstein, P., Getz, T., Ratener, R., *et al.*, 1982b, Dentists' responses to fear- and nonfear-related behaviors in children, *J. Am. Dent. Assoc.* **104:**38–40.

CHAPTER 14

Office Screening for Communicative Disorders in Young Children

JERRY L. NORTHERN,
DEWEY WALKER,
MARION P. DOWNS,
AND SUSAN GUGENHEIM

1. Introduction

Problems in childhood speech–language development and educational retardation, associated with recurrent otitis media during the initial 2 years of life, continues to be confirmed in research publications. Since Eisen (1962) first described the effects of early hearing deprivation on behavior in 1962, numerous studies have confirmed the deleterious results of conductive hearing loss on auditory function. The classic study of Holm and Kunze (1969) on the effect of otitis media on speech and language development has been replicated with similar results in countries around the world, from New Zealand to Alaska. These studies generally demonstrate that many children with an early history of recurrent otitis media manifest a variety of educational problems including delayed speech and language development, auditory processing deficits, disturbance of auditory–visual interpretation, reading disorders, poor spelling skills, as well as classroom lack of attention and behavior troubles (Zinkus *et al.*, 1978).

JERRY L. NORTHERN, DEWEY WALKER, MARION P. DOWNS, and SUSAN GUGENHEIM • Department of Otolaryngology, University of Colorado Health Sciences Center, Denver, Colorado 80262.

Admittedly, research efforts in the area of otitis media associated with speech, language, and educational delay are especially difficult to conduct, and results are not easily generalized (Bluestone *et al.,* 1986). Critics of published studies in this area point out that most data reported are limited by retrospective design, small sample size, inadequate documentation of disease diagnosis, treatment and duration, as well as too many uncontrolled variables, making it difficult to reach supportive conclusions. In particular, Paradise (1981) has been an outspoken critic of published research in this area. Although Paradise notes that it is reasonable to assume a causal relationship between the presence of chronic and continuous middle ear disease with impairment of children's speech, language, and cognition, he states that no convincing evidence of adverse developmental outcome has been proved.

Nonetheless, the current overwhelming mountain of data supports the view that minimal auditory deficiency causes educational and developmental problems in some children. The exact etiology of this effect is still open to question. Lewis (1976) suggests that these problems are due to "inefficient listening strategies that persist beyond the episodes of active ear disease." Skinner (1978) published an excellent essay on the hearing of speech during language acquisition. She points out that even mild hearing loss will cause unstressed words and less-intense speech sounds (voiceless stops and fricatives) to be inaudible, and it is this loss of auditory cues that creates delay in the normal acquisition of language.

The audiogram in Fig. 1 includes frequency and intensity information for "average" spoken English. Obviously, the 20–30 dB hearing loss often caused by middle ear effusion puts the level of spoken English at only 5–10 dB above auditory threshold. The preferred listening level for speech is +30 dB above auditory threshold. The audiogram of Fig. 1 also demonstrates that the unvoiced speech consonants (s, p, t, k, th, f, sh) contain so little energy that they often fall below even normal hearing thresholds in average conversation. As adults with normal hearing, our listening strategies for understanding speech enables us to "fill in" automatically for the missing sounds, but the child who is just learning speech relationships has a critical need to hear all sounds clearly in order to implant the perceptions solidly.

From an educational point of view, successful intervention is dependent on early identification of the problem. Early identification of nonsymptomatic middle ear effusion in young children, however, is not an easy task. There are those who argue that to search for these children serves no useful purpose, since the condition usually subsides by itself and/or the treatment is of dubious value. Although there is certainly controversy about the management of children with chronic, fluctuat-

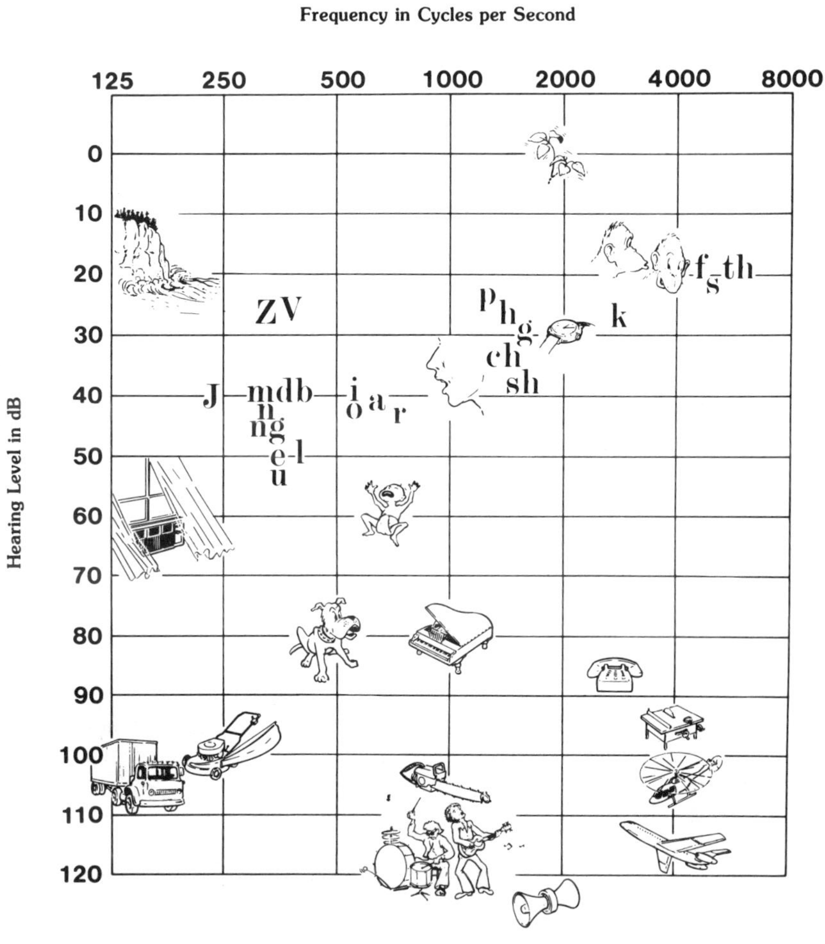

Figure 1. Audiogram of familiar sounds with English phonemes at average conversational level. (With permission from Northern and Downs, 1984.)

ing, mild hearing loss associated with speech and language deviations, one cannot help but be impressed with the large number of studies that have concluded that otitis-prone children experience difficulties in a variety of psychoeducational areas. Whether or not the association between speech–language development and recurrent otitis media in early life is real has often been questioned. To wait for a definitive answer while the suspicion remains, however, is an untenable position. Certainly a positive action step is to develop screening procedures that will be useful to primary-care physicians in identifying children as early as possible who have communication disorders.

The importance of otitis media and its sequelae has drawn attention from the Committee on Early Childhood, Adoption, and Dependent Care of the American Academy of Pediatrics (1984). The Committee issued a policy statement in 1984 as follows:

> There is growing evidence demonstrating a correlation between middle ear disease with hearing impairment and delays in the development of speech, language, and cognitive skills. A parent or other caretaker may be the first person to detect such early symptoms as irritability, decreased responsiveness, and disturbed sleep. Middle ear disease may be so subtle that a full evaluation for this condition should combine pneumatic otoscopy, and possible tympanometry, with a direct view of the tympanic membrane. This is not meant to be a recommendation for specific treatment methods. When a child has frequently recurring acute otitis media and/or middle ear effusion persisting for longer than three months, hearing should be assessed and the development of communicative skills must be monitored.
>
> The Committee feels it is important that the physician inform the parent that a child with middle ear disease may not hear normally. Although the child may withdraw socially and diminish experimentation with verbal communication, the parent should be encouraged to continue communicating by touching and seeking eye contact with the child when loudly and clearly speaking. Such measures, along with prompt restoration of hearing whenever possible, may help to diminish the likelihood that a child with middle ear disease will develop a communicative disorder. Middle ear disease can occur in the presence of sensory neural hearing loss. Any child whose parent expresses concern about whether the child hears should be considered for referral for behavioral audiometry without delay.

2. Otitis Media in Children

Otitis media is one of the most common disorders in children. Otitis media is defined as an inflammation of the middle ear that may or may not be infectious in origin. At any specific point in the continuum, a definite clinical entity can be identified, and at another time a different clinical entity may be present in the same patient.

The general categories of otitis media include: (1) otitis media without effusion; (2) otitis media with effusion; and (3) otitis media with perforation. Each of these categories may be further classified by duration into: (1) acute, 0–21 days; (2) subacute, 22 days to 8 weeks; and (3) chronic, over 8 weeks. In otitis media with effusion and otitis media perforation, the fluid or discharge may be characterized as: (1) serous; (2) purulent; or (3) mucoid (Bluestone *et al.*, 1983).

2.1. General Epidemiological Considerations

Otitis media occurs most frequently during the first 2 years of life, and decreases in incidence thereafter. The incidence of otitis media has been studied by many investigators and found to be a function of age, sex (more otitis media in boys), race (whites have a higher incidence than blacks), genetic factors, socioeconomic status, season, and climate (Giebink, 1984). According to Teele *et al.* (1984), children living in households with many members are more likely to have otitis media than are children living in households with fewer members, and children with siblings or parents who have a history of otitis media have a higher incidence of otitis media than children with parents or siblings without a history of the disease. The statistics concerning the incidence of otitis media are impressive: 76–95% of all children have had at least one episode of otitis media by age 6 years; approximately 50% of all children have had one episode of otitis media by age 1 year and by age 2 years, the incidence increases to 75%. Thus children may be divided into three general groups with regard to otitis media: approximately one third of all children have no episodes, one third may have an occasional episode, and the remaining third have frequent episodes.

Of particular importance is the "otitis-prone" child described initially by Howie *et al.* (1975). An otitis-prone child had otitis media six or more times before the age of 6 years, or whose initial episode of otitis media was due to *Pneumococcus* and occurred before the age of 1 year. It appears that otitis-prone children are at increased risk for speech–language delay perhaps due to their loss of auditory speech models during a "critical" language-learning period.

2.2. Middle Ear Effusions in Neonates

Middle ear effusion occurs commonly in neonates, both in the outpatient population and in the intensive care nursery. In spite of numerous well-documented studies, otoscopy is not routinely performed on neonates because the infant's tympanic membrane is difficult to visualize. In an infant, the external ear canal is distensible and often collapsed, and the tympanic membrane lies in a horizontal plane. Balkany *et al.* (1978) reported the results from examination of 125 consecutive infants from the neonatal intensive care unit and found middle ear effusion in approximately 30% of their sample. The investigators suggested this finding was often overlooked but was especially important since unrecognized middle ear effusion may act as a focus for dissemination of bacteria into the circulation and/or central nervous system. They also found that nasotracheal intubation for longer than 7 days is highly associated with the presence of middle ear effusion.

2.3. Persistent Middle Ear Effusion

An extremely important finding was reported by Teele and his associates (1980) concerning persistence of middle ear effusion following medical treatment. After an episode of otitis media, 70% of the children in the study had persistent middle ear effusion at 2 weeks, 40% at 1 month, 20% at 2 months, and 10% at 3 months. These statistics confirm the importance of careful and thorough medical follow-up for all children identified as having otitis media.

Considerable controversy and confusion exists concerning the treatment of otitis media. Tremendous benefits would be gained if recurrences of otitis media could be prevented or the number of episodes could be substantially reduced.

3. Normal Speech Development

Language competence is the most sensitive indicator of overall development in children and the best predictor of school success (Shapiro *et al.*, 1984). Physicians who manage the medical care of children are in a unique and key position to identify language delay at the earliest possible age. A majority of physicians use parental recall of developmental milestones or they judge a child's developmental level through the use of informal techniques during the routine physical examination. Obviously these techniques lack accuracy and objectivity, which suggests the need for a simple, standardized language-screening tool.

Concurrent with the maturation of auditory functions are the development of speech and language skills. Although an infant is able to differentiate sounds in the first few months of life, the production of sounds does not develop at the same rate. By the first month, the normal infant "coos" and "gurgles," in addition to crying. By 2 months of age, the infant begins to emit specific sounds more than others. Between the ages of 2 and 4 months, the infant seems to focus on the production of vowel-like sounds and true babbling begins. At 5 months the infant sound emissions include consonant–vowel combinations. Glottal and labial sounds enter into the infant vocalizing pattern by the age of 6 months. At 9 or 10 months, the glottal sounds decrease and alveolar sounds are frequently used.

Babbling ceases at about 6 months of age and during the next few months there is undistinguished progress in vocalizing speech sounds. During this period, the mother's feedback of the child's sounds provides the groundwork for the first production of a word. Initially, vocalizations of profoundly deaf infants are identical with those of normal-hearing infants until about the age of 5 or 6 months. However, the lack of auditory feedback in the deaf infant soon causes vocalization to cease.

During the second 6 months of life, the normal-hearing infant continues to mimic sounds vocalized by the mother. The sounds of the child are further imitated by the mother, who in turn adds additional speech improvisations. Soon thereafter the child imitates the mother's imitation, and speech shaping is underway. Occasionally the comprehension of the sound sequence precedes the imitation; sometimes imitation precedes understanding of the meaning of the sound sequence.

The child's first meaningful word is usually uttered around the first birthday and is dependent on a full year of attentive listening activity. Many children can repeat "ma-ma" or "da-da" by the age of 9 months. Soon after utterance of the initial word, the child should begin to build vocabulary. By 18 months the child should have at least a six-word vocabulary and by age 2 years should be able to occasionally express himself in two-word sentences. At 2½ years, a child should be able to point to parts of his body on command and by the age of 3 years should know his own first name. By the age of 3 years, the normal child should be able to begin identifying simple toys on command. Matkin (1984) published a valuable article directed at helping primary-care physicians in making appropriate referrals for communicatively disordered children. He points out the importance of early referral of the child who does not speak, in order to identify the presence of hearing loss, emotional disturbance, social deprivation, or specific language disability. Matkin further suggests that three questions should be included in the preschool medical history: (1) How many words do you estimate your child uses? (2) How many words does your child use in a typical sentence? and (3) How clear is your child's speech to a friend or neighbor? A useful guide for referral of children with "speech delay" is outlined in Table 1.

The main reason for the identification of hearing loss present at birth is to insure that training can begin as soon as possible. Early identification and intervention would allow the hearing-impaired child the maximum opportunity to attain his or her potential communication and intellectual function. The benefit of early habilitation has been substanti-

Table 1. Referral Guidelines for Children with "Speech" Delay

Age	Guideline
12 months	No differentiated babbling or vocal imitation
18 months	No use of single words
24 months	Single-word vocabulary of ≤10 words
30 months	Fewer than 100 words, no evidence of 2-word combinations, unintelligible
36 months	Fewer than 200 words, no use of telegraphic sentences, clarity <50%
48 months	Fewer than 600 words, no use of simple sentences, clarity <80%

[a]From Matkin (1984).

ated by a number of studies, demonstrating that hearing-impaired infants whose hearing habilitative training was initiated before 16 months of age have significantly superior speech and language skills by age 3 and 4 years compared with hearing-impaired infants whose habilitative training was begun later than 16 months of age.

4. Screening Speech, Language, and Hearing

The present state of the art of screening for communicative disorders in the young child is not sophisticated. Screening tools are available, however, which if applied at appropriate ages would constitute an adequate screening program. A protocol utilizing such tools has been developed through the Robert Wood Johnson Foundation project in Colorado. For 4 years the staff of the project screened more than 800 children under 36 months of age for speech, language, and hearing. The screening was conducted in the offices of primary-care physicians, Health Maintenance Organizations, neighborhood health clinics, and university health clinics. During the course of the project the team determined that the brief screening protocol could be effectively incorporated into a busy office schedule. The protocol will be described in detail.

Before the screening was initiated, the Colorado project assessed the current state of speech, language, and hearing screening in the office of the primary physician. In a response to a questionnaire, 484 primary-care physicians, who manage the medical care of children under age 3 years, indicated that they screened language skills with a wide variety of methods. Most of the physicians reported informal screening of language through patient history (parental report) and listening to and observing the child. Many cited use of the Denver Developmental Screening Test (DDST) as a language-screening tool, although this test is a general child development tool and not specifically intended to be a speech and language screen. The DDST may identify language problems in the older child, but it is noted to be weak in screening language skills in the young child (Borowitz and Glascoe, 1986). A small percentage of the survey respondents listed other tests, none of which adequately screens the language of the birth-to-3-years population.

The majority of the primary-care physicians in the Colorado survey reported that they screen hearing in young children through use of parental report. Some clinicians reported using noisemakers to screen hearing. Others cited the use of a watch-tick or a whispered voice, methods which audiologists deem inadequate. A few physicians indicated the use of audiometry; however, audiometric testing of children who are 3 years or younger is extremely difficult even under the best of circumstances.

Estimates of the national prevalence of speech and language disorders among children range between 5 and 10%. Hearing disorders in young children may approach 30–35% prevalence when conductive hearing loss due to middle ear effusion is included. In contrast to these national figures, the physicians in the Colorado survey refer 0.4% of children under 3 years of age to speech–language pathologists, 0.6% to audiologists, and 0.6% to otolaryngologists. These referral figures are strikingly low when compared with the estimated national prevalence.

The lack of uniformity in language and hearing screening procedures and the discrepancy between referral rates to prevalence figures underscored the need for establishing guidelines for routine use by physicians in their offices. This need led to the development of an age-oriented protocol for routine pediatric screening of communicative disorders (Fig. 2). The guidelines include efficient and discriminating procedures that take into account the time constraints of a busy practice, and may be administered by trained office staff.

5. Guidelines for Hearing and Language Screening of Young Children in Physicians' Offices

The protocol described in Fig. 2 has been in use for more than 3 years in a number of offices of Colorado primary-care physicians. In many office situations, the screening procedures are conducted by allied

a

AGE RANGE OF TEST	RECOMMENDED AGES TO TEST	SCREENING TEST	APPROPRIATE RESPONSE	RULES OUT	MANAGEMENT REFERRAL
Any age after birth	Neonatal period	Review child's history for these high risk factors for deafness: **A**sphyxia or anoxia **B**acterial Meningitis **C**ongenital perinatal infections **D**efects of head or neck **E**levated bilirubin **F**amily history of childhood deafness **G**ram birthweight less than 1500g.	No high risk factors in history	Most congenital hearing losses	If any factor is positive, refer for audiological testing
1-4 months	1-2 months	Loud horn 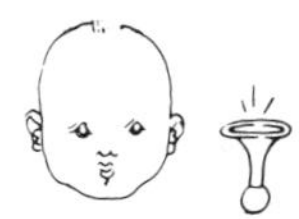	Eye Blink or Startle	Severe to profound loss	For failed screening tests, rescreen in 2 weeks If rescreen is failed, refer for audiological testing
4-36 months	6-9 months and after each middle ear effusion	1. Soft noisemakers (Bell, squeeze toys, rattles, or keys) → 2. Loud horn → 3. Tympanometry for children 7 months and older →	See chart on back for age appropriate response Eye blink or startle Normal tympanogram →	Moderate to severe loss Effusion	
36 months and older	4 - 5 years	Pure-tone audiometry* screen at 20 dBHL at 1000, 2000, 4000 Hz	Finger Raising 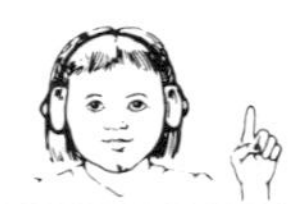	Mild loss and greater	

* Play conditioning may facilitate testing the younger children in the 3-5 age range.

b

AGE RANGE OF TEST	RECOMMENDED AGES TO TEST	SCREENING TEST	APPROPRIATE RESPONSE	RULES OUT	MANAGEMENT REFERRAL
0 - 36 months	13 - 36 months Best Age Range 24 - 30 months	Early Language Milestone Scale (ELM)	Pass Test at appropriate age level	Significant Language Delay	For failed screening tests, rescreen in 1 - 2 weeks If rescreen is failed, refer for audiological and language testing

c

CRITERIA FOR ADDITIONAL FOLLOW-UP	MANAGEMENT		
	HEARING	LANGUAGE	MEDICAL
3 episodes of otitis media in 3-6 months or Persistent middle ear effusion for 3 months or more §	Refer for audiological testing regardless of age	Under 3 yrs: Screen every 6 mos. with ELM	Consider other medical management to interrupt cycle of disease

§ Tympanometry is useful to document the duration of middle ear effusion.

Figure 2. Guidelines for hearing (a) and language (b) screening of young children in physicians' offices. (c) Additional guidelines for following children with ear disease.

health personnel or office assistants. The screening test battery takes approximately 4 minutes to administer. The screening test battery includes the Early Language Milestone (ELM) scale (Coplan *et al.*, 1982), hearing screening with noisemakers, and tympanometry. This screening package has been developed specifically for children between birth and 3 years of age.

5.1. Hearing Screening

The essence of early identification of congenital deafness is to be vigilent in the review of each child's medical history for the high-risk factors of hearing loss. The seven factors to be described have been recommended by the Joint Committee on Infant Hearing (1982), so that when any one factor is positive, the child has a higher probability of hearing loss than other children. Knowledge of these factors is important at any age. The need for early identification of deafness, however, makes screening of these high-risk elements most appropriate during the neonatal period. The high-risk factors include: (1) *severe asphyxia,* which may include infants with Apgar scores of 0 to 3, infants who fail to institute spontaneous respiration by 10 minutes, and those infants with hypotonia persisting for at least 2 hours; (2) *bacterial meningitis,* especially due to *Hemophilus influenzae;* (3) *congenital perinatal infection* including the toxoplasmosis–other infections–rubella virus–cytomegalovirus–herpex simplex (TORCH) complex; (4) *anatomical defects of the head or neck,* including pinna abnormalities, preauricular tags, cleft lip and/or palate; (5) *hyperbilirubinemia* at a level exceeding indications for an exchange transfusion; (6) *family history* of childhood hearing impairment; and (7) *low birthweight* less than 1500 g. This high-risk register for hearing impairment will involve 9–11% of a general nursery population, and from this group severe-to-profound deafness is expected to be about 1 in 70 babies (Gerkin, 1984).

Newborns may exhibit a positive element among the high-risk factors and still have normal hearing. Physicians must be alert to the fact that some congenital hearing losses may have late onset or be progressive in nature. Therefore, careful and routine observation of responses to behavioral hearing screening is justified. When screening test results are questionable or parental concern about the infant's hearing is mentioned, referral to an audiologist for a thorough hearing evaluation is necessary. Together, the primary-care physician and the audiologist can evaluate and monitor an infant's hearing at any age.

During the first 4 months of life, the newborn's behavioral responses to auditory stimuli are limited. Although in-depth auditory testing may be accomplished through electrophysiological techniques, such as auditory evoked potential measurement (Auditory brainstem response audiometry, ABR), office auditory screening can be accomplished with the presentation of a quick-onset loud sound [at least 85 dB sound pressure level (SPL)], such as a toy horn. The appropriate response is a brisk eye blink or body startle. This technique is designed to identify only those infants with severe to profound hearing loss.

Between the ages of 4 and 16 months of age, the baby with normal hearing goes through an orderly auditory maturation process (Fig. 3). During this age period, behavioral responses to quiet auditory noisemakers are seen as localization, i.e., head turns for visual observation of the noisemakers. The tester presents a quiet auditory stimulus, below or above the infant, but well out of the infant's sight. A normal response is for the baby to visually search out the source of the sound to either side in the early months, or a brisk head localization directly toward the sound source as the auditory response matures. The absence of this auditory localization response constitutes a failed screening test and raises the question of a hearing deficit. Although this procedure typically rules out moderate-to-severe hearing loss, experienced examiners with quiet noisemakers can often identify unilateral or bilateral mild hearing loss due to middle ear effusion.

The hearing screening should be done in a sound-treated room in which noise and visual distraction are at a minimum. Failure of a child to localize properly to an auditory signal does not indicate that the child did not hear it. The absence of a response may be due to lack of interest in the sound, delayed auditory maturation, or mental and/or physical impairment. The use of noisemakers, in accordance with expected auditory maturation responses, is intended to be a screening technique only. Additional evaluation by an experienced audiologist is recommended for any child who repeatedly fails to produce appropriate auditory-orienting responses.

Auditory evaluation of a child cannot be considered complete without inclusion of tympanometry. Tympanometry is an objective method of determining the status of the middle ear space and tympanic membrane compliance. It is particularly useful in identifying the presence of middle ear effusion or documenting the duration and number of episodes of otitis media. Tympanometry can detect the presence of middle ear pathology in some young children who are able to hear well enough to pass the behavioral auditory noisemaker screening. The usefulness of tympanometry cannot be overstated. Primary-care physicians who routinely use tympanometry often comment that their diagnostic accuracy

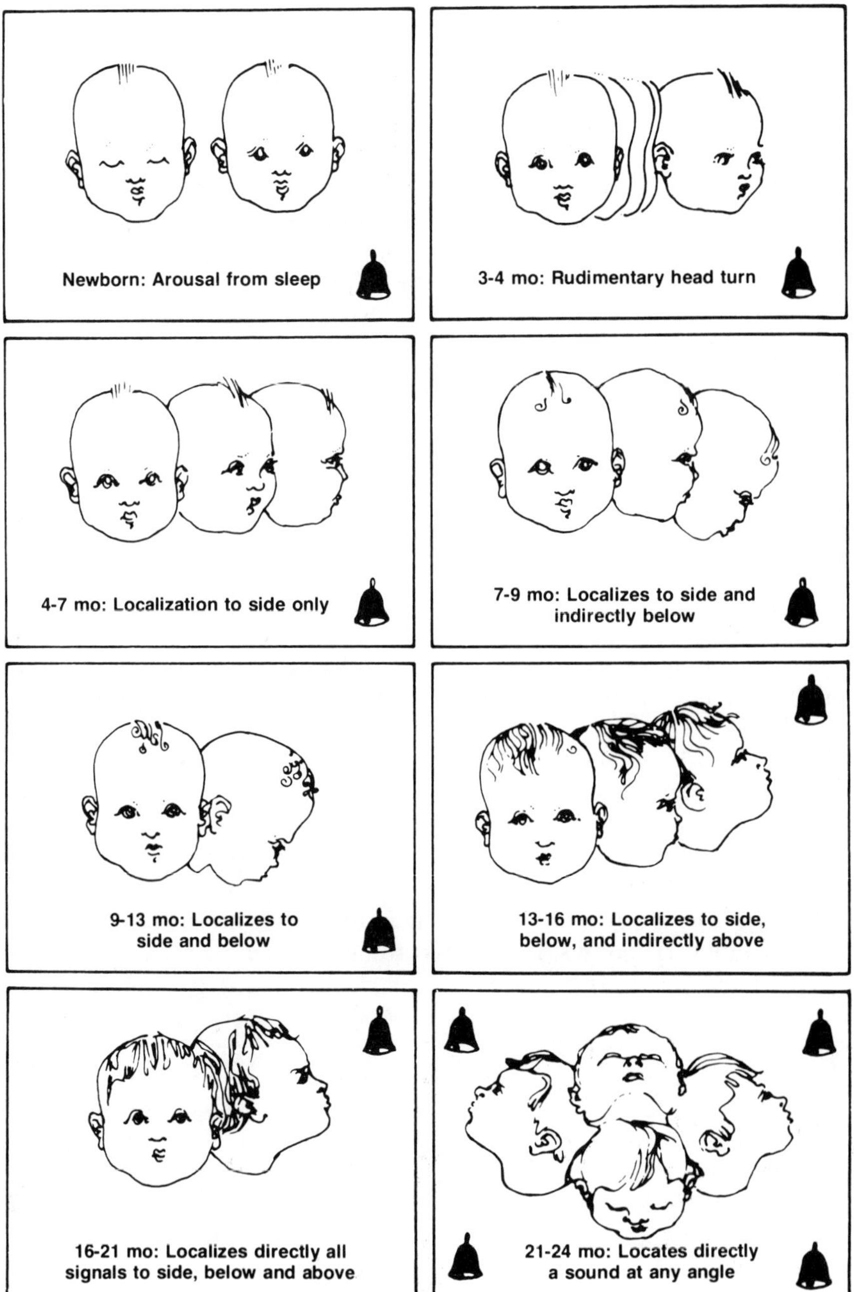

Figure 3. Normal development of auditory behavior a function of age. (With permission from Northern and Downs, 1984.)

with otoscopy is greatly enhanced. Tympanometry in infants less than 7 months of age is *not* recommended because of high false-negative rates.

Children with a mental age of 36 months are often able to comply with traditional pure-tone hearing tests. Techniques of play conditioning may facilitate hearing testing in children between 3 and 4 years of age. Hearing screening is recommended for all children at about the age of 4 years, or prior to their entering preschool. Hearing screening is performed, as recommended by the American Speech–Language–Hearing Association (1985), with pure tones of 1000, 2000, and 4000 Hz at 20 dB hearing level (HL) in each ear, with a finger-raising response by the child as each tone is heard. Failure of the hearing screening test occurs when any of the tones in either ear is not heard. This technique may identify even mild hearing loss in one or both ears. Children who fail the hearing screening test should be rescreened within 2 weeks. If the rescreen is also failed, the child should be referred to an audiologist for further hearing evaluation.

A more detailed and comprehensive discussion of all aspects of childrens' hearing, including auditory maturation, hearing screening, auditory threshold evaluation techniques, as well as medical aspects of hearing loss and syndrome accompanied by hearing loss, has been published by Northern and Downs (1984).

5.2. Language Screening

The Guidelines for Language Screening in Physician's Office (See Fig. 14.2) recommends the use of the Early Language Milestone scale (ELM). The ELM is a well-normed language-screening instrument designed to be a rapid means of evaluating language development of children under 3 years of age. The test addresses both receptive and expressive language through parent report and direct testing of the child. The test format is similar to the Denver Developmental Screening Test (Frankenburg and Dodds, 1967). The administration time of the ELM is 1 to 4 minutes. Each child's ELM profile is scored as "pass" or "fail."

Following 2 years of our experience administering the ELM in physicians' offices, an overall failure rate of 8% was noted. Children who failed an initial ELM screening, as well as a randomly selected sample of children who passed the ELM screening, were subsequently evaluated with a more sophisticated language test, the Sequenced Inventory of Communication Development (SICD). Based on an analysis of this evaluation procedure, it was determined that the best age range for ELM administration is between 24 and 30 months of age. Because the ELM is quickly and easily administered and because of improvement in the accuracy of parental report during a second ELM screen, it is recommended that children who fail to pass the ELM at their appropriate age level should be rescreened with the ELM within 1 to 2 weeks. If the ELM rescreen is also failed, referral to a speech–language pathologist is recommended. All children with language delay should also be referred for a hearing test to rule out the possibility of hearing impairment as a cause of language problems.

6. Additional Guidelines for Following Children with Middle Ear Effusion

Regardless of particular opinions on the relationship between otitis media and language delays, physicians must be sensitive to the identification of communication disorders in children with recurrent middle ear effusion. The criteria presented for additional follow-up implicate those children with three episodes of otitis media within a 3- to 6-month period or those children who present with persistent middle ear effusion for 3 months or longer. It is important for physicians to maintain written notations of each episode of middle ear effusion, from the initial diagnosis to the complete resolution of the problem. Children identified by these criteria should be: (1) referred for audiological evaluation, regardless of age; (2) screened with a formal, standardized language development assessment tool such as the ELM every 6 months to insure adequate language appropriate for age level; and (3) some means other than continued medical treatment management to interrupt the cycle of the middle ear disease.

7. Home Language Stimulation

Screening without follow-up is of no benefit to the child. Providers of health care must assume the responsibility for arranging definitive diagnostic evaluations for suspect patients and providing for remediation when appropriate and possible.

Children who exhibit mild language delay on the screening test may be enrolled in a home language enrichment program. Materials may be recommended for the parents that can be used in the home to enhance the child's speech and language. It is generally accepted that working with parents and instituting a home-based, moderately structured program can produce impressive short- and long-term gains for children.

Table 2. Suggestions for Parents of Children with Middle Ear Problems

The importance of talking

Talking to your child is necessary for his/her language development. Since children usually imitate what they hear, how much you talk to your child, what you say, and how you say it will affect how much and how well your child talks.

Look

Look directly at your child's face and wait until you have his/her attention before you begin talking.

Control distance

Be sure that you are close to your child when you talk (no farther than 5 feet). The younger the child, the more important it is to be close.

Loudness

Talk slightly louder than you normally do. Turn off the radio, TV, dishwasher, etc. to remove background noise.

Be a good speech model

Describe to your child daily activities as they occur

Expand what your child says. For example, if your child points and says "car," you say "Oh, you want the car."

Add new information. You might add, "That car is little."

Build vocabulary. Make teaching new words and concepts a natural part of every day's activities. Use new words while shopping, taking a walk, washing dishes, etc.

Repeat your child's words using adult pronunciation.

Play and talk

Set aside some times throughout the day for "play time" for just you and your child. Play can be looking at books, exploring toys, singing songs, coloring, etc. Talk to your child during these activities, keeping the conversation at his/her level.

Read

Begin reading to your child at a young age (under 12 months). Ask a librarian for books that are right for your child's age. Reading can be a calming-down activity that promotes closeness between you and your child. Reading provides another opportunity to teach and review words and ideas. Some children enjoy looking at pictures in magazines and catalogs.

Don't wait

Your child should have the following skills by the ages listed below:

18 months: 3 word vocabulary.

2 years: 25–30 word vocabulary and several 2-word sentences.

2½ years: At least a 50 word vocabulary and 2-word sentences consistently.

If your child doesn't have these skills, tell your doctor. A referral to an audiologist and speech pathologist may be indicated. Hearing and language testing may lead to a better understanding of your child's language development.

[a]Adapted from "Suggestions for Parents . . ." Noel Matkin, Ph.D., Professor of Audiology, University of Arizona, 1980.

In addition to specific suggestions for parent–child interactions, home programs may positively affect the parents' attitudes toward the child's problems.

At the most basic level, the parent may be provided with a handout that outlines easy suggestions for increasing communication with their child. Table 2 is a reproduction of a handout developed for parents of children with mild language delay due to recurrent middle ear effusion.

Another home stimulation approach to improve the child's language skills is based on an inexpensive paperback book, *Learning Games for the First Three Years* (Sparling and Lewis, 1976). This book suggests 100 age-appropriate parent–child activities, many of which involve language-based interactions. Feagans (1986) suggests a number of simple procedures to be instituted in day-care settings, pediatric and family offices, and community school programs.

8. Hearing Aid Placement

A mild ear-level hearing aid, with appropriate limitations on maximum saturation and gain, can be considered even for young infants. The obvious drawbacks are that (1) it is difficult to convince parents of the necessity for such an extreme antidote; and (2) there may be problems in keeping such an instrument on an infant. Hearing aid placement is a feasible procedure only if (1) the parents are highly motivated, (2) continual guidance by an audiologist or speech therapist is obtained, (3) a total support system by doctor, parent, and therapist is in effect, and (4) a period of diagnostic therapy with a "loaner" hearing aid is initiated to judge the effectiveness of the aid.

The real impact of a hearing aid is that amplification increases the signal of choice (parent or teacher's voice) over the background noise. Actually, if parents and teachers could project their voices 10–15 dB louder, the hearing loss in the child might be compensated for. At any rate, the child enrolled in a home language enrichment program should be given routine language development tests every 6 months until the child functions at the appropriate age level.

ACKNOWLEDGMENT. This manuscript was prepared as part of a project sponsored by The Robert Wood Johnson Foundation.

References

American Academy of Pediatrics, 1984, Middle ear disease and language development, *News & Comment* **35**:9.

American Speech–Language–Hearing Association, 1985, Guidelines for identification audiometry, *Asha* **27:**49–52.

Balkany, T. J., Berman, S. A., Simmons, M. A., *et al.*, 1978, Middle ear effusion in neonates, *Laryngoscope* **88:**398–405.

Bluestone, C., Klein, J. L., Paradise, J., *et al.*, 1983, Workshop on effects of otitis media on the child, *Pediatrics* **71:**639–652.

Bluestone, C., Fria, T., Arjona, S., *et al.*, 1986, Controversies in screening for middle ear disease and hearing loss in children, *Pediatrics* **77:**57–70.

Borowitz, K., and Glascoe, F., 1986, Sensitivity of the Denver Developmental Screening Test in Speech and Language Screening, *Pediatrics* **78:**1075–1078.

Coplan, J., Gleason, J. R., Ryan, R., *et al.*, 1982, Validation of an early language milestone scale in a high-risk population, *Pediatrics* **70:**677–683.

Eisen, N. H., 1962, Some effects of early sensory deprivation on later behavior: The quondom hard-of-hearing child, *J. Abnorm. Soc. Psychol.* **65:**338–342.

Frankenburg, W. K., and Dodds, J. B., 1967, The Denver Developmental Screening Test, *J. Pediatr.* **71:**181–191.

Feagans, L., 1986, Otitis media: A model for long-term effects with implications for intervention, in: *Otitis Media and Child Development* (J. Kavanagh, ed.), pp. 192–208, York Press, Parkton, MD.

Gerkin, K. P., 1984, The high-risk register for deafness, *Asha* **26:**17–23.

Giebink, G. S., 1984, Epidemiology and natural history of otitis media, in: *Recent Advances in Otitis Media with Enfusion* (D. Lim, C. Bluestone, J. Klein, J. Nelson, eds.), pp. 5–9, B. C. Decker, Inc., Toronto.

Holm, V., and Kunze, L., 1969, Effects of chronic otitis media on language and speech development, *Pediatrics* **43:**833–840.

Howie, V., Ploussard, J., and Sloyer, J., 1975, The "otitis-prone" condition. *Am. J. Dis. Child.* **129:**676–679.

Joint Committee on Infant Hearing, 1982, Statement, *Asha* **24:**1017–1018.

Lewis, N., 1976, Otitis media and linguistic incompetence, *Arch. Otolaryngol.* **102:**387.

Matkin, N., 1984, Early recognition and referral of hearing-impaired children, *Pediatr. Rev.* **6:**151–154.

Northern, J., and Downs, M., 1984, *Hearing in Children,* 3rd ed., Williams and Wilkins Co., Baltimore.

Paradise, J. L., 1981, Otitis media during early life: How hazardous to development? A critical review of the evidence, *Pediatrics* **68:**869–873.

Shapiro, B. K., Palmer, F. B., Wachtel, R. C., *et al.*, 1984, Issues in the early identification of specific learning disability, *J. Dev. Behav. Pediatr.* **5:**15–20.

Skinner, M. W., 1978, The hearing of speech during language acquisition, *Otolaryngol. Clin. North Am.* **11:**631–650.

Sparling, J., and Lewis, I., 1976, *Learning Games for the First Three Years,* Berkley Books, New York.

Teele, D. W., Klein, J. O., and Rosner, B., 1980, Epidemiology of otitis media in children. Proceedings of 2nd International Symposium on Current Advances in Otitis Media with Effusion, *Ann. Otol. Rhinol. Laryngol.* **89**(Suppl 68):5–6.

Teele, D. W., Klein, J., Rosner, B. A., *et al.*, 1984, Otitis media with effusion during the first three years of life and the development of speech and language, *Pediatrics* **74:**282–287.

Zinkus, P. W., Gottlieb, M. I., and Shapiro, M., 1978, Developmental and psychoeducational sequelae of chronic otitis media, *Am. J. Dis. Child.* **132:**1100–1104.

CHAPTER 15

Relaxation Imagery Training

Applications to Developmental–Behavioral Pediatrics

KAREN N. OLNESS

1. Introduction

Relaxation mental imagery (RMI) training is a tool of cyberphysiology, which refers to those self-regulatory processes that are mediated by consciousness in living organisms. The prefix "cyber" is derived from the Greek word *kybernētēs,* which means "helmsman" or "steersman." Greater understanding of cyberphysiology with respect to children has major implications for health, including treatment of acute and chronic diseases, public health programs, and health care costs. Of particular interest to those who work with children is how early training in self-regulatory abilities may affect adult life, particularly with respect to health.

Schwartz (1971) first documented that adults could regulate certain autonomic processes through a method popularly known as biofeedback. It soon became evident that children were able to learn self-regulation of various autonomic processes more quickly than adults. From 1975 to 1987 more than 30 English-language articles appeared in pediatric journals, documenting clinical applications of cyberphysiological controls in children. Training in such controls was mediated principally through relaxation imagery training or "self-hypnosis." While various feedback machines facilitate such training, they are not essential to suc-

KAREN N. OLNESS • Division of General Academic Pediatrics, Case Western Reserve University School of Medicine, and Department of Pediatrics, Rainbow Babies and Childrens Hospital, Cleveland, Ohio 44106.

cess. Although mechanisms of cyberphysiological skills remain unknown, research has now provided ample evidence that neurally mediated autonomic responses, usually viewed as reactive reflexes, can be modified by learning that is significantly dependent on image design or modification of figures of thought. Children not only learn more quickly than adults but demonstrate remarkable creativity and variability in the images they describe as related to their successes.

The word "hypnosis" has an unfortunate mystique and is both over- and underrated. A primary misconception concerning its use is that someone with magical powers, that is, the hypnotist, imposes behaviors onto a subject who is unaware of what is going on and is not in control. This misconception may derive from egocentricity on the part of some therapists and wishful thinking on the part of some patients. In fact, *all* hypnosis is self-hypnosis. Successful application of hypnotherapy requires coaching or training by a competent person and rigorous practice by the learner. A useful clinical definition of hypnosis is "an altered state of awareness in which the person is able to accept suggestions from himself to use his mental and physical skills in optimal fashion." (Gardner and Olness, 1981). The effective and appropriate use of hypnotherapeutic techniques, like other therapies, requires careful analysis of the problem and patient. Although children learn and use hypnotherapeutic techniques such as relaxation imagery exercises more readily than adults, they must also practice in order to achieve desired facility (Gardner and Olness, 1981).

As the behavioral pediatric medicine research model seeks to understand how behavioral factors may contribute to or cause diseases or how compliance with treatment is mediated, hypnotherapeutic techniques provide excellent research tools. They can be used in various ways: (1) to document and explain which biological processes can be directly modified; (2) to what degree cyberphysiological controls are possible and predictable; (3) what knowledge is state specific; (4) whether or not certain therapeutic regimens must be state specific; (5) how learning abilities and styles as well as genetics relate to self-regulatory abilities; and (6) whether the state of the therapist affects patient responses.

2. The New Pediatrics and Self-Regulation Strategies

Children and their families may have had greater psychosocial, behavioral, and/or developmental problems and stress deriving from such problems in past times than at present. They may have experienced more sorrow and more days of acute illness, and society paid less attention to their suffering. Today's greater focus by child health professionals on behavioral and developmental issues probably reflects: (1) improved methods of recognition; (2) increased time for intervention; and (3) the availability of some resources to assign to them. For the most part, however, professionals concerned with developmental and behavioral problems still lack precise interventions that can act as predictably as the Sabin polio vaccine or an antibiotic such as ampicillin.

Children (and their families) now live through malignancies and more than half survive; yet the sword of Damocles hangs ever over them. Sophisticated biochemical or immunologic analyses make it possible to diagnose diseases that are chronic and ultimately fatal such as muscular dystrophy and AIDS. The stress of knowing that the disease is long, inexorable, and without cure may cause psychophysiological disease in parents or other family members. *What can we offer for these types of problems?* Green (1985) noted that "today adaptation must be added to the traditional pediatric agenda, highlighting the special opportunities that pediatricians and their child health colleagues have to help children and families adapt to crucial life events and psychosocial stressors."

The recent, albeit early, research in cyberphysiology suggests that training children and their families in self-regulation of some physiological responses may provide important therapeutic and preventive interventions. Although such strategies may not be curative, they provide self-managed techniques that give a sense of mastery to children who have little control over most diagnostic and treatment interventions. Research has demonstrated that children take pride in being able to demonstrate, through use of biofeedback, control of various physiological responses. Families are similarly benefited. There are data to support the benefit derived from training in relaxation with mental imagery techniques as soon as possible after diagnosis of a chronic illness such as hemophilia, sickle cell disease, malignancies, rheumatoid arthritis, or juvenile migraine (Zeltzer and LeBaron, 1982; Hilgard and LeBaron, 1984; Kohen, 1986; Olness *et al.*, 1987; Erickson, 1987).

2.1. Applications to Child Health Professionals

Although the overall working hours and call schedules have become less exhausting for house officers and pediatricians, the demands during actual working times have increased. Patients in the hospital are sicker and the technology utilized in their treatment is much more complex.

Message-delivering beepers and car telephones allow no respite. Patients and families survive complex illnesses for longer periods with increasing stress for them and for the caretakers involved. Competition, regulations, insurance company demands, and paperwork affect each patient–caregiver interaction. The pediatrician generally must juggle dozens of problems concurrently. Unfortunately, the coping methods used by caregivers have increasingly become "second careers," "early retirement," or alcohol and drug abuse.

While not a panacea, nonpharmacological strategies for self-regulation and relaxation are certainly helpful to many therapists. Excellent results with relaxation imagery or self-hypnosis are possible if: (1) time is expended in developing practice modes that are individualized to the child health professional's personal interest, likes, learning styles, and imagery; and (2) the child health professional is willing to invest 30 minutes of practice time daily for 2 months. They can learn to relax voluntarily and quickly when they have a short break or prior to an anticipated stressful patient encounter. They can solve problems of insomnia, muscle tension, or chronic pain. Professionals can learn to concentrate more effectively in reading journals or charts. Similarly, they can learn voluntary control of physiological responses such as perspiration, blood pressure, peripheral skin temperature, and galvanic skin resistance. In so doing, child health care professionals may find work more enjoyable and may also increase their abilities to teach similar strategies to their patients.

Ideally, all children should have the opportunity to demonstrate to themselves their potential in cyberbiological controls. With respect to child health professionals, they should also have the opportunity to learn and practice self-regulatory skills early in training in order to improve learning efficiency, to increase enjoyment, and to live an overall healthier life.

2.2. Applications in Hospital Settings

During the past decade numerous clinical and research studies have confirmed the value of self-regulatory strategies for children who are hospitalized. Reported training procedures have ranged from prospective training for groups of hemophiliac boys to bedside training for acutely ill children. A 5-year prospective study involving 61 children with malignancies concluded that these children benefited most from self-hypnosis training when it was accomplished within the first 4 days after diagnosis (Olness, 1985). Olness (1981), Hilgard and LeBaron

(1984), and Kuttner (1988), have documented that children can benefit from training in methods to reduce pain and anxiety after they have become negatively conditioned to diagnostic and treatment procedures. The most efficient training and optimal responses occur, however, if children have not suffered from previous negative experiences (e.g., multiple uncomfortable bone marrow procedures).

Children hospitalized with chronic conditions including asthma, cystic fibrosis, rheumatoid arthritis, and lupus erythematosus have benefited from training in self-regulation strategies. These conditions may lead to loss of self-control, dependency, and anxiety; however, training in self-hypnosis provides children with at least one component of a treatment regimen that is under their own control. Some children seem to tolerate procedures very well for months or years after diagnosis and then suddenly lose coping skills. Prospective training in self-regulation may avoid this and also may lead to reduction in frequency of hospitalizations.

Members of child treatment teams may benefit directly (and their patients indirectly) from personal acquisition of skills in relaxation and/or pain control in the stressful situations that they frequently encounter.

2.3. Applications in School Settings

There are several anecdotal reports with respect to application of relaxation imagery techniques in the classroom, including: (1) group relaxation methods such as those described in *The Centering Book* (Hendricks and Wills, 1975); (2) special language training methods such as the Lozanoff methods (Ostrander and Schroeder, 1979); (3) training for specific controls in physical education (Swedish system); and (4) training for creativity in pilot projects (the Whole Mind Learning Project completed in a Minneapolis grade school). While prospective, long-term outcome studies have not been reported, there are a few cross-sectional studies that demonstrate short-term changes in children or adolescents who have learned and practiced self-regulation techniques. These approaches enhance the child's personal sense of mastery and coping ability and are well-suited to training in health classes or in physical education settings.

It would seem useful to provide a few simple biofeedback machines in order to give each child the opportunity to learn that changes in thinking can effect changes in body responses, and that these responses can be voluntary changes. Incorporation of this type of learning into a child's knowledge base may have a significant impact on the child's personal body awareness, self-esteem, interpretation of symptoms (e.g., perspiration or blushing), and possible avoidance of psychophysiological illnesses. If children learn to recognize a link between their mental images and physiological responses, they may be able to learn to control both images and responses (e.g., magazines may contain pornographic photos or photos of food, both of which trigger mental images that lead to physiological responses). A creative teacher or coach can provide many examples of mental images and body response connections, allowing the students practice in learning to control these connections.

Rusin and Wynne (1987) recently provided a 10-week stress reduction program in a Minnesota school, at the request of a school social worker. Two sixth-grade classes, one a traditional classroom and one a classroom for boys with behavior problems, were compared. Over a 10-week period both groups participated in sessions devoted to discussion of stress, images, feelings, and behavior. After several sessions, each child was provided with an opportunity to monitor his peripheral temperature and galvanic skin resistance (GSR). It was of interest that the children identified as having behavior problems had high baseline GSR, and with relaxation training they were able to effect more dramatic changes in both skin temperature and GSR.

In Vermont, a group of learning-disabled college students were offered group training in self-hypnosis (Gilmore, 1987). Those students who learned self-regulation strategies through self-hypnosis performed much better than those who did not learn self-hypnosis.

2.4. Applications in Athletics, Arts, and Music

During the past decade professional sports teams and Olympic competitors have retained sports psychologists to train them in RMI techniques in order to improve physiological controls and reduce anxiety, thereby enhancing performance. For example, biathlon competitors can be trained to control their cardiac rates so that cardiac rate can be quickly reduced after a burst of skiing and therefore improve accuracy in riflery. Weight lifters utilize imagery rehearsal techniques, as do basketball players. Astronauts have been taught methods of controlling their autonomic responses. While traditional martial arts training includes relaxation-imagery-type exercises for adults and children, it is only recently that some attention has been given to teaching children such strategies in physical and/or in individual sports training in the Western world. Children and adolescents who develop performance anxiety have benefited from relaxation imagery training to undo these problems. Research studies, however, have not adequately looked at potential benefits from teaching these strategies prospectively to child competitors. Although children have been referred for therapy to undo conditioned anxiety responses associated with musical performance, studies have not been conducted involving prospective training in self-regulation for enhancing musical skills or reducing performance anxieties.

Artists have often described spontaneously the perception of an altered state or imagery changes while in creative modes. This is also true for scientists and inventors. There may be increased efficiency and productivity in persons who regularly spend time in planned or unplanned RMI practice. Bronowski (1974) referred to the value of imagination in his statement from *The Ascent of Man,* "All great civilizations have failed in one regard; they have limited the freedom of imagination of the child."

2.5. Applications in Third-World Child Health

Eighty-five percent of children are born into the Third World; demographic projections are that the percentage will be even higher by the end of this century. Current resources cannot provide externally mediated interventions such as highly trained subspecialists, medications, and/or machines for a majority of acute or chronic problems. Early training in cyberbiological methods is especially relevant in the absence of alternatives such as tranquilizers, psychotherapy, pain medications, worker's compensation, disability coverage, physical therapy, and so forth. Providing children of the Third World with strategies for self-regulation and coping might counteract some of the deprivation they suffer. Such training might be directed by village health workers or by school teachers. The potential for video letter communication from schools in Western countries to schools in Third-World villages may allow transfer of many cyberbiological methods ranging from handwashing to pain control. Clinically, cyberbiological research in these settings is urgently needed.

3. Methods

Training in cyberphysiological controls may be mediated through self-hypnosis training or relaxation imagery training (virtually indistinguishable from self-hypnosis). Concurrent provision of machine feedback may be provided by simple temperature monitors or complex computer game feedback. Although provision of such feedback is not essential to acquisition of voluntary control over certain autonomic processes, this type of feedback raises the interest level of some children and increases the speed of learning.

Acquisition of these skills requires training time for child health professionals. Ideally, the learner should begin with a 3-day intensive workshop, such as that provided by the American Society of Clinical Hypnosis, the Society of Clinical and Experimental Hypnosis, or the Society for Behavioral Pediatrics (see Section 7 for addresses). These workshops provide the learner with practice in developing skills in a comfortable setting. Following the initial workshop, the student should begin applying acquired skills in clinical settings, if possible, with a mentor available. Many areas of the United States have component sections of the American Society of Clinical Hypnosis where one may seek out child health professionals who are members and may be available as a mentor. The Society for Behavioral Pediatrics can provide names of members who are skilled in teaching cyberphysiological training strategies. Initially the student should work only in problem areas with which he/she is very familiar in terms of diagnosis and treatment. Sessions should be audio- or videotaped and the learner should review these to improve skills. Training to develop skills in the use of various biofeedback units may take considerable time, depending on how many computers, connections, and dials are involved.

It is also important that families be aware of the need for practice and reinforcement of those training strategies that have been employed. Olympic competitors from Sweden are asked to practice cyberphysiological training 30 minutes for 9 weeks before it can be assumed that acquisition of desired controls is sufficient for competition. Children learn more quickly than adults and many studies indicate that they can learn pain control strategies in one or two practice sessions. Children with juvenile migraine have demonstrated, in prospective studies, that four training sessions with daily practice in between is sufficient to acquire pain control. Except in situations in which the child is very weak, it is recommended that parents not remind children to practice cyberphysiological strategies, although they may discuss a reminder system, such as a sign on the door, red yarn around the toothbrush handle, and so forth. Because training emphasis is on self-control and coping ability, it is counterproductive for parents or other adults to remind or insist on practice.

4. Decision Making Regarding Appropriate Therapy

Before recommending that a child learn cyberphysiological strategies, one must make several judgments about: (1) the underlying problem; (2) motivation of the child and family; and (3) strategies appropriate for a particular child.

1. *Have diagnostic efforts been sufficient? Is the basis for the child's problem sufficiently established?* We have published a study that reviews 80 consecutive referrals for hypnotherapy in children of whom 20 had previously unrecognized biological bases for their symptoms. For example, one child referred with intractable headaches had carbon monoxide poisoning. (Olness and Libbey, 1987)

2. *What is the setting for training? How may a treatment team facilitate or sabotage training efforts?* A therapist may be very competent and a child may not respond if other members of the treatment team are uninformed about cyberphysiological methods. It is important to spend time with colleagues prior to embarking on a course of treatment, which has as its goal the development of some self-regulated skills in control of physiological responses.

3. *What is the influence of age and development of the child?* The therapist must decide whether or not the child is capable of learning a self-regulation strategy. Some bright 2-year-olds can learn self-hypnosis, but generally these strategies are more appropriate after age 3 years. Very young children may learn very well in a group setting, which is less intimidating. It is important to consider the "goodness of fit model" as a conceptual framework from which to determine what, if any, therapy is appropriate for a given child (Chess and Thomas, 1984). The characteristics and capacities of the child must be carefully considered with respect to how that child may handle specific demands and expectations.

4. *What are the effects of learning styles, strengths, and learning handicaps?* It is helpful to question parents about how they believe their child learns best. Some children do not follow verbal instructions well, or forget them quickly. Others learn best by reading or watching video examples or by using computers. Strategies utilizing computer games may be preferable for some children. Verbal coaching may be inappropriate for some children. Parents can usually provide helpful insights with respect to the temperament of the child, how he or she handles new situations, and what kind of people he or she likes.

5. *What are the influences on the child's interests, likes, and dislikes?* It is essential to spend time learning from the child and/or parents what he is like. It is important to determine the child's strengths, interests, fears, and dislikes. Does the child like music? Does he or she like basketball? What is the child afraid of? With this information, the therapist can develop a practice plan that includes concentration on activities or situations that are pleasant for the child, e.g., "imagine yourself at the top of a ski run on a day in which the snow is perfect, the sky the way you like it, and your equipment exactly as you like."

6. *What are the effects of varying cultural backgrounds?* Cultural backgrounds are important in explaining and planning training strategies. Symptoms such as pain may be handled differently depending on the individual's cultural experience. Temperamental differences may be viewed differently depending on the cultures. In some cultures, e.g., Thai, it is inappropriate to express feelings directly. One may induce significant stress by asking specific questions about how the child is feeling.

7. *Does the therapist's state of mind influence outcome?* If the therapist is anxious or fatigued, this may have a negative effect on the training session. A few seconds of rapid self-relaxation may help the therapist. The therapist should develop a personal expectation of success and use the occasion to enhance the child's sense of self-esteem and personal mastery.

5. Research Findings

Unfortunately, most child health professionals are trained with "lip service" to the concept of mind–body connections. This concept remains, for the majority, a commonsense notion validated for some when they observe their own tachycardia or perspiration in association with anxious thoughts. Many professionals have searched for predictable ways of providing therapy that relate to the important connections between the mind and physiological changes. Some degree of amazement is experienced by the professional who learns techniques such as self-hypnosis and is then able to observe evidence in self and in others that changing mental images (whether visual, auditory, olfactory, or tactile) can result in measurable changes in body functions, and that some of these changes occurred within seconds of the thought change.

Various controlled studies have documented the ability of children to self-regulate peripheral temperature, brain stem auditory evoked potentials, electromyographic responses, transcutaneous oxygen, and salivary immunoglobulins (Dikel and Olness, 1980; Hogan *et al.*, 1985; Olness and Conroy, 1985; Olness and Culbert, 1987). These studies suggest that it is important to document these skills, to sort out associated factors or traits that may be predictive of success or failure, and to compare strategies and times in order to determine optimal teaching methods.

Children demonstrate individual patterns with respect to autonomic responses and the ability to regulate them. For example, one child may have an elevated GSR and normal peripheral temperature during waking hours, while others may have the opposite. Cyberphysiological monitoring for children has become increasingly sophisticated and is a noninvasive intervention. Monitoring during normal activities can provide information for child health professionals concerning: (1) responsiveness of specific autonomic processes to mental and/or physical activities or to medications; (2) feedback to children regarding how their thinking affects body responses; and (3) evidence of specific stressors that may produce inappropriate or undesirable physiological responses in certain individuals, e.g., labile blood pressures or cardiac arrhythmias.

The new area of psychoneuroimmunology, which provides evidence that self-regulation of specific immune responses is possible, is important and exciting (Ader, 1981; Mayer and Haggerty, 1962; Schleifer *et al.,* 1986). A few case reports in children and some adult laboratory experiments have led to pilot studies in children where changes in salivary immunoglobulins and lymphocyte function in association with relaxation imagery practice for a short period of time were demonstrated. Animal studies have amply demonstrated that immune processes can be conditioned. If similar conditioning occurs in humans, it is conceivable that relaxation imagery exercises may mediate deconditioning of undesirable immune responses or enhance desirable responses. Advances in this important area within the next decade may lead to practical clinical applications.

6. The Future

Although adults recognize various physiological responses to stress for both peers and themselves, there are few data to guide anticipatory advice regarding stress for children and their families. Most adults recognize the usual physiological responses to stress or anxiety, such as epigastric pain, blushing, tachycardia, or anorexia. Yet few know how and when these responses began or were conditioned. Anecdotal evidence supports the idea that a classical conditioning paradigm is associated with the onset of many psychophysiological responses. For example, a child was nauseated because of a viral gastroenteritis and concurrently experienced an anxiety-producing situation; subsequently, she became nauseated whenever she was anxious. It is well-documented that these responses can be extinguished through training in self-hypnosis. If the symptom has been reinforced over years, this process may require weeks or months of training. If teachers, parents, or coaches are alert to the onset of undesirable physiological responses to stress in their charges, with self-hypnosis therapy perhaps years of discomfort and possible risks to ultimate good health can be avoided.

It appears that there is a state specificity of learning and reestablishment of that same state for optimal recall of learned material. There are data that support the concept that the release of peptides that mediate learning is specific to specific states. For example, studies indicate that memory processing in mice is positively affected by peptide release during feeding. If, indeed, learning is so dependent on the concurrent peptide release associated with it (or replication of the same peptide release state as was present when the original release occurred), it would seem reasonable to use self-regulation strategies that duplicate the same state at each training session. It is interesting to speculate that rituals prior to sermons in church or karate or biofeedback training may lead to replication of state and therefore enhanced learning. Controlled studies will be necessary in order to document whether or not children learn more quickly if efforts are made to replicate the same state during each training session.

As research continues in these important areas, more precise assessments of genetic or intrinsic learning styles and patterns will develop that will allow more useful and efficient choice of self-regulation methods.

Current knowledge of cyberphysiology in children suggests that it will become important to consider a child's self-regulation abilities at many junctures of diagnosis and treatment. How do they affect the expression of symptoms? How do they relate to laboratory measures? How do they affect the transport of intravenous or intramuscular or oral medications? Do they relate to the shortening or prolongation of symptoms? Do physicians and nurses inadvertently suggest negative images that trigger negative responses? Most important, perhaps: can more information enable the child health professional to facilitate adaptation in children and families not only to illness but to success, to stress, to family changes, and to societal changes?

In summary, advances in cyberphysiology have major implications for and applications to developmental and behavioral pediatrics. These will relate to self-control and stress reduction for the adults who work with children in the home, at school, at play, and in health care settings. They will relate to the development of cyberphysiological controls early in life, with reductions in requirements for medications and other treatments, greater feelings of comfort and self-control, and possibly less need for hurtful behaviors such as drug abuse, overeating, and/or crime. Early training in cyberphysiological controls may reduce acquisition of certain chronic diseases or reduce morbidity from them.

Both Jacob Bronowski and William Blake spoke and wrote of the importance of the imagination and how it should be nurtured in children. Perhaps adults will learn to do that more effectively and perhaps the next generation of adults will retain more imagery skills with significance for adaptation, for health, and for happiness.

7. Appendix

1. The American Society of Clinical Hypnosis
   2250 East Devon Avenue, Suite 336
   Des Plaines, IL 60018
   (312) 297-3317

2. Society for Behavioral Pediatrics
   241 East Gravers Lane
   Philadelphia, PA 19118
   (215) 248-9168
   (Ms. Noreen Spota, Business Administrator)

3. Society for Clinical and Experimental Hypnosis
   128-A Kings Park Drive
   Liverpool, New York 13090

References

Ader, R. (ed.), 1981, *Psychoneuroimmunology,* Academic Press, New York.

Bronowski, J., 1974, *The Ascent of Man,* Little Brown, Boston.

Chess, S., and Thomas, A., 1984, The goodness of fit model: Theoretical and practical implications, in: *Origins and Evolution of Behavior Disorders from Infancy to Early Adult Life,* pp. 20–23, Brunner and Mazel, New York.

Dikel, W., and Olness, K., 1980, Self-hypnosis, biofeedback, and voluntary peripheral temperature control in children, *Pediatrics* **66:**335–340.

Erikson, C., 1987, Hypnotherapy is a successful adjunct intervention in children with sickle cell disease, presented at the Society for Behavioral Pediatrics, Washington, D.C., May, 1987.

Gardner, G. G., and Olness, K. N., 1981, *Hypnosis and Hypnotherapy with Children,* Grune and Stratton, New York.

Gilmore, L., 1987, Hypnosis and learning-disabled college students, presented at the American Society of Clinical Hypnosis Scientific Meetings, April, 1987, Las Vegas.

Green, M., 1985, The adaptation of children and families; the new pediatric agenda, in: *The Psychosocial Aspects of the Family; The New Pediatrics* (M. Green, ed.), pp. 1–12, Lexington Books, Lexington, MA.

Hilgard, J. R., and LeBaron, S., 1984, *Hypnotherapy of Pain in Children with Cancer* (W. Kaufman, ed.), Los Altos, CA.

Hendricks, G., and Wills, R., 1975, *The Centering Book,* Prentice-Hall, Inc., Englewood Cliffs, N.J.

Hogan, M., Olness, K., and MacDonald, J., 1985, The effect of hypnosis on brain stem auditory responses in children, *Am. J. Clin. Hypn.* **27:**91–94.

Kohen, D., 1986, Relaxation mental imagery (self-hypnosis) in the management of asthma: Preliminary report of pulmonary function studies and behavioral outcomes in a prospective long-term study with 28 children (abstract), *Am. J. Dis.* **140:**297–298.

Kuttner, L., 1988, Favorite stories: A hypnotic pain reduction technique for children in acute pain, *Am. J. Clin. Hypn.* **30:**289–295.

Mayer, R., and Haggerty, R., 1962, Streptococcal infections in families: Factors altering individual susceptibility, *Pediatrics* **29:**539–549.

Olness, K., 1981, Imagery (self-hypnosis) as adjunct therapy in childhood cancer: Clinical experience with 25 patients, *Am. J. Pediatr. Hematol. Oncol.* **3:**313–321.

Olness, K., 1988, A five-year prospective study of relaxation mental imagery as adjunct therapy in 61 children with malignancies, *Topics in Pediatrics* (in press).

Olness, K., and Conroy, M. M., 1985, Voluntary control of transcutaneous oxygen flow in children, *Int. J. Clin. Exp. Hypn.* **3:**1–5.

Olness, K., and Culbert, T., 1988, Voluntary control of salivary immunoglobulins in children, *Pediatrics* (in press).

Olness, K., and Libbey, P., 1987, Unrecognized biologic bases of behavioral symptoms in patients referred for by hypnotherapy. *The Amer. J. of Clin. Hyp.* **30:**1–8.

Olness, K., MacDonald, J., and Uden, D., 1987, Comparison of propranolol, placebo, and self-hypnosis in management of juvenile classic migraine, *Pediatrics* **79:**593–597.

Ostrander, S., and Schroeder, L., 1979, *Super Learning,* Dell Publishing Co., New York.

Rusin, W., and Wynne, E., 1987, A classroom stress reduction program using computor game feedback (abstract), *Ambulatory Pediatr. Assoc.*, p. 20.

Schleifer, S. J., Scott, B., Stein, M., *et al.*, 1986, Behavioral and developmental aspects of immunity, *J. Am. Acad. Child Psychiatry* **26:**751–763.

Schwartz, G. E., 1971, Cardiac responses to self-induced thoughts, *Psychophysiology* **8:**462–467.

Zeltzer, L., and LeBaron, S., 1982, Hypnosis and nonhypnotic techniques for reduction of pain and anxiety during painful procedures in children and adolescents with cancer, *J. Pediatr.* **101:**1032–1035.

Chapter 16

Graduates of the Neonatal Intensive Care Unit

HAROLD PERL

1. Introduction

Over the past century the management of sick and premature newborns has progressed dramatically. The field of newborn care has benefited from technological advances far beyond any other field of medicine. What was originally a sideshow at various World's Fairs and Expositions (supported by admission charges to viewers) has flourished into the present-day high-technology tertiary centers known as neonatal intensive care units. The role of health care provider for the newborn has also experienced its own evolution. Initially it was the obstetrician who was responsible for the well-being of the newborn after birth. Gradually, a specialist in newborn and infant care, the *pediatrician,* assumed this role. Presently, the *neonatologist,* a pediatric subspecialist, has assumed the management of the sickest newborns.

2. Incidence

It is estimated that over 100,000 infants are admitted each year to intensive care nurseries. The discharge of these patients from the intensive care nursery marks the resolution of their "acute" illness. Their return to primary pediatric care, however, may be only the beginning for a host of possible long-term complications.

HAROLD PERL • Neonatal Intensive Care Unit, Hackensack Medical Center, Hackensack, New Jersey 07601.

Advances in neonatology have dramatically improved the survival rates of very-low-birthweight (VLBW) infants under 1500 g and especially those "micropreemies" with birthweights of 500 to 1000 g. A recent study from the University of Pennsylvania revealed an increase in survival rates of micropreemies from a rate of 26% during the 1978–1980 period to 64% in 1982–1984 (Gerdes *et al.,* 1986). The survival rates for this population rise markedly with increasing gestational age and birthweight, from 20% at 24 weeks to 83% at 27 weeks' gestation.

3. Sequelae

Along with increased survival of the tiny infant comes the need for the neonatologist to monitor the long-term outcome of these infants. From the inception of neonatology, there has always been concern about propagating a generation of severely handicapped infants and children. This has never materialized. In the study cited from the University of Pennsylvania, the incidence of moderate or severe handicaps was only 15% (Gerdes *et al.,* 1986). The percentage of infants with long-term complications has either remained stable or has actually decreased. The absolute number has increased, however, as a result of the significant increase in survival rates. We will therefore briefly review the most common complications of the neonatal intensive care graduate.

3.1. Intraventricular Hemorrhage

Intraventricular hemorrhage (IVH) occurs in approximately 30–40% of preterm infants. The periventricular vasculature sits in a loose lattice work of connective tissue with very little support to existing arteries and veins. Risk factors such as hypoxia, shock, pneumothorax, and mechanical ventilation may result in rupture of these fragile vessels. Surveillance with cranial ultrasonography of premature infants less than 34 weeks' gestation and follow-up for those affected have become routine. The most widely accepted classification is that of Papile *et al.* (1978):

- Grade I: isolated subependymal hemorrhage
- Grade II: IVH without ventricular dilatation
- Grade III: IVH with ventricular dilatation
- Grade IV: IVH with parenchymal extensions

Cranial ultrasound has been extremely useful in the acute management of premature infants. As experience broadens, it has become a powerful prognostic indicator of neurodevelopmental complications. Several studies have revealed a direct relationship between grades III and IV, IVH, and major handicaps (Papile *et al.*, 1983). The long-term significance of other ultrasonographic findings such as periventricular leukomalacia and cystic changes is still being evaluated.

3.2. Bronchopulmonary Dysplasia

The clinical definition of bronchopulmonary dysplasia (BPD) has evolved over the past 20 years. It is now defined as a chronic lung disease of infancy in which lung parenchyma at 30 days of age shows any radiologic abnormality in addition to ventilator dependence. The incidence of BPD among infants weighing 700–1500 g ranges from 7 to 35%. The major factors contributing to BPD are (1) immaturity, (2) barotrauma, and (3) oxygen toxicity. Which of these is the major factor has been a source of controversy for years in the pediatric literature. A recent study of eight academic centers revealed that Columbia Presbyterian Babies Hospital had a dramatically reduced incidence of chronic lung disease (Avery *et al.*, 1987). This has been at least partially attributed to their efforts in avoiding intubation and mechanical ventilation, using only nasal continuous positive airway pressure (CPAP) and allowing PCO_2 levels of 60 torr or more. This suggests that the major contributing factor is barotrauma induced by mechanical ventilation.

The successful management of BPD can be divided into two major goals:

1. Gradual but persistent weaning from mechanical ventilation, while maintaining acceptable blood gases and pH. Bronchodilators, steroids, and diuretics have all been used with varying success. Persistent O_2 therapy is becoming a common practice.
2. Provide adequate nutrition to enhance healing and growth of new lung tissue. The development of total parenteral nutrition has made a significant contribution to the improved outcome for patients with BPD.

The most common problem encountered in the follow-up of infants with BPD is bronchospasm. It is often triggered by viral infections, environmental irritants, or dehydration. Despite classical teaching, affected infants do have bronchial smooth muscle that is responsive to bronchodilators such as theophylline. The use of furosemide has received greater acceptance because of its diuretic effect and its possible direct effects on pulmonary lymph flow or vascular capacitance.

3.3. Retinopathy of Prematurity

Improved survival among low-birthweight infants has resulted in an increased number of infants with retinopathy of prematurity (ROP). Occurrence of active disease is reported to be 38–54% in newborns under 1000 g and roughly 5–15% in 1000- to 1500-g infants. More than 500 infants in the United States are estimated to be blinded from ROP each year and about 2100 will have reduced vision. The precise etiology of ROP remains unclear, but several risk factors have been identified:

1. Degree of prematurity. Prematurity and low birthweight have been identified most frequently with the increasing incidence of ROP. The smaller the newborn, the more immature is the retinal vasculature and the larger the retinal vascular area.
2. Duration of oxygen. Increased oxygen concentration and prolonged oxygen treatment places infants at greater risk for ROP. As a result, meticulous care is taken to monitor arterial blood gases and continuous transcutaneous PO_2 levels. A definite safe range for arterial PaO_2 is unknown. Similarly, the critical duration of oxygen exposure for the development of ROP is unknown. Until such guidelines are established, the accepted recommendations are for PaO_2 levels between 50 and 70 mm Hg.
3. Other reported associated factors have been hypercapnea, septicemia, apnea, exchange transfusions, patent ductus arteriosus (PDA), indomethacin, and genetic factors.

A uniform classification or grading system was adopted at the Retinopathy Conference in Washington, D.C. in 1981:

- Grade I: the peripheral retinas are gray and avascular
- Grade II: retinal vascular engorgement with dilated and tortuous terminal vessels
- Grade III: extra retinal vascular proliferation with possible hemorrhage or exudates
- Grades IV and V: peripheral and complete retinal detachment

All infants less than 36 weeks or weighing less than 2000 g who have received oxygen therapy should be examined by a person experienced in recognizing ROP at 6 to 8 weeks of age.

Medical treatment of ROP remains controversial. Vitamin E has been used both prophylactically and in the early acute stages. Recent reports by Hittner *et al.* have shown vitamin E to be effective in reducing the severity of ROP (Hittner *et al.*, 1981). The exact dosage, though, and the incidence of severe side effects remain to be clarified. An alternative treatment for severe ROP is the use of cryosurgery. Cryotherapy attempts to induce remission by interrupting the process of neovascularization and to prevent further detachment by inducing scarring at the periphery thereby reducing the amount of traction on the retina. Treatment of late cicatricial disease includes scleral bucking and at times vitrectomy.

3.4. Hearing Problems

The incidence of neurosensory hearing loss in premature infants has been reported to be approximately 1–3%. The risk factors to which these infants are exposed include hypoxia, hyperbilirubinemia, environmental noise levels, antibiotic therapy, and congenital infections. The American Academy of Pediatrics (1988) recommends hearing screening for all infants with birthweights less than 1500 g. A list of all groups at risk for hearing impairment is provided in Table I.

It has been well-documented that the earlier hearing loss is identified, the better the outcome for these infants. Screening should be performed by 3 months of age for high-risk patients, using a behavioral screening test. If the behavioral response to sound is equivocal or nonresponsive, the patient should be screened with brain stem evoked response audiometry. Comprehensive audiologic evaluations should be repeated as the patient gets older and testing becomes more reliable.

4. Summary

Some of the more common long-term medical problems encountered by the neonatal intensive care unit graduate have been reviewed. Other areas of neurodevelopmental delay and learning disabilities are beyond the scope of this review. As the survival rate of critically ill

Table 1. Infants at Risk for Hearing Impairment

Family history of hearing loss
Congenital infections (TORCH[a])
Anatomic malformations involving the head and neck
Birthweight less than 1500 g
Hyperbilirubinemia
Bacterial meningitis
Severe birth asphyxia

[a]Toxoplasmosis–other infections–rubella virus–cytomegalovirus–herpes simplex.

infants continues to improve, primary pediatricians will encounter increasingly patients with chronic illnesses. These children will become an integral part of their general practice. The neonatal intensive care unit graduate often requires the follow-up care of many subspecialties. However, it is crucial for the primary physician to become familiar with these problems in order that the family be prepared and directed appropriately. It is also helpful to obtain the support of a multidisciplinary neonatal follow-up program.

References

American Academy of Pediatrics, 1988, *Guidelines for Perinatal Care*, 2nd ed., American Academy of Pediatrics and the American College of Obstetrics and Gynecology, pp. 106–107.

Avery, M. E., Tooley, W. H., Keller, S. B., *et al.*, 1987, Chronic lung disease in low-birthweight infants, *Pediatrics* **79:**26–31.

Gerdes, J. S., Abbasi, S., Bhutani, V. K., *et al.*, 1986, Improved survival and short-term outcome of inborn "micropreemies," *Clin. Pediatr.* **25:**391–394.

Hittner, H. M., Godio, L. B., Rudolph, A. J., *et al.*, 1981, Retrolental fibroplasia: Efficacy of vitamin E in a double-blind clinical study of preterm infants. *N. Engl. J. Med.* **305:** 1365.

Papile, L. A., Burstein, J., Burstein, R., *et al.*, 1978, Incidence and evolution of subependymal and intraventricular hemorrhage: A study of infants with birth weights less than 1,500 gm. *Pediatrics* **92:**529–534.

Papile, L. A., Musich-Bruno, G., and Scaefer, A., 1983, Relationship of cerebral intraventricular hemorrhage and early childhood neurologic handicaps, *J. Pediatr.* **103:** 273–277.

Suggested Reading

Bancalari, E., and Gerhardt, T., 1986, Bronchopulmonary dysplasia, *Pediatr. Clin. North Am.* **33:**1–23.

Bernbaum, J., and D'Agostino, J., 1986, The NICU graduate: Managing the major complications, *Contemp. Pediatr.* **3:**69–82.

Christophersen, E. R., (ed.), 1985, *Dev. Behav. Issues Perinatol.* **12:**307–474.

Eviatar, L., 1984, Continuing care of the high-risk infant: Evaluation of hearing in the high-risk infant, *Clin. Perinatol.* **11:**1–10.

Kingham, J. D., 1985, Classification of retinopathy of prematurity, in: *Retinopathy of Prematurity: Current Concepts and Controversies* (A. R. McPherson, H. M. Hittner, and F. L. Kretzer, eds.), pp. 17–25. B. C. Decker, Philadelphia.

Kurban, K., and Teale, R. L., 1984, Rationale for grading intracranial hemorrhage in premature infants, *Pediatrics* **74:**358–363.

Lucey, J. F., and Dungman, B., 1984, A re-examination of the role of oxygen in retrolental fibroplasia, *Pediatrics* **73:**82–96.

Northway, W. H., Jr., Rosen, R. C., and Porter, D. Y., 1967, Pulmonary disease following respirator therapy of hyaline membrane disease: Bronchopulmonary dysplasia, *N. Engl. J. Med.* **276:**367–368.

Porat, R., 1984, Continuing care of the high-risk infant: Care of the infant with retinopathy of prematurity, *Clin. Perinatol.* **11:**123–151.

Chapter 17

Pediatrics, Neurology, and Psychiatry—A Common Ground

The Child Who Fails to Speak

N. PAUL ROSMAN

1. Introduction

Speech and language difficulties (delays, disorders, deficits) are among the more frequently encountered developmental problems of early childhood. These difficulties may have pediatric, neurologic, and/or psychiatric origins. The child who fails to speak represents an excellent example of a developmental problem in which these medical disciplines share a common ground.

A few basic definitions are in order. *Language* refers to a system of symbols used for communication. These symbols can be written, gestured, or spoken. On the other hand, *speech* is the physical production of spoken language, i.e., articulation. Speech requires the integration of oral, respiratory, and laryngeal movements.

This chapter will review some of the causes of speech disturbances in children.

N. PAUL ROSMAN • Departments of Pediatrics and Neurology, Tufts University School of Medicine, and Division of Pediatric Neurology, Floating Hospital for Infants and Children, New England Medical Center Hospitals, Boston, Massachusetts 02111.

2. Levels of Language

In order to appreciate the problem of the child who fails to speak, it is first necessary to define levels of language and to review several basic principles of speech per se.

Phonemes are the smallest components of language. There are 46 phonemes in English: 9 vowels and 37 consonants. When combined, vowels and consonants form words. The speech system can produce 12–14 phonemes and 3–5 syllables of speech per second. As an example, "well and will" are differentiated by vowel phonemes, whereas "but and cut" by consonant phonemes. *Syntax* is the grammatical organization of words to form sentences. *Semantics* is the structuring of words, phrases, and sentences to convey a meaningful message. *Pragmatics* is the use of language, both verbal and nonverbal, for the purposes of communication. A useful means of assessing a child's language and cognitive development is through the strategy of "pretend play." This technique may reveal weaknesses and/or disorders in the child's communication system.

3. Speech

Speech (verbalization) is one of the major language forms by which humans communicate. Although we listen more than we talk, the average individual speaks approximately 18,000 words each day. As an average, a person spends 13 years of their life talking, which ranks second only to sleeping.

In written language there are only 26 letters (the written symbol is called a *grapheme*), however, in spoken English there are 46 sounds (phonemes), including diphthongs (which do not appear in written English). It is of interest that in no language in the modern world (of which there are about 3000) do we find more than 70 phonemes.

3.1. Normal Speech Development

The maturation of sequential development of speech is summarized in Table 1. This table provides a guideline for estimating rate and competency of the maturational process, and a basis of cause for concern when delays are noted. Delays and disorders in speech development may predict subsequent problems in cognitive and educational development.

The general order in the normal sequence of grammatical development is first the acquisition of nouns and verbs, followed by adjectives

Table 1. Sequential Development of Speech

Age	Speech
Birth	Undifferentiated cry and coo
2–3 months	Differentiated cry; responsive cooing
3–4 months	Random babbling
5 months	46 sounds used in (later) speech
5–7 months	Rhythmic babbling
6–8 months	Self-imitation
8–10 months	Echolalia
1 year	1–2 words
11/2 years	5–50 words
2 years	2- to 3-word combinations; 200–300 words
3 years	3- to 4-word combinations; 1000 words
4 years	5-word combinations; 1500–2000 words
5 years	6-word combinations
6 years	More than 7500 words
7 years	7-word combinations; 20,000(±10,000) words
8 years	8-word combinations

and adverbs, and finally prepositions, pronouns, and conjunctions. As a rule, speech development is more rapid in females than in males. This may explain the greater frequency of most speech disorders among males.

3.2. Speech Delay and Deficits

Speech *delay* is generally defined as a failure in the acquisition of *words* by 18 to 24 months, and/or of *phrases* by 3 years of age. Approximately 50 out of 1000 children who are beginning school speak so poorly that they cannot be understood by strangers. About 10 of every 1000 children exhibit severely retarded speech development. Speech and language *deficits* are present in more than 5% of children in the United States.

3.3. Speech Disorders Sometimes Associated with Speech Delay

There are a variety of speech disorders that may be associated with delays in acquisition of speech, including dysphonia, dysrhythmia, structural dysarthria, and neurological dysarthria. *Dysphonia* is basically a disorder of voicing and is generally associated with abnormalities of the larynx or the respiratory pathway. Disorders of respiratory coordination, *dysrhythmia,* are often seen as stuttering and stammering. This phenomenon is frequently seen as a transient episode in children 2 to 5 years of age. It occurs twice as frequently among boys. Dysrhythmias have been seen also in association with dichotic listening difficulties. *Dysarthria* generally relates to disorders of speech sound production. Structural causes of dysarthria include abnormalities of the lips, tongue, palate (e.g., submucous cleft), nose (e.g., obstructions), pharynx (e.g., velopharyngeal insufficiency), vocal cords (e.g., paralysis), and the jaw (e.g., mandibular hypoplasia). Neurological causes of dysarthria include lesions of the upper motor neuron structures (e.g., corticobulbar (pyramidal) tracts, basal ganglia, cerebellum) or of the lower motor neuron (e.g., medulla). It is necessary to look for other associated signs that can assist in the clinical localization of the lesion, such as volitional palatal movements, tongue bulk, jaw-jerk, and oral–facial dyspraxia.

3.4. Major Causes of Speech Delay in Children

3.4.1. Psychosocial Stressors

A variety of psychosocial stressors may cause a speech delay in children. Generally, psychosocial causes are as frequent in girls as they are in boys. Among the more common psychosocial causes of speech delay are ordinal position in the family (e.g., the second child), multiple children in the family, and twin gestations. Speech development may also be slower with depressed socioeconomic environments, institutionalized children, and offspring of deaf-mute parents. Children exposed to two languages may be delayed in speech, if the introduction of the second language is delayed.

3.4.2. Mental Retardation

Approximately 3% of all children are mentally retarded and more than half of these have significant difficulties with speech. Thus, mental retardation joins hearing loss as one of the two major contributors to speech delay. Speech development correlates well with level of intelligence:

- With an IQ of 50–70, speech delay is frequent (but not invariable)

- With an IQ of 20–50, speech development is nearly always delayed
- With an IQ of 20 or less, very few children communicate by speech

At the other end of the spectrum, above-average intelligence correlates with advanced speech development.

When assessing mentally retarded children with speech delay, it is essential to exclude coexisting factors that may be contributing to the child's speech retardation. Examples include deafness, articulatory difficulties (structural and/or neurological), and environmental deprivation.

It is important to identify cases of speech delay in which the presence of mental retardation has been *misdiagnosed* because of poor selection of psychological test instruments; tests in which there is a heavy emphasis on items dependent on language should not be used.

3.4.3. Seizures

It has been known for more than 30 years that seizures in childhood can result in delayed speech development or loss of previously acquired speech. The seizures can be of varying types and either antedate the speech difficulty (so that the child will fail to acquire speech normally) or, if the seizures develop later, speech can first develop normally and then regress. Not uncommonly, such children are misdiagnosed as deaf. Infrequently, the seizures are not manifested clinically and are evidenced only on an electroencephalogram (EEG).

Different EEG abnormalities have been found in these cases; most often there are bilateral seizure discharges, maximal in the temporal regions. Seizure activity in such cases may produce a "functional ablation" of the cortical language area or, and perhaps more likely, may represent a cortical manifestation of a subcortical deafferenting process. In either case, speech could be impaired. Clinical control of seizures in such cases is often reasonably easy, but normalization of the child's EEG is more difficult; such improvements may or may not be paralleled by improvement in the child's speech. On the other hand, speech can sometimes improve in the absence of an unchanged EEG. Thus, the prognosis is variable. Mental subnormality may be an accompaniment of the seizure disorder, contributing to the speech delay.

3.4.4. Disordered Acoustic Input

The normal auditory system has the capacity to handle sounds ranging in intensity up to 140 dB and sound frequencies ranging from 20 to

20,000 Hz or cycles per second (cps) of sound. The system can distinguish 350 different intensities and 1600 frequencies, handling 20 to 30 segments of sound per second. A person is felt to have normal hearing if he is able to detect pure tones between 500 and 4000 cps at levels of 20 dB or less.

A bilateral loss of more than 25 dB, in the range of 1000–3000 cps, will cause some impairment in perception of speech. About 5% of school-age children suffer chronically from such a deficit; about 20% of school-age children suffer from middle ear infections causing some hearing impairment for some part of their lives. About 2 in 1000 children require a hearing aid and 1 in 1000 children show marked language retardation secondary to deafness.

Acoustic input can be disordered with *hearing loss, impaired auditory discrimination,* or with *impaired decoding of speech* (verbal auditory agnosia).

3.4.4a. Hearing Loss. Hearing impairment is the most frequently overlooked but the most indentifiable disorder affecting language development. Childhood deafness may be conductive or sensorineural in type. Of the conductive causes of hearing loss, most are related to recurrent middle ear infections and/or effusions (submucous cleft palate and eustachian tube dysfunction may be important contributors).

Middle ear disease may cause persistent deafness or, more often, intermittent hearing loss. While there are unquestionable adverse effects on speech (and learning) if such hearing impairment is persistent, this association is less certain in instances of intermittent hearing loss. There are a wide variety of causes for sensorineural deafness. These include congenital infections (e.g., rubella), neonatal meningitis (e.g., group B streptococcus), kernicterus, ototoxic drugs (e.g., kanamycin, gentamicin), aseptic meningitis (e.g., mumps), bacterial meningitis (e.g., *Hemophilus influenzae*), and genetic disorders (e.g., Wardenberg's, Usher's, and Alport's syndromes).

Clearly, hearing should be tested in every speech-delayed child. There are two basic approaches to such testing: *behavioral tests* and *physiological tests.* The former, in which the child is required to produce a specific gesture when he hears a certain sound, has the advantage of testing the *entire* acoustic system, including the processing of the acoustic message and use of that message to program a specific output. Such techniques may be unreliable in young children, however, and especially in those with language disorders.

When behavioral audiometry is impossible or unreliable, one must turn to physiological measures of hearing, such as reflex contraction of the stapedius muscle in response to sound, cochleography, and particularly brain stem auditory-evoked responses. These techniques do not require cooperation of the child and therefore are applicable to infants and to children who are multiply-handicapped or otherwise uncooperative. They provide no information, however, on the child's ability to process sound and use it to program behavior.

At a minimum, tympanometry should be done in all children with established or suspected chronic middle ear effusions.

If a child is born congenitally deaf, speech development will progress to the stage of babbling, and then regress because of lack of "feedback." Echolalia will fail to develop and by age 1 year, the child may be mute. With a high-tone hearing loss, the child will have difficulty producing sounds such as "f, th, sh." Such a hearing loss may be missed since the child may be responsive to lower frequency sounds and may compensate by visual cues. With a more severe hearing loss affecting all frequencies, the child will produce only those sounds that he can see, i.e., those associated with much lip movement such as "o, m, w, u." The child who is deaf from early life characteristically watches the faces of others closely.

In the speech-delayed child determined to be hearing-impaired, the earliest possible intervention is critical.

3.4.4b. Impaired Auditory Discrimination. Here, the child has normal hearing but has difficulty differentiating between similarly sounding words (bat/pat; tan/tam; bow/thou). In such children, perception of dichotic auditory stimuli may be altered (normally, the ear contralateral to the dominant temporal lobe is the preferred ear).

3.4.4c. Impaired Decoding of Speech (Verbal Auditory Agnosia). In this disorder, also called "word deafness," children are unable to decode speech sounds. Thus, they understand little of what is said to them and their speech is rudimentary, distorted, and quite often absent. Such children are often considered to be deaf. Visual processing of language with communication by manual techniques (finger spelling, gestural language, sign language), however, is available to these children.

The syndrome may be congenital or acquired; brain pathologies, if demonstrable, vary (e.g., infarction, angioma). In such cases, there is often an accompanying seizure disorder. These seizures are usually manifested clinically and most often are of partial complex type. Occasionally, they are seen only on EEG. Electroencephalographically, the seizure is usually bilateral; less often, it is present only on the left side. With anticonvulsant treatment, the seizures are often well controlled, with improvement in EEG less consistently achieved. Unfortunately, such improvements are not necessarily accompanied by improved language function; thus, the prognosis is guarded.

3.4.5. "Pathological" Left-Handedness

It has long been known that lesions in the left cerebral peri-Sylvian and/or peri-Rolandic regions, acquired before 6 years of age, may "displace" speech and language representation to the right cerebral hemisphere or to both hemispheres. Since speech "resides" in the left hemisphere in 95% of right-handers and 70% of left-handers (in 15% of left-handers it is right-sided and in 15%, bilateral), early left cerebral lesions not uncommonly produce speech delay and "pathological" left-handedness (definite left-handedness that appears too early, e.g., in the first year, and/or in the absence of left-handedness in other family members). Underdevelopment of the right limbs may be an accompanying feature.

3.4.6. Aphasia

Aphasia is the *loss* of previously acquired, linguistically correct speech; thus, by definition, it is never a congenital disorder. As elaborated by Geschwind (1972), childhood aphasia contrasts in several important ways with that seen in adults. Speech output in the aphasic child is reduced and mutism is relatively common, whereas speech output in the aphasic adult can be considerable and mutism is rare. In childhood aphasia, speech is characteristically nonfluent, while in the adult aphasic it is usually fluent. Further, recovery from aphasia is much better in children than in adults.

The aphasic child's recovery of speech can be so rapid that it cannot be attributed to "relearning" by the right cerebral hemisphere. Thus, when a child learns to speak, he very likely learns with both cerebral hemispheres. When the (normally dominant) left hemisphere is injured, the right one "takes over," but usually at the expense of nonverbal functioning (normally resident in the right hemisphere); thus, impaired visual–motor functioning (with or without accompanying loss of intelligence) not uncommonly will be seen in the child recovering or recovered from aphasia.

Writing difficulty (dysgraphia) always accompanies aphasia, and usually is more severe than the difficulty with speech. If such is not the case, a hearing loss should be suspected.

Although the prognosis in childhood aphasia is generally good, and full recovery may occur, perceptual handicaps, intellectual impairment, and speech difficulties not uncommonly persist. The speech difficulties can be assisted by ongoing speech therapy (which ideally is first introduced as the child begins to recover from his acute brain insult).

3.4.7. Developmental

Synonyms have included developmental aphasia, word deafness, central deafness, and auditory imperception. The frequency of this disorder is uncertain, but in severe form approximates 1 in 1000; the frequency of less severe cases doubtlessly is much greater. The clinical patterns vary with the severity:

1. Mild. A number of word sounds are defective (dyslalia); there are particular difficulties with consonant production (wada/water; dere/there; free/three); spoken language and language comprehension are normal
2. Moderate. Word sounds are moderately impaired and spoken language is impaired; language comprehension is normal
3. Severe. Word sounds are severely impaired and both spoken language and language comprehension are impaired
4. Very severe. There is gross failure in development of both spoken language and language comprehension; a large percentage of such children are noncommunicative

Factors predisposing to developmental speech delay include sex (male/female: 2.5/1), parity (frequent in second children), gestational and perinatal abnormalities, late development of hand preference, and a family history of speech delay.

The speech of these children tends to be monotonous with little intonation, consonants are omitted or substituted, terminal syllables are dropped, and single words are articulated more clearly than connected speech. Such children are usually of (low) average intelligence and on examination may show a lack of hand preference, visual–motor difficulties, and dyslexia.

3.4.8. Disordered Emotionality

When a child fails to develop speech, secondary behavioral problems are an almost invariable result, complicating the diagnostic assessment and treatment. There are, in addition, several disorders with speech delay in which emotional upset is a striking accompaniment. Examples include elective mutism and autism.

3.4.8a. Elective Mutism. Children with elective mutism speak only with a small group of intimates in very specific situations, usually with family members at home. In contrast with many disorders associated with speech delay, elective mutism occurs at least as often in girls as in boys. Such mutism usually develops at about age 3 to 5 years after a period of normal speech development.

Elective mutism should be distinguished from *transient mutism,* seen in many 3- to 4-year-old children who may be fully fluent at home, but in a new setting, such as at school or in a doctor's office, they may talk little, rarely, or only in a whisper. Such transient mutism is probably caused by normal separation anxiety; as anxiety diminishes with familiarity, talking begins.

Many electively mute children are shy from early in life. A number appear to have abnormally strong ties to their mothers. These mothers are often described as anxious, domineering, and overprotective. Such families sometimes show increased frequencies of depression, neurosis, and marital problems.

Some workers have found elective mutism to be associated with other developmental disorders: delayed speech development, enuresis, encopresis, and lowered nonverbal intelligence. About one child in five has an underlying speech or other language handicap; here, the mutism appears to develop as a secondary reaction to the communication difficulty. Other causes of elective mutism include instances that are reactive to traumatic events (psychological, physical) and those where the mutism is used as an attention-seeking or passive–aggressive device (with silence used as a "weapon").

In addition to shyness, electively mute children are often oppositional, with poor malleability. A number are aggressive at home and sulky with strangers. Some show excessive and unusual motor activities.

The ultimate prognosis in elective mutism is generally good, with improvement normally before 10 years of age; in a minority, the difficulty persists. As mutism improves, so do the accompanying behavioral upsets.

3.4.8b. Autism. Autism is a rare disorder (2–4 cases per 10,000), but a serious one. Unfortunately, the term "autism" has come to mean different things to various professionals and parents. To date, the diagnosis remains a clinical one. The criteria for diagnosis are not uniformly agreed upon; further, there is no one pathognomonic clinical feature. Thus, the situation is rather like that in Tourette's disease or common migraine. Nonetheless, there are certain features without which the diagnosis should not be made, namely: it is a disorder affecting multiple brain-related functions, with abnormalities seen that are not normal for *any* stage of a child's development. Thus, development is *deviant,* not merely delayed.

DSM-III criteria for diagnosis are useful. These include:

- Onset before 2½ years
- Pervasive lack of responsiveness to others

- Grossly deficient language
- Peculiar speech patterns (if speech is present)
- Bizarre response to aspects of the environment
- Absence of delusions and hallucinations

Though there may be occasional instances in which autism seems to be of "psychogenic" origin, developing after some environmental stress (e.g., birth of a sibling), even in such circumstances one cannot exclude an underlying brain abnormality (predisposing the child to decompensation after exposure to the stressor). The data supporting an *organic basis* for autism are many. In fact, such a basis was emphasized by Kanner when he first described the syndrome in 1943. He viewed these children as coming into the world with *"innate inability to form the usual, biologically provided affective contact with people."*

Many diseases have been implicated in specific cases of autism, disorders as diverse as congenital rubella, phenylketonuria, and fragile X syndrome, with a clinical picture that is often identical to cases where there is no definable cause. Even in the latter cases, however, there is much to implicate an organic etiology: the increased incidence of pre- and perinatal complications; the high frequency of mental retardation (at least 70%), the prominence of EEG abnormalities (20–80%), and tendency to develop seizures (25%); the high frequency of abnormal neurological signs including nonright-handedness; abnormalities on neurophysiological testing; abnormalities found on pneumoencephalograpy, cranial computed tomography and magnetic resonance imaging; and neuropathological alterations in brain.

About 50% of all autistic children do not develop useful speech by age 5 years, and in such children the prognosis is uniformly poor. In the 50% in whom some useful speech development is achieved by 5 years of age, the prognosis is somewhat better. Overall, one autistic child in six makes an adequate social adjustment and can do some regular work by adulthood; one child in six makes a fair adjustment; while four in six remain severely handicapped and unable to lead independent lives. Patients with higher IQs and those in whom language has developed do best.

4. Summary

This chapter has highlighted various organic and psychological causes of why children fail to speak at expected ages, i.e., stages of anticipated developmental maturation. The emphasis on early detection should lead to early and meaningful intervention strategies. Delays in providing early assistance may have an impact on the child's overall psychosocial and educational development.

References

American Psychiatric Association, 1980, Pervasive developmental disorders in *Diagnostic and Statistical Manual of Mental Disorders,* 3rd ed., pp. 86–92, Washington, D.C.

Bauman, M., and Kemper, T. L., 1985, Histoanatomic observations of the brain in early infantile autism, *Neurology* **35:**866–874.

Courchesne, E., Hesselink, J. R., Jernigan, T. L., *et al.,* 1987, Abnormal neuroanatomy in a nonretarded person with autism: Unusual findings with magnetic resonance imaging, *Arch. Neurol.* **44:**335–41.

Eimas, P. D., and Kavanagh, J. F., 1986, Otitis media, hearing loss, and child development: A NICHD conference summary, *Publ. Health Rep.* **101:**289–293.

Ferry, P. C., and Cooper, J. A., 1978, Sign language in communication disorders of childhood, *J. Pediatr.* **93:**547–552.

Garvey, M., and Gordon, N., 1973, A follow-up study of children with disorders of speech development, *Br. J. Disord. Commun.* **8:**17–28.

Gascon, G., Victor, D., Lonbroso, C., *et al.,* 1973, Language disorder, convulsive disorder, and electroencephalographic abnormalities, *Arch. Neurol.* **28:**156–162.

Geschwind, N., 1972, Disorders of higher cortical function in children, *Clin. Proc. Child. Hosp. Natl. Med. Cent.* **28:**261–272.

Gordon, N., 1986, Intermittent deafness and learning, *Dev. Med. Child Neurol.* **28:**364–369.

Gottlieb, M. I., Zinkus, P. W., and Thompson, A., 1979, Chronic middle ear disease and auditory perceptual deficits. Is there a link? *Clin. Pediatr.* **18:**725–731.

Hayden, T. L., 1980, Classification of elective mutism, *J. Am. Acad. Child. Psychiatry* **19:**118–133.

Hier, D. B., and Rosenberger, P. B., 1980, Focal left temporal lobe lesions and delayed speech acquisition, *J. Dev. Behav. Pediatr.* **1:**54–57.

Kanner, L., 1943, Autistic disturbances of affective contact, *Nerv. Child.* **2:**217–250.

Kolvin, I., and Fundudis, T., 1981, Elective mute children: Psychological development and background factors, *J. Child Psychol.* **22:**219–232.

Landau, W. M., and Kleffner, F. R., 1957, Syndrome of acquired aphasia with convulsive disorder in children, *Neurology* **7:**523–530.

Landau, W. M., Goldstein, R., and Kleffner, F. R., 1960, Congenital aphasia. A clinicopathologic study, *Neurology* **10:**915–921.

Rapin, I., Mattis, S., Rowan, A. J., *et al.,* 1977, Verbal auditory agnosia in children, *Dev. Med. Child Neurol.* **19:**192–207.

Roberts, J. E., Sanyal, M. A., Burchinal, M. R., *et al.,* 1986, Otitis media in early childhood and its relationship to later verbal and academic performance, *Pediatrics* **78:**423–430.

Satz, P., Orsini, D. L., Saslow, E., *et al.,* 1985, The pathological left-handedness syndrome, *Brain Cognit.* **4:**27–46.

Shoumaker, R. D., Bennett, D. R., Bray, P. F., *et al.,* 1974, Clinical and EEG manifestations of an unusual aphasic syndrome in children, *Neurology* **24:**10–16.

Teele, D. W., Klein, J. O., Rosner, B. A., *et al.,* 1984, Otitis media with effusion during the first three years of life and development of speech and language, *Pediatrics* **74:**282–287.

Zinkus, P. W., 1986, Perceptual and academic deficits related to early chronic otitis media, in: *Otitis Media and Child Development* (J. E. Kavanagh, ed.), pp. 107–116, York Press, Parkton, MD.

Suggested Reading

Bradford, L. J., 1980, Understanding and assessing communicative disorders in children, *J. Dev. Behav. Pediatr.* **1**:89–95.

Cantwell, D. P., and Baker, L., 1985, Speech and language: Development and disorders, in: *Child and Adolescent Psychiatry: Modern Approaches,* 2nd ed. (M. Rutter and L. Hersov, eds.), pp. 526–544, Blackwell Scientific, London.

Herskowitz, J., and Rosman, N. P., 1982, Learning disbilities and disorders of speech and language, in: *Pediatrics, Neurology and Psychiatry—Common Ground: Behavioral, Cognitive, Affective and Physical Disorders in Childhood and Adolescence,* pp. 480–511, Macmillan, New York.

Ingram, T. T. S., 1969, Developmental disorders of speech, in: *Handbook of Clinical Neurology,*vol. 4 (P. J. Vinken and G. W. Bruyn, eds.) pp. 407–442, Elsevier, New York.

Rapin, I., and Wilson, B. C., 1978, Children with developmental language disability: Neurological aspects and assessments, in: *Developmental Dysphasia* (M. A. Wyke, ed.), pp. 13–41, Academic Press, London.

Resnick, T. J., 1986, A practical approach to children with speech and language disorders, *Int. Pediatr.* **1**:40–45.

Rutter, M., 1977, Speech delay, in: *Child Psychiatry: Modern Approaches* (M. Rutter and L. Hersov, eds.), pp. 688–716, Blackwell Scientific, Oxford.

Rutter, M., and Martin, J. A. M., 1972, The child with delayed speech, in: *Clinics in Developmental Medicine,* No. 43, pp. 1–268, J. B. Lippincott Co., Philadelphia.

CHAPTER 18

Developmental–Behavioral Disorders

Need the Geriatrician Be Concerned?

FREDRICK T. SHERMAN

1. Aging of America

1.1. Demographic Changes of All Populations

The graying of America occupies the minds of congressmen, social scientists, health planners, fiscal intermediaries, and physicians. In 1900, 3 million people, or about 4% of the United States population, was 65 years of age and older. By 1986, the total had risen to 26 million, representing 11% of the population. Not only have the absolute number and percentage of older adults markedly increased, but changing mortality trends have effected longevity patterns as well. In 1900, approximately 25% of the population could expect to live more than 65 years, and less than 4% could expect to survive until age 85. In 1980, however, 70% of the population could expect to survive to age 65, and over 17% will live to age 85. The demographic trends will lead to 16% of the population being over the age of 65 in the year 2020, with the most rapidly growing segment of the elderly being those over age 85.

While 95% of older adults live in the community, most in families typically consisting of an elderly married couple with no children or

FREDRICK T. SHERMAN • Department of Medicine, Health Sciences Center, State University of New York at Stony Brook, Stony Brook, New York 11794; and Huntington Hospital, Huntington, New York 11743.

other relatives residing in their home, 5% live in nursing homes. The median age of nursing home residents is 81 compared with a median age of 75 for all adults 65 years of age and older.

With increased longevity comes the onset and accumulation of chronic medical and psychiatric disorders, as well as chronic disabilities. Acute illnesses, i.e., pneumonia, urinary tract infections, and falls, often interact with existing disabilities leading to disease–disability interactions that can further worsen overall function. The five most-common chronic conditions among the elderly include arthritis (38%), hearing impairment (27%), vision impairment (20%), hypertension (20%), and heart conditions (20%). While these chronic conditions can be minimally and episodically symptomatic, serious deterioration can occur in the elderly patient when a fall, acute confusional syndrome, urinary and/or fecal incontinence, or an adverse drug reaction interacts with any of these conditions.

With the increase in chronic disabilities, the utilization of health care resources also increases. While comprising 11% of the population, the elderly account for 30% of total personal health care expenditure. At least 40% of patient visits to internists are by people over age 65 compared with 20% to family practitioners.

1.2. Demography of Developmentally Disabled Populations

Like all segments of the adult population, those with mental retardation and developmental disabilities (MR/DD) are living longer. It is estimated that between 200,000 and 1.2 million persons in the United States with MR/DD are over the age of 55. Like all adult populations, generations of MR/DD people are growing older, and these older disabled persons will have a greater life expectancy. Approximately 40% of mentally retarded people will survive to age 60. In the past, working with MR/DD patients was the work of pediatricians. Now, with the graying of the MR/DD adult, we must consider whether the fields of gerontology (i.e., the study of aging) and geriatrics (i.e., the medical, psychiatric, and social care of the elderly) need to pay attention to this small but growing population with needs that approach those of the geriatric population.

2. Normal Senescence

While growth and development concern the pediatrician, senescence occupies the mind of the geriatrician. It has long been thought that after the relatively brief phase of growth and development, ending about age 20, the longest phase of our life cycle, maturation, begins, lasting until age 65 when senescence starts its natural decline until death. On the contrary, all of the studies of normal aging populations have shown that after the phase of growth and development comes a brief phase of maturation and then the longest phase of our life, senescence, usually beginning about age 35 or 40. While many normative age-related changes occur in a deteriorating fashion during senescence, these changes are often slight and certainly never produce symptoms that bring an older patient to the physician's office. Also, during senescence there is increased physiological, anatomic, and psychological heterogeneity among individuals as they grow older. In fact, many of these age-associated declines may be modified by exercise, diet, personal habits, or psychosocial factors (Rowe and Kahn, 1987).

The older adult has decreasing organ reserve and is less likely to handle physiological stress at the same rate and degree of response as the young or middle-aged individual. For example, when functional aerobic capacity is tested in normal male adults, maximum oxygen uptake (V_{O_2} max) decreases by 0.46 ml/kg per min per year and the maximum heart rate decreases by 1.04 beats/min per year (Bruce, 1985). There are also decrements in total body height secondary to narrowing of the intervertebral disks, usually in middle age, as well as loss of height of individual vertebrae that occurs mainly in old age. Body composition changes as well, with an increase in total body fat and a decrease in lean body mass; the latter is characterized by decreasing size of muscle, e.g., psoas and sacrospinalis, as well as decreasing muscle density (Rossman, 1986). These normal age-related changes interact with diseases in late life and lead to acute and chronic disabilities that present unique challenges to the geriatrician.

3. Common Geriatric Problems

3.1. Ageism

Ageism is a prejudice against an elderly person merely because of his chronological age. Inexperienced junior clinicians, biased senior clinicians, or busy practitioners may label older MR/DD individuals as a "crock" or a "gomer" because of negative attitudes toward old age, chronic illness, developmental disabilities, or mental retardation. It is certainly possible that a newly graduated physician may never have cared for a mentally retarded individual during his entire career. The older patient may appear confused, chronically and irreversibly ill, and be socially and financially dependent. These negative biases may lead to a cursory history and physical and neurological examinations and ultimately to poor care.

3.2. Underreporting and Nonreporting

Elderly MR/DD people have frequently been shown to underreport or fail to report symptoms and illness to their physician. In part, this may be due to the impossibility of recounting 50 years of medical and surgical history, especially when most of the information may never have been conveyed to the patient by the physician or comprehended by the patient. Also, the elderly individual may think that breathlessness, weakness, falls, dizziness, visual and hearing loss, vague muscle or joint pains, leakage of urine, constipation, depression, and memory loss are part of normal aging and therefore not worthy of reporting to their physician. Caregivers, both lay, semiprofessional, and professional, may have similar misconceptions. None of these symptoms should be attributed to normal aging; all are potentially reversible. "What can you expect at my age?" or "I guess I'm getting old!" are expressions that should prompt further questioning to determine the duration, severity, and etiology of the functional change.

3.3. Nonspecific Indicators of Serious Illness

The older MR/DD adult may present with nonspecific signs of serious illness. Table 1 lists these nonspecific signs and symptoms. Any of these signs or symptoms should prompt an immediate and thorough

Table 1. Nonspecific Signs and Symptoms of Serious Disease in the Elderly

Weakness
Taking to bed
Anorexia
Falling or unsteady gait
Dyspnea, tachypnea
Weight loss
Urinary and/or fecal incontinence
Confusion

evaluation of the older patient including history, physical, and neurological examinations and laboratory and mental status testing.

4. Clinical Problems in Aging MR/DD Populations

4.1. Medical Problems

If gerontologists and geriatricians are to contribute to the well-being of the aging MR/DD population, it is important to determine whether the kinds of chronic conditions that exist are similar to those of aging non-MR/DD populations (Janicki and Wisniewski, 1985; Walz *et al.,* 1986).

An extensive client registry data base of mentally retarded adults aged 45 to 90 years has been established in New York State (Janicki and Jacobson, 1986). Approximately half of the sample had intellectual skills in the mild to moderate range and the other half were severely to profoundly retarded. Data on physical, functional, and adaptive behavior characteristics were collected to determine whether there were identifiable patterns of chronic disease conditions and declining sensory and behavioral capabilities among aging retarded adults. As expected, with increasing age a greater percentage of retarded adults, irrespective of intellectual level, was affected by individual conditions and a greater number of conditions were present in each individual. At age 45, the mean number of impaired body systems was 0.5, while at 85 to 90 it was 2.0. Specifically, cardiovascular, musculoskeletal, respiratory, digestive, genitourinary, endocrine, and hearing and vision conditions significantly increased between ages 45 and 80.

In addition, significantly more community-residing mentally retarded adults had cardiovascular conditions than those in institutions, while fewer community residents had musculoskeletal conditions. Mobility and sensory dysfunction (i.e., hearing and vision) also increased with aging, particularly among the severe to profoundly retarded adult. Motor activity and cognitive practical skills were also assessed. Among the mildly to moderately retarded group, cognitive skills did not decline until age 70, while motor skills began to decline at age 50 with the rate of decline increasing with age.

Among the severely retarded, motor skills were stable until age 70, while cognitive skills actually showed a slight increase through the early 70s and declined thereafter. These latter results are probably due to the cross-sectional nature of the study with a greater mortality rate among the more profoundly retarded. Functional skill losses were most prominent in mobility and fundamental activities of daily living.

Overall, sensory capabilities were lost gradually and not precipitously. Therefore, mental retardation, by itself, should not be considered a reason for decline in vision or hearing and it is likely that the same causes for loss of vision in the older general population, i.e., cataracts, glaucoma, and senile macular degeneration, apply to the aging MR/DD population. Fortunately, with proper diagnosis at least the first two are treatable. Further, these data suggest that the decline in certain skills, particularly mobility and gross motor abilities, may start in the mid-50s, suggesting 55 as the age for defining the aging mentally retarded populations.

This study also showed major differences between community-residing and institutionalized mentally retarded populations. Consequently, each of these populations has different needs, and health care generalizations about one group cannot necessarily be extended to the other. This is similar to the large gap between the needs of community-residing older adults and those in nursing homes.

It is interesting to note that when activities of daily living and gross motor skills were analyzed in the profoundly to severely retarded groups, there was maintenance of skills for dressing/grooming, language, and independent living to age 70 to 74; for eating and reading/writing to age 75 to 79; and for toileting to age 80 to 84. For those with mild to moderate impairment, there was a decline in gross motor and independent living skills starting at age 50 to 54. In contrast, all other domains remained stable through age 70 to 74 and declined thereafter. In general, there was more marked decline in those with greater intellectual abilities, i.e., the mild to moderately retarded group showed greater loss over time of skills and capabilities than the severely to profoundly retarded, whose life skills and capabilities were less developed.

In a recent survey of general health characteristics of adult developmentally disabled persons, primarily community dwelling, a variety of secondary medical problems such as obesity, chronic skin conditions, hygiene-related problems, and onset of Alzheimer's disease were noted (Buehler *et al.*, 1985). The developmentally disabled have been shown to have access problems to health care and it is likely that some of their health problems could have been prevented if diagnosed and treated earlier by interested and expert medical practitioners.

4.2. Psychiatric Problems

4.2.1. IQ Changes

Studies that longitudinally assess IQ in mentally retarded adult populations have shown varied results, the majority showing either no significant change or a slight decrement. IQ testing, however, does not tell us about overall activities of daily living (ADL) function, and based on previously cited studies, ADL function can be maintained; albeit, at a lower level, well into late life even in the profound to severely retarded.

4.2.2. Prevalence of Mental Illness

While there is little prevalence data, mental illnesses that effect the MR/DD who live into late life include behavioral disorders, dementia, depression, delirium, paranoid states, and anxiety neuroses. Clearly, any prevalence data must differentiate between community-residing and institutionalized individuals.

In a study of long-stay institutionalized mentally retarded individuals over age 40, 30% were found to have a psychiatric disorder (Day, 1985). Eighty percent were aged 40 to 65 years and two thirds were moderately or severely retarded. The prevalence of various disorders was: (1) behavioral disorders (50%), e.g., explosive behavior with aggression toward others, self-aggression and verbal abusiveness, sex offenses, and petty theft; (2) psychoses (28%), e.g., bipolar disorders and schizophrenia, including paranoid state; (3) neuroses (4%); (4) undiagnosable but probably psychotic (9%); (5) and organic states (9%), e.g., senile and presenile dementia and acute confusional states.

There was a progressive fall in the prevalence of hospitalized residents with any form of psychiatric illness with increasing age, decreasing from 49% in the 40- to 49-year-old group to 17% in the over-70 group. This trend held true for behavioral disorders, the neuroses, and the psychoses, but with organic states the trend was reversed with the highest prevalence in the over 70s. A simultaneous study of first admissions of adults age 40 and over to a psychiatric unit for the mentally handicapped showed the following prevalence rate: behavior disorders (36%); psychoses (22%); neuroses (33%); and organic states (4%). Once again, there is a difference between community-residing and institutionalized populations with regard to the prevalence of the various types of psychiatric disorders in middle-aged and elderly mentally retarded populations. While behavioral disorders continue to be common, neuroses (e.g., reactive depression and anxiety state) increase in prevalence compared with the institutionalized long-stay patients.

4.2.3. Dementia

As populations of MR/DD live longer, they enter the age range when dementia becomes more common. Dementia, a symptom complex, is characterized by global intellectual deterioration in an adult severe enough to interfere with occupational or social performance. Cognitive changes include disturbance in memory, language use, perception, constructional abilities and other praxis, and the ability to learn new skills, solve problems, think abstractly, and make judgments (Katzman, 1986).

Studies of mentally retarded populations over age 50 and over age 65 reveal a prevalence of dementia of 12% and 13.6%, respectively. These prevalence figures are similar to the 15% figure quoted for the general community-residing population over age 65 years. At age 80, approximately 20% of older adults are affected by some degree of dementia. In nursing homes, dementias affect at least 50% of the residents, with Alzheimer's disease being the most common cause, accounting for 60 to 75% of all cases.

In a study of 200 older adults presenting with memory loss for an outpatient evaluation, intensive study revealed that 75% had Alzheimer's disease (Larson *et al.*, 1985). One third of the patients, however, had medical and/or psychiatric problems that were contributing to their dementia. The most common secondary diagnoses were depression and drug-induced or exacerbated dementia. Furthermore, evaluation revealed 278 additional medical diagnoses, of which 115 led to treatment recommendations. Overall, 55 patients (27.5%) experienced improvement in cognitive function of at least 1 month's duration. In 28 patients (14%), the improvement lasted for at least a year. Only two patients who presented with dementia completely reversed, one for the withdrawal of cimetidine and the other who had mild dementia from chronic alcoholic abuse.

The differential diagnosis of dementia includes over 70 disorders. Diagnosis is aided by history, physical examination, neurological examination, including mental status and psychiatric testing, laboratory tests and computerized tomography or magnetic resonance imaging studies, and specialized neuropsychological tests, if needed. Of interest to the geriatrician are the reversible, treatable, or arrestable causes of dementia. Table 2 uses the mnemonic DEMENTIAS for remembering the most common reversible causes of dementia.

Alzheimer's Disease and Down's Syndrome. The interrelationship between Down's syndrome (DS) and Alzheimer's Disease (AD) is of particular interest to the clinician caring for the MR/DD population. Extensive clinical and neuropathological observations suggest that an additional risk factor for the onset of AD is the presence of DS. The hallmark of AD is the neuropathological changes of senile plaques and neurofibrillary tangles. The senile plaque, which is found mainly in the cerebral cortex, consists of a central core of amyloid encircled by degenerative neuronal terminals and reactive cells. Neurofibrillary tangles, composed of helically twisted pairs of filament, are located in the cere-

Table 2. Arrestable and Reversible Causes of Dementia in the Elderly

D	*D*elirium/*d*rugs
E	*E*yes/*e*ars/*e*nvironment
M	*M*etabolic/*m*ultiinfarct/*m*ultiple
E	*E*KG/*e*ndocrine/*e*thanol
N	*N*utritional/*n*ormal pressure hydrocephalus
T	*T*rauma, *t*umor
I	*I*nfection
A	*A*ffective disorders/*a*ngular gyrus syndrome
S	*S*ubacute arteriopathic encephalopathy/*s*urgery

bral cortex and hippocampus. In two large consecutive series of autopsies in DS patients, senile plaques with or without neurofibrillary tangles were found in all brains examined above the age of 40 years.

In addition to the increased number of plaques and tangles seen in older DS patients, the activity of the cerebral cholinergic and hypothalamic noradrenergic neurotransmitter systems is decreased as is typical in AD (Karlinsky, 1986).

While there appears to be a strong correlation between the presence of Alzheimer's type neuropathology in older DS patients, the clinical diagnosis of AD in DS was made in only about 25 to 45% of DS patients in both retrospective and prospective studies (Dalton and Crapper McLachlan, 1984).

A longitudinal clinicopathological study of seven severely retarded DS patients above age 40 revealed that a clinical diagnosis of AD could be made in all by using periodic cognitive assessments, neurological examinations, and laboratory tests (Wisniewski *et al.*, 1985). The cognitive deficits of AD appeared at about age 51 ± 6.2 years. Learning capacity, visual memory loss, and decreased occupational and social functioning were demonstrated in all DS patients with onset of AD. The duration of cognitive and behavioral deficits from onset until death was 5.6 ± 2.2 years, with death occurring at an average of 56.6 ± 6.5 years. Urinary incontinence developed in four of seven and seizures occurred in six of seven patients before death. Amyloid angiopathy was observed in five of seven patients and small infarcts were detected in four of seven DS brains.

5. Prevention

While the prevention of childhood infectious diseases, dental caries, periodontal disease, scoliosis, and maintenance of ideal body weight and normal cholesterol has been the realm of the pediatrician, the prevention of illness and disability in late life occupies the practice of the geriatrician. Like all aging patients, mentally retarded and developmentally disabled patients require preventive care. In addition, they may suffer from congenital defects, altered diet, and growth impairment that necessitates further preventative steps.

Specific preventative steps in the aging MR/DD population include:

1. Routine annual examinations. While the utility of an annual examination with selected laboratory tests has a low yield in nursing home patients in terms of new treatable diagnoses, similar studies in aged MR/DD populations do not exist. Hence, it would seem reasonable to perform a comprehensive yearly examination including breast, pelvic, oral, and rectal examinations, if possible, as well as functional assessments of gait, mental status, and activities of daily living status.
2. Infectious diseases. Institutionalized elderly people with mental retardation should receive a yearly influenza vaccination. Those who have not received a vaccination should be chemoprophylaxed with amantadine if an outbreak should occur. While no data exist on mentally retarded individuals with regard to pneumococcal vaccination, it would seem prudent to administer this one-time dose of vaccine, especially to those with chronic illness including cardiopulmonary disease, neurological disease affecting the gag reflex, or a seizure disorder. Immunizing all residents of group homes or institutions with developmentally disabled patients against hepatitis B is recommended by the Communicable Disease Center. Finally, tetanus is a disease that occurs predominantly among the elderly, and a routine booster should be given every 10 years after the initial basic series.

6. Conclusion

The accumulation of years of chronic medication usage, compounded by alterations in pharmacodynamics and pharmacokinetics that are a part of normal senescence, make the drug management of the geriatric MR/DD patient challenging. Body composition, nutrient needs, and caloric expenditure in late life are also altered and must be tempered by existing disabilities and activity levels in the older MR/DD patient. Finally, the geriatrician, with the tools of interdisciplinary team meetings and family conferences, and the skills of resource utilization and disease prevention, is in an excellent position to advise primary-care physicians, institutional decision makers, and governmental agencies about place of residence, use of valuable resources, and rehabilitation potential of the older MR/DD population.

References

Bruce, R. A., 1985, Functional aerobic capacity, exercise and aging, in: *Principles of Geriatric Medicine* (R. Andres, E. L. Bierman, and W. R. Hazzard, eds.), pp. 87–103, McGraw Hill Book Company, New York.

Buehler, B., Smith, B., and Fifield, M., 1985, *Medical Issues in Serving Adults with Developmental Disabilities,* Technical Report #4, Utah State University Developmental Center for Handicapped Persons, Logan, UT.

Dalton, A. J., and Crapper McLachlan, D. R., 1984, Incidence of memory deterioration in aging persons with Down's syndrome, in: *Perspectives and Progress in Mental Retardation,* Vol. 2: *Biomedical Aspects* (J. M. Berg, ed.), pp. 55–62, University Park Press, Baltimore.

Day, K., 1985, Psychiatric disorder in the middle-aged and elderly mentally handicapped, *Br. J. Psychiatry* **147:**660–667.

Janicki, M. P., and Jacobson, J. W., 1986, Geriatric trends in sensory, physical and behavioral abilities among older mentally retarded persons, *Am. J. Ment. Defic.* **90:**490–500.

Janicki, M. P., and Wisniewski, H. M. (eds.), 1985, *Aging and Developmental Disabilities,* Paul H. Brookes Publishing Co., Baltimore, MD.

Karlinsky, H., 1986, Alzheimer's disease in Down's syndrome: A review, *J. Am. Gerontol.* **34:**728–734.

Katzman, R., 1986, Alzheimer's disease, *N. Engl. J. Med.* **314:**964–973.

Larson, E. B., Reifler, B. V., Sumi, S. M., *et al.,* 1985, Diagnostic evaluation of 200 elderly outpatients with suspected dementia, *J. Gerontol.* **40:**536–543.

Rossman, I., 1986, The anatomy of aging, in: *Clinical Geriatrics,* 3rd ed. (I. Rossman, ed.), pp. 3–22, J. D. Lippincott Company, Philadelphia.

Rowe, J. W., and Kahn, R. L., 1987, Human aging: Usual and successful, *Science* **237:**143–149.

Walz, T., Harper, D., and Wilson, J., 1986, The aging developmentally disabled person: A review, *Gerontologist* **26:**622–628.

Wisniewski, K. E., Dalton, A. J., Crapper McLachlan, D. R., *et al.,* 1985, Alzheimer's disease in Down's syndrome: Clinicopathologic studies, *Neurology* **35:**957–961.

Index

Acting-out depression suicide, 127, 128
Adaptation and pediatrics, 159, 160
Adjustment disorder
  with depressed mood, 6
  and temperament, 54, 58, 59
Adolescent
  and child depression, 1–12; *see also* Depression
  noncompliance with medical regimens, 195, 196, 205–208
Adolescent crisis, 112–114
Affective disorders and depression, 8, 116
Aggression and television, 93, 94, 98, 99
Agreement, temperament and diagnostic process, 55, 57, 58
AIDS
  embryopathy, 29–31
  teenage, 114
AIDS-related complex, 29
Alcohol abuse, 112, 135, 136, 144
Alternative, nonstandard therapies, learning disabilities, 88
Alzheimer's disease and Downs syndrome, 274, 275
Amitriptyline, 9
Anorexia nervosa, 155
  and depression, 11
  and temperament, 59
Antisocial behavior
  and depression, 11, 113
  and temperament, 59
Anxiety disorders and depression, 6, 9
Anxiety reduction, 238
Apgar scores (low) and asphyxia, 16–19, 25
  and seizures, 20
Aphasia, 260
Asphyxia, outcome, 16–19, 25
  hypoxic–ischemic encephalopathy, 22
  variables, 18
  and very low birthweight, 25
Audiogram, familiar sounds, 214, 215
Auditory behavior, normal development, 226
Auditory deficiency, educational and developmental problems, 214
Auditory discrimination, and speech delay, 259
Auditory function and speech development, 218
Autism and speech delay, 262, 263
Autistic behavior, 155
  fragile X syndrome, 34

Baby Doe, 173, 174
Barotrauma, 249
Bayley Scales of Infant Development, and asphyxia, 17, 18
Beck Depression Inventory—Adolescents, 3
Behavior adjustment problems
  minor, 59, 60
  moderate, 60–62
  severe, 59
Behavior difficulties and learning disabled, 82
Behavior modification, learning disabled, 88
Bereavement and depression, 6
Biobehavioral pediatrics, 154, 156, 159, 165

Biochemical treatment of depression, 9, 10
Biofeedback, 233, 237
Biological indicators of depression, 8, 9
Bronchopulmonary dysplasia, 249, 250

Cerebral giantism, 31–33
Cerebral palsy
  and asphyxia, 17
  and seizures, 20
Child abuse and suicide, 115, 142
Child/adolescent depression, 1–12; *see also* Depression
Child advocacy, pediatricians, 77
Child developmental associate, 163, 164
Childhood Depression Inventory, 2, 3
Children's Depression Rating Scale, 2, 3, 9
Children's Depression Scale, 2, 3
Choroid plexus bleeding, 21
Chronic illness and self-regulating strategies, 235–237
Clinical correlates, learning disabilities, 79–82, 90
Clinical importance of temperament, 53, 54
Clumsiness and cerebral giantism, 31, 32
Cluster suicide, 114, 120–123
Cognitive deficits and seizures, 20
Cognitive styles, 184
Cognitive thought deficits and learning disabilities, 82
Communicative disorders, office screening, 213–230
  guidelines for screening in physician's office, 221–228
    children with middle ear effusion, 228
    hearing, 224–227
    language, 227, 228
  hearing aid placement, 230
  home language stimulation, 228–230
  normal speech development, 218–220
  otitis media, 216–218
  screening speech, language and hearing, 220, 221
Community residential program, 170
Community service, juvenile delinquents, 42
Compliance, enhancement in pediatric primary care, 193–208
Compliance (*cont.*)
  compliance with medical procedures, 194, 195
  improving compliance with medical procedures, 196–205
  improving compliance with medical regimens, 205, 206
  noncompliance with medical regimens, 195, 196
  suggestions for medical community, 206, 207
Conceptual thought deficits and learning disabilities, 82
Concern, temperament and diagnostic process, 55–57
Confrontation of adverse witnesses, juvenile offenders, 46
Congenital anomalies and learning disabilities, 80
Conversion symptoms, 59
Coprolalia, 37
Cortisol hypersecretion and depression, 8
Counseling, learning disabilities, 85, 86, 88, 90
Court-appointed expert witness, 44, 45
Cranial ultrasound, 248
Craniofacial abnormalities
  AIDS embryopathy, 29, 30
  cerebral giantism, 31
Crisis suicide, 127, 128
Cyberphysiology, 233, 239, 240, 243
Cyclothymic disorders, 8

Deinstitutionalization, 171
  philosophical and ethical considerations, 171–174
  strategies, 174, 175
Dementia, and causes, 273–275
Demographic changes in populations, 267, 268
Denver Developmental Screening Test (DDST), 221
Depression, child and adolescent, 1–12, 113, 156
  biochemical treatment, 9, 10
  biological indicators, 8, 9
  developmental concerns, 10, 11
  diagnosis, 1–5
  differential diagnosis, 5–7
  epidemiology, 7

Depression, child and adolescent (*cont.*)
  office management, 11, 12
  risk factors, 7, 8
  and suicide, 116–120, 126, 127, 129, 131–133, 142
  and temperament, 59
Deprivation syndromes, 10
Developmental aphasia, 261
Developmental–behavioral diagnosis: *see* Temperament and developmental–behavioral diagnosis
Developmental–behavioral disorders and geriatrics, 267–277
  demographic changes in populations, 267, 268
  geriatric problems, 269
    ageism, 269, 270
    clinical problems, 271–275
    nonspecific indicators of serious illness, 270, 271
    underreporting and nonreporting, 270
  normal senescence, 268, 269
  prevention, 275, 276
Developmental–behavioral implications of television, 97–104
  aggressive/violent behaviors, 98, 99
  health processes, 100–103
  suicide, 99, 100
Developmental–behavioral pediatrics, 153–167
  adaptation, 159–162
  master clinicians, 157, 158
  new ambulatory care models, 162–165
Developmental concerns, depression, 10, 11
Developmental delay, 155
Developmental disabilities, long-term management strategies for adults and adolescents, 169–175
  impact on health care delivery, 171–174
  intermediate care facility, 169
    goals, 170
  resolving problems, 174, 175
Developmental *versus* physical problems, temperament, 58, 59
Dexamethasone suppression test (DST), 8, 9
Diagnosis
  assessment instruments and diagnostic criteria, 3
  depression, 1–7, 10
Difficult temperament, 50, 60
  poor-fit interactions, 51, 52
Directional disorientation and laterality awareness, 81
Disordered acoustic input, speech delay, 257
Dispositional process, juvenile offenders, 47
Distraction and compliance, 197, 198
Divorce and youth suicide, 115, 130
Dominance and laterality, mixed preference and learning disability, 82
Dominance training, 189
Down's syndrome and Alzheimer's disease, 274, 275
Drug abuse, 112, 135, 136, 144
Drug studies, depression, 9, 10
Due process rights, juvenile offenders, 45–48
Dysarthria, 256
Dysgraphia, 260
Dyslexia, 76
Dysphonia, 255, 256
Dysrhythmia, 256
Dysthymic disorder, 4, 5, 8, 9

Early Language Milestone (ELM) scale, 224, 227
Echokinesis, 37
Ecolalia, 37
Educational strategies, management of learning disabilities, 87, 88, 90
Elective mutism, 261, 262
Emotional difficulties and learning disabilities, 82
Enuresis, 9, 54, 155
Epidemiology, depression, 7
Epilepsy and seizures, 20
Ethical considerations, health care delivery, 171–174
Evaluation
  competitive dimensions of private practice, 72, 73
  HMO quality, 71, 72

Familial occurrence
  cerebral giantism, 32

Familial occurrence (*cont.*)
  Tourette's syndrome, 36
Fears about medical procedures, guidelines for coping, 203, 204
Fixed sentencing, juvenile offenders, 41–43
Folic acid treatment, fragile X syndrome, 35, 36
Fragile X syndrome, 33–36
  prenatal diagnosis, 35

Geriatrician and developmental–behavioral disorders, 267–277
  clinical problems, 271–275
  demographic changes in population, 267, 268
  geriatric problems, 269–271
  normal senescence, 268, 269
  prevention, 275, 276
Grief counseling, youth suicide survivors, 146
Growth failure, AIDS embryopathy, 29
Growth hormone
  and cerebral giantism, 32
  and depression, 9

Hallucinations and depression, 7
Haloperidol, Tourette's syndrome, 37
Health maintenance organization, 67, 69, 70
  evaluation of quality, 71, 72
Health practices and television, 94, 100–103
Health promotion, biobehavioral pediatrics, 163–166
Hearing aid placement, 230
Hearing deprivation, early, and speech–language development, 213
Hearing loss
  early identification, 219, 220
  risk factors, 224
  and speech delay, 258
Hearing problems, 251
Hearing screening, 220, 221
  guidelines, 221, 222, 224–227
Hemisphere specialization, 177, 178, 182–184, 186
Hemisphere styles, 185–187
Hemisphericity theory, 180, 182
High-risk infant, outcome, 15–27
  hypoxic–ischemic encephalopathy, 22, 23
  low Apgar scores, and asphyxia, 16–19
  seizures, 19, 20
  subependymal germinal matrix hemorrhage/intraventricular hemorrhage, 21, 22
  very low birthweight, 23–25
Hospitalization, strategies to decrease aversiveness, 207
Human feature argument, handicapped, 172
Human immunodeficiency virus (HIV), intrauterine infection, 29–31
Hydrocephaly, intraventricular hemorrhage, 21
Hyperactivity, 155
  and depression, 11
Hypnosis, 234
Hypoxic–ischemic encephalopathy, 22, 23, 26

Imipramine, 9
Incarceration of juvenile delinquent, 41
Incidence
  of hearing problems, 251
  of neonatal intensive care unit graduates, 247, 248
  of otitis media, 217
  of substance abuse, teenagers, 136, 137
Infancy, depression, 10
Instructions, teaching a child to follow, 198–200
Insurer sponsored PPO, 69
Intellect
  structure, 181, 192
  verbal *versus* visuospatial, 180, 186
Intelligence and asphyxia, 17
Intermediate care facility, 169
  goals, 170
  impact on health care delivery, 171–174
Intersensory integration deficits and learning disabilities, 81, 82
Interviews, diagnosis of depression, 2, 3, 12
Intraventricular hemorrhage, 21, 22, 26, 248, 249
  and very low birthweight, 25

Investor–entrepreneurial-sponsored PPO, 69
IQ changes, mentally retarded, 272, 273
Iron deficiency, 80

Juvenile Court, founding principles, 43, 44
Juvenile delinquency, 41–48, 112, 136, 139–141
  court-appointed expert witness, 44, 45
  due process rights, 45–48
  fixed sentencing, 41–43
  founding principles of juvenile court, 43, 44

Language, 181, 183
  difficulties, 253
  levels, 254
  screening, 220, 221
    guidelines, 223, 227, 228
  and speech difficulties and learning disabilities, 80, 81
  stimulation at home, 228–230
Lateral orientation, 187
Lead poisoning, 80
Learning
  passive *versus* active and television, 95
  state specificity, 244
Learning disabilities
  definitions, 75, 76
  and depression, 7
  pediatric training, 78
  suicide, 128
  temperament, 58
Learning-disabled child, pediatric assessment and management, 75–90
  definitions, 75, 76
  factors of pediatric roles, 77, 78
  management, 85–89
  pediatric assessment, 78–85
    clinical correlates, 79–82
    guidelines, 82, 83
    model, 83–85
Learning skills and television, 103–105
Learning style, 178
Loner suicide, 127, 128
Loss, personal and suicide, 115

Macrocephaly, cerebral giantism, 31
Macroorchidism, fragile X males, 34
Managed-care plan, 67–74
  evaluating competitive dimensions of private practice, 72, 73
  evaluation of quality, 71, 72
  of HMO, 69, 70
  preferred provider organization, 67–69
  selection by physician providers, 70, 71
Management of learning disabilities, pediatric roles, 85–89
  behavior management, 88, 89
  counseling, 85, 86
  educational strategies, 87, 88
  intervention strategies, 87–89
  medical intervention, 86
  referrals, 86
Management strategies, adolescents and adults with developmental disabilities, 169–175
  impact on health care delivery, 171–174
  intermediate care facilities, 169
    goals, 170
  resolving problems, 174, 175
Management structure, HMO, 71, 72
Manic–depressive illness and depression, 7
Masked clinical depression, 117
Masked depression, 4, 5
Master clinicians, 157, 158
McCarthy Scales of Children's Abilities, 21
Measurement, of temperament, 52, 53
Medical intervention, learning disabilities, 86, 90
Medical problems, mentally retarded/developmentally disordered populations, 217, 272
Medical procedures, compliance, 194–205
Medical regimens, compliance, 195, 196, 205, 206
Megavitamin therapy, learning disabilities, 89
Mental abilities, hemispheric profiles, 187–189
Mental illness prevalence, 273
Mental retardation
  cerebral giantism, 31, 33
  fragile X syndrome, 33, 34
  intraventricular hemorrhage, 21

Mental retardation (*cont.*)
  seizures, 20
  speech delay, 256, 257
  temperament, 58
  very low birthweight, 23
Microcephaly, AIDS embryopathy, 29, 30
Middle ear effusions, neonates, 217, 218
  guidelines for screening children, 228
  persistent, 218
  speech delay, 258
Minimal brain dysfunction, 76
Minnesota Multiphasic Personality Inventory, 21
Misconceptions and myths, youth suicide, 122–124
Mortality rates, infants
  asphyxia, 18
  very low birthweight, 24
Motor abnormalities and learning disabilities, 80
Motor activity, abnormalities and depression, 11
Motor vehicles
  reckless operation, 112
  single vehicle fatalities, 115, 120, 121

National Collaborative Perinatal Project data
  asphyxia, 17, 18
  hypoxic–ischemic encephalopathy, 23
  seizures, 20
Necrotic cortical lesions, 21, 26
Neonatal intensive care unit graduates, 247–252
  incidence, 247, 248
  sequelae, 248–251
    bronchopulmonary dysplasia, 249, 250
    hearing problems, 251
    intraventricular hemorrhage, 248, 249
    retinopathy of prematurity, 250, 251
Neurodevelopmental deficit and high-risk infant, 16
Neurologic abnormalities and learning disabilities, 80
Neurologic disorders, very low birthweights, 24, 25
Neuromotor impairment
  hypoxic–ischemic encephalopathy, 23
  intraventricular hemorrhage, 21
  seizures, 20
Noncompliance, pediatric, 193, 195, 196
Nonspecific indicators of serious illness in elderly, 270, 271
Nonverbal learning disability, 188

Obesity, and television viewing, 94, 95, 102, 105
Ocular hypertelorism, AIDS embryopathy, 29, 30
Oculomotor deficits and learning disabilities, 81
Office management, depression, 11, 12
Optometric training, learning disabilities, 89
Otitis media, 79, 213, 216–218
  incidence, 217
Oxygen treatment and retinopathy of prematurity, 250

Pain, strategy for coping, 197, 198
Parental compliance, 193
Parental descriptions, validity, 84, 85
Parental misconceptions of behavior, 63
Parental report, screening hearing, 221
Parents
  effect on child's compliance, 194, 202
  role in self-destructive behavior intervention, 141–143
Pathology left-handedness and speech delay, 260
Patient demographics, private practice, 72, 73
Pediatric assessment of learning disabilities, 78–85
  clinical correlates, 79–82
  guidelines, 82, 83
  model, 83–85
Pediatric Early Elementary Examination, 84
Pediatric Evaluation of Educational Readiness, 84
Pediatric role in learning disabilities, 77, 78
Pediatric training
  learning disabilities, 78
  about television viewing, 105

Pediatrics, neurology, and psychiatry, children with language and speech difficulties, 253–264
  causes of speech delay, 256–263
    aphasia, 260
    autism, 262, 263
    disordered acoustic input, 257, 258
    elective mutism, 261, 262
    hearing loss, 258, 259
    impaired auditory discrimination, 258
    impaired decoding of speech, 259
    mental retardation, 256, 257
    pathological left-handedness, 260
    psychosocial stressors, 256
    seizures, 257
  levels of language, 154
  normal speech development, 254, 255
  speech delay, deficits and disorders, 255, 256
Pediatrician
  and pediatric compliance, 206, 207
  personal qualities, 157
Peers, role in self-destructive behavior intervention, 143, 144
Peer influence, adolescent crisis, 114
Peer modeling and compliance, 196, 197
Perceptual handicap, 76
Perceptual training, 89
Perinatal complications and high-risk infant outcome, 16, 26, 27
Periventricular leukomalacia, 21
Phobic disorder, 59
Physician
  role in self-destructive behavior intervention, 144–146
  selection of managed care plan, 70, 71
Physician-sponsored PPO, 68, 69
Pills, teaching child to accept, 199, 202
Planning for death, 132, 133
Preferred provider organization (PPO), 67–69
Pregnancy, teenage, 114, 135, 138, 139
Prejudices, against handicapped, 172–174
Prenatal diagnosis, fragile X syndrome, 35
Prevalence
  of hearing disorders, 221
  of speech and language disorders, 221
Privacy of juvenile records, 47
Private practice, evaluating competitive dimensions, 72, 73
Problem solving and television, 95
Proof of guilt beyond a reasonable doubt, juvenile offender, 46, 47
Prospective adaptation, pediatrics, 160
Psychiatric problems, mentally retarded/developmental disordered populations, 272–274
Psychogenic pain and depression, 11
Psychoneuroimmunology, 243
Psychosocial risk factors, depression, 8
Psychosocial stressors and speech delay, 256
Psychostressors, adolescent crisis, 113
Psychotic suicide, 127, 128

Rates
  depression, 7
  youth suicide, 115, 125
Reading, 81
  impact of television viewing, 94, 103, 104
Rehabilitation of juvenile delinquent, 41, 42
Rehearsal and compliance, 196
Relaxation imagery training, developmental–behavioral pediatrics, 233–245
  appropriate therapy decision, 240–242
  methods, 239, 240
  research findings, 242, 243
  self-regulation strategies: *see* Self-regulation strategies, pediatrics
Retinopathy of prematurity, 250, 251
Right to counsel, juvenile offender, 46
Right-hemisphere style of thinking, 177, 183
Right–left brain theory, 177–189
  hemispheric profiles of mental abilities, 187–189
  hemisphere styles, 185–187
  specializations of hemispheres, 182–184
  structure of the intellect, 181, 182
  two intelligences, 180, 181
  use of hemispheres as a whole, 184, 185
Right to life, handicapped, 172, 175
Right to notice, juvenile offender, 45
Risk factors
  of depression, 7
  of drug and substance abuse, 137
  of juvenile delinquency, 140

Rose Institute Study, Advisory Board on Missing Children, 42
Running away, 112, 141

School performance
  behavioral adjustment problems, 60
  learning disabilities, 76, 85
Screening
  speech, language and hearing, 220, 221
    guidelines, 221–228
Seizures
  neonatal, 19, 20, 26
  and speech delay, 257
Self-destructive behaviors in children and adolescents, 111–147
  adolescent crisis, 112–114
  cluster suicides, 120–122
  depression and suicide, 116–120
  intermediate levels of intervention, 141–146
    parents, 141–143
    peers, 143, 144
    physician, 144–146
  myths and misconceptions, 122–124
  self-destructive behaviors, 135–141
    drug and alcohol abuse, 136–138
    juvenile delinquency, 139–141
    teenage pregnancy, 138, 139
  suicide
    adolescent, 125–132
    childhood, 124, 125
    contributing factors and warning signs, 132–135
    youth, 114–116
  survivors of youth suicide, 146, 147
Self-hypnosis, 236, 239
Self-regulation strategies, pediatrics, 234–239, 244
  athletics, arts, music, 238, 239
  health care professionals, 235, 236
  in hospital, 236, 237
  in school, 237, 238
  third-world child health, 239
Senescence, normal, 268, 269
Sensory integration therapy, and learning disabilities, 89
Separation anxiety disorder, 155
  and depression, 6
Sequenced Inventory of Communication Development, 227
Sleep disturbance, 155
  and temperament, 54
Slow-to-warm child, 52, 53, 60
Somatization disorders and depression, 11
Soto's syndrome, 31–33
Speech
  decoding impairment, 259
  normal development, 254, 255
  screening, 220, 221
Speech delay, 255
  causes in children, 256
Speech disorders associated with speech delay, 255, 256
Speech disturbances, 253
Speech–language delay, 219, 220, 228
  "otitis-prone" child, 217
Speech–language development, 213
  effect of mild hearing loss, 215
  normal, 218–220
Speech–language difficulties, learning disabilities, 80, 81
Stanford-Binet Intelligence test and asphyxia, 17
Star chart and compliance, 205
Stressors, children and adolescents, 161
Stress reduction, 243, 244
  program in school, 238
Subependymal germinal matrix hemorrhage, 21, 22
Substance abuse and television, 94, 95, 101, 102, 105
Suicidal ideation, 119, 125, 128, 131, 142
Suicide, 111, 112, 114–116
  adolescent, 124–132
  categories, 128, 129
  childhood, 124, 125
  cluster, 120–122
  contributing factors and warning signs, 132–135
  and depression, 116–120
  misconceptions, 122–124
  survivors, 146, 147
Suicide and television, 99, 100
Symptoms of depression, 6
Syndromes
  AIDS embryopathy, 29–31
  cerebral giantism, 31–33
  fragile X syndrome, 33–36
  Tourette's syndrome, 36, 37

Television viewing, child and adolescent development, 93–107
  developmental–behavioral implications, 97–104
    aggressive/violent behavior, 98, 99
    health practices, 100–103
    suicide, 99, 100
  epidemiological considerations, 94–96
  management, 104, 105
  quantitative considerations, 96, 97
Temperament and developmental–behavioral diagnosis, 49–64
  clinical importance, 53, 54
  definitions, 49–52
  in diagnostic process, 55–63
    agreement, 57, 58
    behavioral adjustment problems, 59–62
    concern, 56, 57
    developmental or physical problem, 58, 59
    management problems, 62, 63
  measurement, 52, 53
  origins and stability, 53
Temperamental risk factors, 51, 52, 60
Temperament–environment interactions, 61, 62
Temporal–sequential deficits and learning disabilities, 81
Therapeutic intervention, depression, 2
Thinking style, hemisphere, 177, 183
Third-world child health, 239
Tic syndrome, 36
Tourette's syndrome, 36, 37
Tricyclic antidepressants, 9, 10
Tympanometry, 225, 227, 259

Underreporting, mentally retarded/developmental disordered, elderly, 270

Verbal auditory agnosia, 259
Verbal specialization, left hemisphere, 182, 183
Very low birthweight, 23–26, 248
Viewing time, television, 96
Violence and television viewing, 93–95, 98, 99, 104–106
Visuoperceptual deficits and learning disabilities, 81

Warning signs, suicide, 132–135
Wechsler Intelligence Scale for Children
  asphyxia, 17
  seizures, 20
Werther effect, 94, 99, 100, 120–122
Women, fragile X syndrome, 35